TERRORISM AND WAR

TERRORISM AND WAR
UNCONSCIOUS DYNAMICS OF POLITICAL VIOLENCE

edited by
Coline Covington, Paul Williams, Jean Arundale and Jean Knox

Introduction by
Lord Alderdice

KARNAC
LONDON   NEW YORK

First published in 2002 by
H. Karnac (Books) Ltd.
6 Pembroke Buildings, London NW10 6RE

A subsidiary of Other Press LLC, New York

Arrangement copyright © 2002 Coline Covington, Paul Williams,
Jean Arundale, Jean Knox and to the edited collection and the
individual authors to their contributions.
All photographs copyright © 2001 Justin Beal.

The rights of the contributors to be identified as the authors of this work
have been asserted in accordance with §§ 77 and 78 of the Copyright Design
and Patents Act 1988.

All rights reserved. No part of this publication may be reproduced, stored in
a retrieval system, or transmitted, in any form or by any means, electronic,
mechanical, photocopying, recording, or otherwise, without the prior written
permission of the publisher.

British Library Cataloguing in Publication Data

A C.I.P. for this book is available from the British Library

ISBN 1 85575 942 X

10 9 8 7 6 5 4 3 2 1

Edited, designed, and produced by The Studio Publishing Services Ltd,
Exeter EX4 8JN

www.karnacbooks.com

CONTENTS

ACKNOWLEDGEMENTS ix

FOREWORD
   Coline Covington xi

CONTRIBUTORS xiii

Introduction
   Lord Alderdice 1

TERRORISM

Introduction
   Coline Covington 19

CHAPTER ONE
Thoughts and photographs, World Trade Centre:
11th September 2001
   Justin Beal 23

CHAPTER TWO
The eleventh of September massacre
   Ron Britton 31

v

CHAPTER THREE
Thoughts on September 11th, 2001
  Philip A. Ringstrom   35

CHAPTER FOUR
Beyond bombs and sanctions
  Aleksander Vucho   51

CHAPTER FIVE
From containment to leakage, from the collective to the
  unique: therapist and patient in shared national trauma
  Dvora Miller-Florsheim   71

CHAPTER SIX
The psychodynamic dimension of terrorism
  Salman Akhtar   87

CHAPTER SEVEN
Reflections on the making of a terrorist
  Stuart W. Twemlow and Frank C. Sacco   97

HATRED, ENMITY AND REVENGE

Introduction
  Jean Arundale   127

CHAPTER EIGHT
On hatred: with comments on the revolutionary, the saint,
  and the terrorist
  K. R. Eissler   131

CHAPTER NINE
The role of hatred in the ego
  Ping-Nie Pao   151

CHAPTER TEN
Fundamentalism and idolatry
  Ronald Britton   159

CHAPTER ELEVEN
The benign and malignant other
  Coline Covington   175

WHY WAR?

Introduction
    Paul Williams   185

CHAPTER TWELVE
Freud/Einstein correspondence   187

CHAPTER THIRTEEN
Jung correspondence: letter to Dorothy Thompson   203

CHAPTER FOURTEEN
Thoughts for the times on war and death: a psychoanalytic address on an interdisciplinary problem
    Donald M. Kaplan   209

CHAPTER FIFTEEN
Psychoanalysis and war
    Diana Birkett   229

Psychoanalysis and war—response to Diana Birkett
    Isobel Hunter-Brown   239

CHAPTER SIXTEEN
Psychological defence and nuclear war
    Robert D. Hinshelwood   249

CHAPTER SEVENTEEN
Silence is the real crime
    Hanna Segal   263

THE AFTERMATH OF WAR

Introduction
    Jean Knox   287

CHAPTER EIGHTEEN
Destructiveness, atrocities and healing: epistemological and clinical reflections
    Renos K. Papadopoulos   289

CHAPTER NINETEEN
Omagh: the beginning of the reparative impulse?
    Raman Kapur   315

CHAPTER TWENTY
The transgenerational transmission of holocaust trauma:
Lessons learned from the analysis of an adolescent with
obsessive compulsive disorder
Peter Fonagy 329

CHAPTER TWENTY ONE
The holocaust and the power of powerlessness:
survivor guilt an unhealed wound
Alfred Garwood 353

CHAPTER TWENTY TWO
Exile and bereavement
Barbara Hart 375

Forget
Czeslaw Milosz 391

GLOSSARY 393

BIBLIOGRAPHY AND REFERENCES 407

ACKNOWLEDGEMENTS

Chapter Two (pp. 31–34), Britton, R. (2001), "The 11th of September Massacre". *BPAS Bulletin. Reprinted with the permission of BPAS Bulletin.*

Chapter Six (pp. 87–96), Akhtar, S. (1999), "The Psychodynamic Dimension of Terrorism". *Psychiatric Annals*, 29:6 June 1999: 350–355. *Reprinted with the permission of Slack Incorporated.*

Chapter Eight (pp. 131–150), Eissler, K. R. (2000), "On Hatred: Comments on the Revolutionary, the Saint, and the Terrorist". *Psychoanalytic Study of the Child*, 55: 27–44. *Reprinted with the permission of Yale University Press.*

Chapter Nine (pp. 151–158), Pao, P. (1965), "The Role of Hatred in the Ego". *Psychoanalytic Quarterly*, 34: 257–264. *Reprinted with the permission of Psychoanalytic Quarterly.*

Chapter Twelve (pp. 187–202), "Freud/Einstein correspondence—Why War?" *S.E.*, Vol. 22: 199. Acknowledgments: Freud's letter: © 1950, 1964 Sigmund Freud Copyrights & The Institute of Psycho-Analysis, London, by arrangement with Paterson Marsh Agency. Einstein's letter: Permission granted by The Albert Einstein Archives, The Hebrew University of Jerusalem, Israel.

Chapter Thirteen (pp. 203–208), "Jung correspondence—(Sept. 1949) Letter to Dorothy Thompson", *C. G. Jung Letters*, vol. 1: 534. *Reprinted with the permission of Taylor & Francis Books Ltd.*

ACKNOWLEDGEMENTS

Chapter Fourteen (pp. 209–228), Kaplan, D. (1984). "Thoughts for the Times on War and Death": A Psychoanalytic Address on an Interdisciplinary Problem. *Int. R. Psycho-Anal.*, 11: 131–141. Reprinted with the permission of the International Journal of Psychoanalysis.

Chapter Fifteen (pp. 229–238), Birkett, D. (1992), "Psychoanalysis and War". *BJP*, 8: 300–306. Response to Birkett by Hunter-Brown. Reprinted with the permission of British Journal of Psychotherapy.

Chapter Sixteen (pp. 249–262), Hinshelwood, R. D. (1986), "Psychological Defence and Nuclear War". *Medicine and War*, 2: 29–38. Reprinted with permission of Medicine and War, Frank Cass Publishers.

Chapter Seventeen (pp. 263–286), Segal, H. (2001), "Silence is the Real Crime". *International Review of Psycho-Analysis*, 14: 3–12. Reprinted with the permission of International Journal of Psychoanalysis.

Chapter Eighteen (pp. 289–314), Papadopoulos, R. (1998), "Destructiveness, Atrocities and Healing: Epistemological and Clinical Reflections". *JAP*, 43: 455–479. Reprinted with the permission of Journal of Analytical Psychology.

Chapter Nineteen (pp. 315–328), Kapur, R. (2001), "Omagh: The Beginning of the Reparative Impulse?" *Psychoanalytic Psychotherapy*, 15: 265–278. Reprinted with the permission of Psychoanalytic Psychotherapy, Taylor & Francis Ltd. http://www.tandf.co.uk/journals

Chapter Twenty (pp. 329–352), Fonagy, P. (1999), "The Transgenerational Transmission of Holocaust Trauma". *Attachment and Human Development*, 1: 92–114. Reprinted with the permission of Psychoanalytic Psychotherapy, Taylor & Francis Ltd. http://www.tandf.co.uk/journals

Chapter Twenty One (pp. 353–374), Garwood, A. (1986), "The Holocaust and the Power of Powerlessness: The Unhealed Wound of Survivor Guilt". *BJP*, 13: 243–266. Reprinted with the permission of British Journal of Psychotherapy.

Chapter Twenty Two (pp. 375–392), Hart, B. (1994), "Exile and Bereavement". *Psychoanalytic Psychotherapy*, Vol. 8, No. 3. Reprinted with the permission of Psychoanalytic Psychotherapy, Taylor & Francis Ltd. http://www.tandf.co.uk/journals

Milosz poem, © 2000 by Czeslav Milosz. *Permission of The Wylie Agency and Penguin UK Ltd.*

FOREWORD

Coline Covington

The idea for this collection was born a month after the terrorist attack of 11th September. The British Psycho-Analytical Society was holding a reception to celebrate the opening of its new premises in Maida Vale, London. Amongst the historical displays in its impressive new library was a notice of a lecture given by Edward Glover to The Federation of League of Nation's Societies in Geneva in 1931, entitled, "War, Sadism and Pacifism". On seeing this timely notice from the past, I turned to my colleague, Paul Williams, joint editor-in-chief of the International Journal of Psycho-Analysis, and said that it would be interesting to bring together a historical collection of psychoanalytic papers on war and terrorism. A month later, we had asked Jean Knox, editor of the Journal of Analytical Psychology, and Jean Arundale, editor of the British Journal of Psychotherapy, to join us as editors and we had obtained a contract from Karnac Books. These three journals are representative of the different strands of depth psychology that the British Confederation of Psychotherapists incorporates, namely: psychoanalysis, analytical psychology, and psychoanalytic psychotherapy.

In the wake of 11th September, there was a widespread reaction of shock, disbelief and outrage. People also felt frightened and helpless. Above all, such questions were asked as, "How could this happen?" and "What kind of person (or group) would do such a thing?" While politicians, the media, historians, social commentators, and many others presented their views and theories, there was also an overwhelming response to one particular internet discussion held by PsyBC on the events of 11th September amongst practitioners in the mental health field. However, even this wealth of knowledge and research into human aggression and its consequences within the field of psychoanalytic psychotherapy remained behind relatively closed doors. As chair of the BCP, I felt that this was an opportunity on behalf of the profession to demonstrate the thinking that has gone on within psychoanalytic psychotherapy over the last century about war, terrorism, and the generations of survivors of terror.

The collection of papers we have selected has been drawn from our professional journals, starting with Freud's correspondence with Einstein on "Why War?" in 1932 and extending into the present to include unpublished papers from a wide circle of authors. The book is divided into four sections: "Terrorism", "Hatred, Enmity and Revenge", "Why War?", and "The Aftermath of War". These headings broadly reflect the way in which the papers selected fell into these categories. The papers were selected for their insight and quality of writing, and they represent a range of psychoanalytic and analytical psychology perspectives. We have also included a glossary of psychoanalytic terms at the end of the book in the hope that all the papers will be accessible to those who are interested in the unconscious dynamics of mass destruction.

We would like to give special thanks to the following people for their help: Stan Ruszczynski, editor of the British Association of Psychotherapy Journal; Marilyn Lawrence, editor of the Psychoanalytic Psychotherapy journal; Pramila Bennett, administrative editor of the Journal of Analytical Psychology; Lyndsay MacDonald, who put this book together from obtaining permissions to the finished product; and Justin Beal, who has generously allowed us to reproduce his photographs and commentary of 11th September.

CONTRIBUTORS

Salman Akhtar, M.D., is a Professor of Psychiatry, Jefferson Medical College, lecturer on Psychiatry, Harvard Medical School, and a training and supervising analyst, Psychoanalytic Centre of Philadelphia. He is the author of *Broken Structures* (1992), *A Quest for Answers* (1995), *Inner Torment* (1999), and *Immigration and Identity* (1999), as well as the editor or co-editor of nineteen other books in psychiatry and psychoanalysis. He has also published five volumes of poetry.

John Alderdice is Speaker of the Northern Ireland Assembly and a Consultant Psychiatrist in Psychotherapy. For eleven years the Leader of Northern Ireland's cross-community Alliance Party and a key negotiator of the Good Friday Agreement, he has substantial experience of political conflict and terrorism. He is also steeped in international affairs as a Vice-President of the European Liberal Democrat Party (a key voting block in the European Parliament) and Deputy President of Liberal International, the world-wide federation of over eighty political parties.

Jean Arundale, Ph.D., is a member and training therapist of the

xiv   CONTRIBUTORS

British Association of Psychotherapists and Editor of the British Journal of Psychotherapy.

Justin Beal works as an artist and an architect in New York City. He is working on a Hays-Brandeis Fellowship researching portable architecture and is enrolled in the Whitney Museum's Independent Study Program.

Diana Birkett trained with the Centre for Psychoanalytical Psychotherapy and works as Counselling Co-ordinator for MIND in Tower Hamlets; as a psychotherapist at the Enid Balint Centre, Barnes Hospital; and in private practice, specializing in eating disorders and alcohol problems. Her work for the Medical Foundation for the Care of the Victims of Torture has contributed to her study of trauma in psychonalysis, and in particular to the effects on the individual psyche of the breakdown of the State.

Ronald Britton, F.R.C.Psych., president, British Psycho-Analytical Society and Vice-President, I. P. A.

Coline Covington, Ph.D., is Chair of the British Confederation of Psychotherapists and consultant editor of the Journal of Analytical Psychology. She is a training and supervising analyst of the Society of Analytical Psychology and a training therapist of the British Association of Psychotherapists (Jungian Section). She is co-editor with Barbara Wharton of *Sabina Spielrein: Forgotten Pioneer of Psychoanalysis* to be published by Routledge (2003).

Kurt Eissler was born in 1908 in Vienna. Eissler was the author of about 100 papers and 12 books, including *A Psychoanalytic Study of Goethe* and *Three Instances of Injustice*, the latter containing a study of the mechanisms of slander. The writing of *Freud and the Seduction Theory: A Brief Love Affair* occupied Eissler for more than 10 years. A custodian of Freud's correspondence following the death of Anna Freud, Eissler himself died in 1998.

Peter Fonagy, Ph.D. F.B.A., is Freud Memorial Professor of Psychoanalysis and Director of the Sub-Department of Clinical Health Psychology at University College London. He is Director of the Child and Family Centre at the Menninger Foundation, Kansas. He is also Director of Research at the Anna Freud Centre, London. He is a clinical psychologist and a training and supervising analyst in the British Psycho-Analytical Society in child and adult analysis. He has written many books, his most recent being *Psychoanalytic Theories: Perspectives from Developmental Psychopathology* (with Mary Target—in press with Whurr Publications).

Alfred Garwood is the founder of the Association of Child Survivors of Great Britain and the co-founder of the Foundation for Holocaust Survivors. He is a practicing general practitioner and a group analyst working in the NHS. He was awarded the 1998 British Journal of Psychotherapy essay prize. He works internationally with the youngest Holocaust survivors born between 1941 and 1945.

Barbara Hart is a psychoanalytic psychotherapist in private practice in London. She is an Associate Member of the Lincoln Centre. She has had extensive experience of working with refugees, both at the Africa Educational Trust and subsequently at the Refugee Support Centre, a counselling and psychotherapy service which she helped to establish in 1989.

Bob Hinshelwood is professor at the Centre for Psychoanalytic Studies, University of Essex. He is a full member of the British Psycho-Analytical Society and for twenty years was a consultant psychotherapist in the National Health Service. He has written *What Happens in Groups* (1987), *A Dictionary of Kleinian Thought* (1989), *Clinical Klein* (1994), *Observing Organisations* (2001), *Thinking about Institutions* (2002) amongst other books. He founded the International Journal of Therapeutic Communities in 1980 and the British Journal of Psychotherapy in 1984.

Isobel H. Hunter-Brown graduated 1940 Hons. English Literature and Language at Glasgow University. She studied Medicine there after the war, qualifying in 1953, and then began training in psychiatry at the Professor's unit. She obtained a D.P.N and qualified as a psychoanalyst. She is a member of the Royal College of Psychiatrists and has worked at the Portman Clinic and the

Cassell Hospital. She was consultant for Leicester University Student Health Service, but is now retired.

Donald M. Kaplan was born in 1927 in New York. Arts and artists were at the centre of his interests, in addition to clinical psychoanalytic issues. He published more than 40 papers, including applied psychoanalytic studies of the American theatre, focusing on issues such as stage fright and homosexuality. Kaplan was an Associate Editor of *American Imago* for 27 years until his death in 1994.

Raman Kapur is Director of Threshold (Richmond Fellowship Northern Ireland), a mental health charity offering therapeutic communities and psychotherapy. He is also a consultant clinical psychologist, formerly Chair of the Division of Clinical Psychology (Northern Ireland) and Course Director of the joint Threshold/ School of Psychology, Queen's University of Belfast training in psychoanalytic psychotherapy. He is also a regular contributor to BBC Radio Ulster.

Jean Knox is a psychiatrist and analytical psychologist in private practice in Oxford. She is a professional member of the Society of Analytical Psychology and the Editor of the Journal of Analytical Psychology. She is also a member of the Executive Committee of the International Attachment Network.

Dvora Miller-Florsheim has been a senior clinical psychologist and supervisor in Psychotherapy and Psychodiagnosis since 1976. She is a supervisor in the post-graduate psychotherapy program in Bar-Ilan University and supervisor and teacher in the Department of Psychotherapy, School of Continuing Medical Education, Tel Aviv University.

Ping-Nie Pao, born 1922, became director of Chestnut Lodge Hospital, Rockville, MD, USA, and was the author of the seminal work, *Schizophrenic Disorders: Theory and Treatment From a Psychodynamic Point of View* (1979). This book and the work it inspired were summarized in *Toward a Comprehensive Model for Schizophrenic Disorders: Psychoanalytic Essays in Memory of Ping-Nie Pao* (1985), edited by David Feinsilver. Pao was also author of studies on self-injury. He died in 1981.

Renos K. Papadopoulos, Ph.D., is professor at the University of Essex, consultant clinical psychologist at the Tavistock Clinic, systemic family psychotherapist, and an Analytical Psychologist. As consultant to the United Nations and other organizations, he has worked with refugees and other survivors of political violence in several countries.

Philip Ringstrom, Ph.D., Psy.D., is a senior Training and Supervising Analyst, Faculty Member, and Member of the Board of Directors of the Institute of Contemporary Psychoanalysis in Los Angeles, CA and is in full time private practice in Encino. He is on the Editorial Board of *Psychoanalytic Dialogues* and in addition to publishing there has published in many volumes. He is also a reviewer for the *Journal of the American Psychoanalytic Association*.

Frank Sacco is President of CSI, a private mental health clinic, in Springfield and Boston, Massachusetts. He is a consultant to the FBI on US school shootings as well as an expert in bully prevention in schools and violent conflict mediation.

Hanna Segal was born in Poland in 1918 and has lived and worked in London since 1940. She is a practising psychoanalyst. She was twice President of the British Psycho-Analytical Society and also served as Vice-President of the International Psycho-Analytical Association. She is a founding member and Fellow of the Royal College of Psychiatry. Hanna Segal was one of the pioneers of the psychoanalysis of psychotics and has written numerous papers on psychoanalysis, collected in two volumes. She has also written extensively on psychoanalysis in the social and political scene and on the psychoanalytic contribution to the understanding of art.

Stuart W. Twemlow, M.D., is in private practice as a psychoanalyst and psychiatrist; Co-director of Peaceful Schools Project, Child & Family Centre, Menninger Clinic, Topeka, Kansas; Clinical Professor of Psychiatry & Behavioural Sciences, University of Kansas School of Medicine, Wichita, Kansas.

Aleksandar Vucho, M.D., Ph.D., is a training analyst, Belgrade Psychoanalytical Study Group. He works full time in private practice.

Paul Williams is a member of the British Psycho-Analytical Society, Joint Editor-in-Chief of the International Journal of Psychoanalysis and Visiting Professor in the School of Community Health and Social Studies, APU, Essex, UK.

Introduction

Lord Alderdice

In the aftermath of the devastating terrorist attacks on the World Trade Centre in New York and the Pentagon in Washington DC on 11 September 2001, we are all struggling to understand the implications of a phenomenon which now dominates serious thought. Psychoanalytically orientated thinkers should not avoid the question. As Moises Lemlij (1992) pointed out, writing of his experiences as a psychoanalyst in Peru during the terrorist campaigns of Sendero Luminoso and the MRTA, the failure to respond to violence and aggression in a community may be a denial of reality.

Terrorism is not a new thing. When a body of people have faced overwhelming odds at almost any time in history it has always been on option. Of course such a group could face the foe in a set piece battle and would almost certainly lose in a crushing defeat. In the absence of an unexpected collapse of the enemy the sustaining hope was that their sacrificial courage would inspire future generations. The 1916 Easter Rising in Ireland is the classic example in recent European history. A community could instead simply knuckle under with or without the belief that in the end the oppressor would face justice at the hands of providence. A third option was to embark on a dangerous campaign of terror that would in the short-term provoke reprisals but might eventually weary or undermine the powerful enemy and bring victory. There are many examples of such campaigns, and during the twentieth century a number achieved signal successes in bringing an end to colonial rule.

If terrorism is not new, what is it about the recent attacks that gives us a sense that something has changed? Is it the scale of the destruction, or the anxiety that we are facing some altogether new uncertainty? Are we in some sense facing a new enemy? Is this sense of dread occasioned by the reawakening of memories of previous catastrophic experiences? Why has the attack on the United States of America provoked such a response? In reflecting on these and other related questions we may be facing a similar watershed of understanding to that faced by Freud at the end of the Great War. He once described himself as "a liberal of the old school" (1930a). While his thinking was not, like that of many other liberal intellectuals of the nineteenth century, characterized by an overweening optimism that education and scientific advancement alone would quickly build a new, free and civilized world, he was nevertheless deeply affected by the catastrophe of the Great War. Science, art, culture, sociology, and even to some extent the study of the mind had suggested that things were evolving for the better, but as the deluge which swamped the world in 1914 subsided four years later, that optimism had been swept away. The old world order had gone. Things had changed and were changing, but was it certain that it was all for the better? Freud embarked on substantial developments in his own thinking to try to come to some better understanding of the terrible events of the war. Similarly we should reflect on the meaning of these recent developments lest we miss a powerful stimulus to our theoretical advancement and practical work.

There is also another wider imperative. The death of the old world order in the trenches of the 1914–1918 War was followed by a century during which Marx's explanation of what motivated man held intellectual political hegemony, not only where communism became the dominant movement, but even in freer democratic socialist societies. Freud was unimpressed with the communist explanation of aggression, describing it as "an untenable illusion" (1930b), but it became a determining force of the twentieth century.

Were the subsequent tragedies of the twentieth century inevitable? Could a better understanding of man have helped ameliorate them? In the absence of progress in our thinking today, political leaders and public opinion will likely turn to previous political or religious ideas, investing them with a fundamentalist certainty that spells disaster. This book is a serious effort to marshal some of the material already at our disposal as an encouragement to serious thought on the subject of Terrorism and War.

Of course while Marxism dominated progressive political thought it was not the only practical political dynamic of the last one hundred years. My generation of young Europeans has come to see the European Union primarily in terms of the Common Market, Monetary Union, and the Euro. In this focus on economic co-operation it is often forgotten that for the original architects of "ever closer union" the driving force was not primarily a commitment to economic liberalism but a reaction to their experience of the horrors of war. Europe had many wars throughout the centuries and the humiliation and misery of conflict had been the common experience of almost every generation, however the unprecedented destruction of not one but two World Wars in a single generation demonstrated that nationalism and imperialism offered no stability to the people of Europe. Worse still, scientific advance had created the frightening prospect that a future war would be even more catastrophic.

Previously the slowness of communication and travel and the limited power of physical force and traditional explosives had confined the capacity for destruction through war. Radio, air travel, nuclear power and other scientific marvels changed all that. The new technologies offered dazzling beneficial opportunities for wealth creation and distribution. Surely if the world's capacity to produce enough food and the other necessities of life could be harnessed to a scientific means of production and social distribution the recipe for a better world was to hand? The speed of change ensured that things could get better more quickly, but to the silver lining there was a dark cloud. They could also deteriorate with terrifying speed. The Second World War ended with the demonstration that man at war could lose all the vestiges of civilization in a Holocaust, and Hiroshima and Nagasaki showed how we could now with certainty destroy not only an enemy but also all life on the planet. Men no longer went off to war. War now visited itself with terrifying results on whole communities through aerial bombardment, biological and chemical weapons, and nuclear attack. The boundaries had gone and the nature and significance of conflict had changed completely and irrevocably. Any local war could now escalate into global destruction.

The belief that wars were primarily caused by the individual vanities and ambitions of monarchs and imperialists was also dealt a blow, for it was democratically elected politicians and communist leaders who had led their countries into the costly blood bath of the Second World War. The events of the twentieth century posed a serious question about the notion that the aggressive drive which results in the violence of war was only a result of an excessive concentration of power, or merely the understandable frustration of the majority of people deprived of their just economic rewards. It is surely, as Freud maintained, something deeper and more essential to the human condition. So profoundly a part of humanity did Freud consider aggression to be, that while not entirely gloomy he was less sanguine than some about the prospects of preventing war, as is shown by his correspondence with Einstein (published later in this volume). His personal experience and observation in the Europe between the wars gave little encouragement to optimism.

After the Second World War, particularly in Europe, which had been the cockpit of both the conflicts, the fear of war was greatest. To the traditional rivalries between France, Britain, and Germany was added the even more terrifying prospect of being the turf upon which a nuclear conflict would be fought out between the USSR and the USA. War was now too terrible to contemplate and so it must at all costs be prevented. Co-operation on the economic reconstruction of a devastated Europe opened the route to new models of cross-border co-operation, and the pooling of sovereignty in an increasing range of competencies. Fifty years later war between historic Western European rivals like Germany and France is unthinkable and the benefits of this international approach may even have manifested itself in the resolution of long-standing small scale conflicts such as that in Northern Ireland. Although there has been less success to date in places like Cyprus and the Balkans, where ancient feuds remain unresolved and dangerous, some believe that it is just a matter of time and effort.

Outside Europe too, world leaders moved beyond placing their hope in the independence of nation states to interdependence through international co-operation. This was the basis for the United Nations and for the rapid development of international law and international economic institutions. The United Nations established various organs whose purpose was to address hunger, disease, underdevelopment, workers rights, and of course the prevention and resolution of conflicts. This was surely recognition that we could no longer depend on the limits of our ability to destroy each other and our environment, to protect us against the excesses of our wars. The Nuremberg Tribunals may have seemed to be "victor's justice" but they proved to be a precedent for the more recent tribunals established after the conflicts in the former Yugoslavia and Central Africa, and they in their turn presaged the establishment of the International Criminal Court. The adoption of the International Declaration of Human Rights showed humanity's realization that if we did not find a way of containing and transforming our aggressive urges there was a real danger that we would simply destroy our race and life on this earth. Without a recognition of and respect for human rights there would be nothing left. Local laws set down the boundaries for acceptable behaviour in a local community, but human rights set down limits and requirements for humanity's survival.

While no reasonable person would dismiss these profound signs of progress, their success in preventing and resolving conflict has been limited. The end of imperialism, the democratization of political power, and the establishment of international and in some cases global institutions of law and co-operation are remarkable and positive achievements in themselves, but we are still threatened by our own capacity for violence. The conviction that man is essentially an economic animal whose desires can be met and aggression controlled by political institutions framed on this basis has proved itself inadequate, but the ending of the Cold War, which divided the world on this very issue, has not brought peace either. The extensive use of terrorism during the second half of the twentieth century could have been interpreted as a kind of protective device. After 1945 the super-powers knew that a direct confrontation could bring a total war and complete nuclear catastrophe and so they diverted their aggression into sponsoring guerrilla wars and terrorist campaigns in various parts of the world. While the collapse of the

Soviet Union led to an end of such hostilities, most notably in South Africa and Northern Ireland, in other places especially in the Middle East there was a further deterioration. Terrorism was not merely a tool of the great powers, an expression of their vicarious struggle. It was a phenomenon in its own right. Indeed after September 11th it is clear that it no longer facilitates a localizing and controlling effect. On the contrary in its use of planes and mobile telephones (two of the symbols of progress and globalization), it globalizes the threat at a stroke.

From a psychoanalytical point of view none of this is surprising. I think that Freud's comment about being a "liberal of the old school" was meant to convey his belief that human beings flourished better if they were free to conduct their lives as they chose and to take responsibility for themselves, within the boundaries of what was legal and acceptable in the society in which they found themselves. An end to empires, the growth of democracy and the clarification of reasonable and fair laws and economic rules are a communal equivalent to the search for personal freedom and boundary setting which is familiar to us in the clinical setting. One of the distinctive contributions of psychoanalysis is the appreciation that congenial social and economic circumstances while helpful, are not in themselves a sufficient protection against mental and emotional disturbance, hence Freud's scepticism about an entirely economic view of man and the causes of aggression. Armed only with non-analytic explanations of violence our world community will not make sense of terrorist attacks like those of September 11th, 2001. President G. W. Bush undoubtedly expresses the views of many people when he denounces the actions of an "Axis of Evil". Terrorism is seen as the successor to communism—an evil belief system against which a war can be waged, and presumably won. It certainly cannot be assumed to be low level war. As the Chief Justice of India, Justice B. N. Kirpal recently pointed out, India lost 5,468 lives in four so-called "high intensity conflicts" it has fought, but 61,013 civilians and 8,706 security personnel in terrorism over the last 15 years. The deterioration in the world-wide situation was noted by the Secretary-General of the Council of Europe, Walter Schwimmer (2002), when he said that more people had died in terrorist attacks in the previous year than in any other year in history. The growth of terrorism is no fringe activity. It affects us all, and will affect us more.

When we are attacked in a substantial way, by something we do not understand, the natural reaction is to attack back and, since we are not certain how to respond, we are likely to resort to old modes of defence, including the moral characterization of the assailing force as "evil". The use by the United States of America of the detention camp in Guantamemo Bay is a case in point. This country normally observes extensive legal protection for suspects. It is now exploring the use of the military commission procedure for prosecution. As far as I know this procedure has only two precedents. It was used in 1776 when John Hickey attempted to assassinate George Washington. (Since the assassination attempt took place some two weeks before Independence it was not thought that the British courts, which still had jurisdiction at the time, would find him guilty.) The second time was after World War II in Germany and Japan. The proposal to adopt unusual procedures in response to the current terrorist threat is not the only measure of the gravity with which the situation is viewed in Washington DC. The previous US foreign policy of "respond to attack" has been replaced by a pre-emptive doctrine of "search them out before they get us".

Perhaps the most dangerous response, however, is the tendency to think and speak of the situation in moralizing terms. A recent tribute to those who died heroically serving and saving others in the aftermath of 11th September 2001, quotes approvingly from an address by President John F. Kennedy to the United Nations almost exactly 40 years earlier on 25th September 1961. He said:

> Terror is not a new weapon. Throughout history it has been used by those who could not prevail, either by persuasion or example. But inevitably they fail, either because men are not afraid to die for a life worth living, or because the terrorists themselves came to realise that free men cannot be frightened by threats, and that aggression would meet its own response. And it is in the light of history that every nation today should know, be he friend or foe, that the United States has both the will and the weapons to join free men in standing up to their responsibilities. [Kennedy, 2000]

It is not hard to imagine the current incumbent of that high office making a similar declaration, and though its truths are no less true in our time, some of its rhetoric is more difficult to believe. Free men can be frightened by threats, and terrorists do not inevitably fail.

8   TERRORISM AND WAR

The question is not whether the United States has the will or the weapons but whether we all have the combined insight to bring the use of terrorism to an end in our time. Merely describing it as an evil has led to the futility and foreign policy inconsistency that "one man's terrorist is man other man's freedom fighter"

President Kennedy's own commitment to a better world was intimately connected during the 1960s with civil rights marches not only in the United States, but also across much of the world, including Britain, Germany, France, Japan, and in Northern Ireland. In each context the campaigners addressed the particular concerns of their own community and in Northern Ireland discrimination against Catholics was centre-stage. The mainly Catholic protestors were joined by a significant number of Protestants who shared their concerns about injustice in Northern Ireland, but many other Protestants were opposed to the civil rights movement, staging counter-demonstrations, which resulted in violence. Vigilante groups emerged in both communities and the situation deteriorated with the appearance of gun and bomb attacks. Terrorism, which had a long history in Ireland, had reappeared. As the situation began to spiral out of control the reaction of the government was predictable and understandable. These were criminal acts to be met by the full force of the law, first by police intervention, then the army called in as back-up and by 1971 normal due process was set aside and hundreds of republicans and loyalists were interned by executive order, without trial. However natural this response the result was not stabilization but further deterioration. What I find very disturbing is that the current response of the "War on Terrorism" reminds me very much of the experience of Northern Ireland at the outbreak of the "Troubles", albeit on a different scale. A "law and order" approach was taken, executive internment without trial used to detain suspects, and while some thought was given to the underlying causes of the violence, it was not successfully applied to the problem. The terrorist campaign became entrenched and my generation lived the whole of its adult life in the shadow of guns and bombs.

It is not just in the United States that robust measures are being taken. In the United Kingdom the recent proposals for anti-terrorist legislation lie in a direct line, not only with the unsuccessful efforts of the 1974 Prevention of Terrorism Act and other reactions to

Provisional IRA terrorism, but with the similar unsuccessful initiatives of the Gladstone cabinet's 1881 Coercion Bill, the Asquith Coalition's response to the 1916 Easter Rising and Lloyd George's use of the Black and Tans. There is no doubt that liberal democracy must be defended against attacks from without and within, just as the therapist must often strive thoughtfully to protect the therapy from the attacks of the resistance. The difficult question is how to conduct that defence and strike the right note. For those who try to understand everyone's point of view there is the danger of the "therapeutic impotence" ascribed to one former Northern Ireland Secretary who, it was said, "argued with his conscience over every decision—and the result was always a draw". While such uncertainty and fear of intervention is unhelpful, it is scarcely less disastrous than the opposite tendency to overreact, often nourishing the very opposition one is trying to suppress.

Sober reflection by the authorities in Northern Ireland over many years led to the adoption of a number of principles in addressing terrorism there. Most fundamentally came the recognition that the purpose of policing is first and foremost the maintenance of the human rights of everyone in the community and that all actions must be measured against this indicator of success. As a result, attempts were made to ensure that all legislation against terrorism was drafted to approximate as closely as possible to ordinary criminal law and procedure and to conform to international law and conventions. It was regarded as crucial to observe due process and maintain scrutiny and control over security operations by civil authorities which were subject to democratic accountability. Any additional offences and powers had to be justified as necessary, proportionate, and balancing security needs and civil rights and liberties. The reason for this painstaking approach arose from the recognition that if it began to appear to the civilian population that the liberal democratic nature of the society was being damaged by the reaction of the government, then the authorities would be blamed for the loss of freedom in the long-term, not the terrorists. Any resort to general repression makes it difficult for a government to demonstrate that it is taking proportionate and properly directed measures only against terrorists and their active collaborators. Such measures usually adversely affect the law-abiding population more than the terrorists. Borders rarely stop criminals, and obvious security operations give advance warning to those they are meant to trap, causing maximum inconvenience only to ordinary civilians. Soon the terrorists are able to present themselves, to at least some sections of the community, as the protectors of civil society against an oppressive regime—exactly the view the terrorists set out to demonstrate and address.

The start of such a road to reflection is the existential commitment to understanding what is going on in the mind of the terrorist and his supporters. This stance is relatively easy to describe in a psychoanalytical text. It is quite another matter to promulgate it in the raging heat of a community torn apart by violence and death, but it is at precisely this level that I believe the creation of psychoanalytical space is most needed. I have come to the view that the psychoanalytic approach can create a space for reflection too valuable to be restricted only to work with individuals and small groups. This is particularly important when political discourse in a community is overtaken by powerful emotions, as is the case during times of crisis, like now. The violence of domestic and international terrorism, which has been experienced by more than half of the countries in the world, provokes particularly strong feelings. The purpose of this book is to create the space to think psychoanalytically about a tactic of war whose very purpose is to provoke powerful feelings and reactions, and to destroy the capacity to reflect.

Given that many of those surrounding President G. W. Bush come from his father's period in office and may wish to accomplish in this term what they did not complete first time around, it is hardly surprising that the "War against Terrorism" tends to be couched in Cold War rhetoric. But terrorism is unlike other "isms", such as nationalism, communism, liberalism or socialism. It is not a belief system but a tactic. It may be used by the left or the right, or by more populist or nationalist extremists. It involves the premeditated use of violence to create a climate of fear, but is aimed at a wider target than the immediate victims of the violence. Count Mikhail Bakunin, the nineteenth century Russian anarchist, called this the "propaganda of the deed"—the target is the audience, not the immediate victims. The victims are commonly civilians. While often arbitrarily chosen they have symbolic significance, but the real target is not the victim. The target is the responsible authority. The purpose of the terrorist act is to provoke. This makes terrorism very different from ordinary crime. While the ordinary criminal generally hopes to avoid detection for as long as possible, the terrorist organization will regularly claim responsibility. As suicide bombers have shown, many terrorists are not so troubled if they are personally punished so long as their campaign is ultimately successful. Stronger penalties may even be welcomed by terrorists, for example the escalating Hunger Strike and dirty protest during Margaret Thatcher's time as Prime Minister, which led to a loss of moral authority by the British Government. (This is a particularly interesting protest from a psychoanalytical point of view, given the struggle between a highly symbolic woman and a rebellious body of men, using various bodily functions for the expression of the struggle.) There are many other differences between terrorists and other prisoners: the relationship between colleagues is more supportive; they survive better in solitary confinement; they use educational facilities better; and they tend to be puritanical, self-sacrificial and less recidivist, for complex and rational military, political and psychological reasons.

Perhaps one of the most interesting features of terrorism is the difference between victim and target. A recent piece of legislation gives recognition to this aspect of the definition of terrorism. In India the Prevention of Terrorism Act (POTA) came into effect on 24th October 2001 with a time limit of three years, taking special measures against terrorism. In Section 3 of the Act it defined terrorism as an action

> ... to strike terror in the people, does any act or thing using bombs ... or detains any person and threatens to kill or injure such person in order to compel the Government or any other person to do or abstain from doing any act ...

This affirms the essential element of attacking a victim in order to affect a target, often, though by no means always a government. The victim may be the terrorist's own community or even his or her own body, but the target is the authority. The mechanism of triangulation and the use of the symbolic are very familiar to psychoanalytically informed thinkers, the Oedipal Complex being one of the most important contexts in which we find them. We are also familiar in working with individuals and families, and from our experience as therapists, how those who are "weak" can provoke the "strong" into counter-productive and pathological reactions. Similarly the organizationally weak terrorist group aims to provoke organizationally strong authorities into a substantial over-reaction that will damage their standing and moral authority both domestically and internationally. To this end the violence is not only intentionally criminal in terms of the domestic law but also of any human code, such that by violating all social norms it provokes outrage and cannot be ignored. We are used to the uncomprehending reaction of those who, without the benefit of a psychoanalytical knowledge, encounter many of our patients, especially those who are suffering from psychosis. It is also my experience that people from a stable law-abiding polity find it almost impossible to comprehend that those who engage in terrorism believe themselves to be entirely justified. Terrorists and their supporters see themselves as righting some terrible wrong, some humiliation, some deep disrespect that has been done them, their community or their nation. They in their weakness are, with great courage and risk to themselves, embarked on the heroic task of righting that wrong. One thing at least is common to both the terrorists and those who are combating terrorism. Both believe that to kill off the "evil thing" is good, and should one die in the attempt it is not only a moral and courageous act but also one which confirms the wickedness of the enemy. Though some may shudder at the thought, the sentiments proclaimed by President Kennedy at the United Nations in 1961 might be shared with remarkable identity, albeit from a radically different perspective, by some of those who espouse terrorism. In this regard I do not make a difference as some commentators do between those who adopt terrorism to achieve a manifest political end, and those whose terrorism is more theological or transcendent. In both cases they are motivated by beliefs rather than by more obvious personal betterment. I think that the difference that some writers observe is more to do with a lack of understanding of the thinking of terrorists. I do however take the view that there is often a fundamentalism about the way in which the beliefs are held, which demonstrates a more primitive mode of thinking, and one which is difficult to engage. It reminds me of the problems of making sense and engaging with psychotic patients. To simply dismiss them as "mad" is to fail to even embark on the road to understanding. A psychoanalytical approach can bring substantial light to bear on the thinking of even the most disturbed patients, so long as one appreciates that their thinking is not secondary process in form. I do however make a differentiation between terrorism, whose purpose is to bring about radical change in a polity, and the tactics of terror used by some dictatorial states to hold on to power and maintain the status quo. I am not making any judgements about moral equivalence or otherwise, but I am differentiating between the two because the mechanisms are different and without some clarity of definition it is hard to come to an understanding of the different mechanisms by which violence is used in the political field.

Returning to Northern Ireland, the application of these principles helped stabilize the situation but it did not resolve it. A stalemate developed where neither side could win militarily. This led to a serious exploration of the political dimension. Initially many different solutions were suggested with the unstated assumption that if the "right plan" could be invented everyone would suddenly grasp it with relief and implement it. Of course this was an illusion. It is not the content of a solution that is critical but the process of achieving it. We know in our clinical work that merely telling the patient where the problem lies, or giving them an analytic text to read, is rarely a healing intervention. It is taking the patient through the analytic process that is transformational.

The political transformation began outside Northern Ireland. We know that when parents bring us a child with symptoms we must address not just the child but also the parental relationship if we are not to have our therapeutic efforts founder. In our clinical work we are aware not only that there will be acting out which needs to be contained and explored but that it will often take a long time for change to take place. It is also important that there are not any "no-go areas" or things that cannot at all costs be spoken about. Our psychoanalytic work must be, in the current political parlance, "inclusive". In the same way it was characteristic of our process and of the South African process that the parties involved were not just the large and law-abiding parties, but all the parties, and that everything was open to be spoken about, without commitment. There is considerable evidence that the importance of these insights is yet to be fully established in international conflict resolution.

While all of this may tell us something about the characteristics of terrorism as a tactic, and may even hint at some of the ways in which we may more appropriately address it, the question remains, "What is the terrorist trying to achieve?" In our psychoanalytic work we know that careful observation of the symptoms often evinces some indications of the underlying motivation. What is so striking about the intensely symbolic events of September 11th is that the mighty intelligence and military apparatus of the United States was humiliated and ineffectual. This result, which left the world's only super-power impotent and uncertain, may convey something of the origins of the aggressor's motivating force.

I have already mentioned how, in my experience, there is always in those who embark on a campaign of terrorism a sense that they are righting some terrible wrong. What is the nature of this injustice? Of course social and economic disadvantage may play a role but it seems to me that this in itself is rarely a sufficient explanation. I have been struck in my dealings with people in all such communities by how much they want to be treated with respect. My experience of politicians is that we have an almost insatiable desire to be respected. Conversely disrespect and humiliation is rarely either forgotten or forgiven. Of course it is not reasonable to expect committed political enemies to feel respect for each other, but unless they are helped through a peace process to find ways of behaving respectfully there is little prospect of even a working arrangement. With respectful behaviour much can be achieved. One of the reasons why conflicts in countries such as mine run so deep and create such violence is because each side treats the most essential features of the other with disrespect. This is true of nationhood. The disregard of my nation's language—even if I myself cannot speak it—is felt as a disrespect of me. The same is true of religion. Religious beliefs fulfil a fundamental need to create order out of the uncertain experiences of life. When our belief structure, religious or otherwise, is attacked it is perceived as a threat to that which protects us from chaos. We defend against the attack for fear of a breakdown of our way of making sense of life, and dealing with the disappointments of the past, the vagaries of the present, and our fears for the future. Such an attack may be overt as in the Crusades and all their more recent counterparts, or it may be the less obviously brutal but none the less threatening march of modernity. Modernity has rarely been sensitive to conservatism; indeed its advocates often proclaim their successes with some arrogance, less in what they say than in how they behave. No surprise then that with a combination of fear and envy almost all the religious families are now seeing fundamentalist wings develop which in their different ways, and sometimes with violence, fight against the very culture that the West sees as offering the best hope for the future. Of course there are issues about world development, inequality, ignorance, disease, and poverty, but these are not the only threats to world order. In his excellent book on the origins of criminal violence Gilligan (1996) reaches similar conclusions about the motivating power of disrespect (he calls it "shame") in his work with individuals convicted of profound violence against others.

In Northern Ireland we have found that patient reflection on the motivations of those who have acted with the extreme violence of terrorism, and positive engagement with their representatives, has taken us as a community towards a hopeful place which is beyond merely economic betterment. In the process we have stretched our capacity to contain our own feelings and responses. We have tried to develop ways in which both sides, and those who do not wish to be described as from either side, are able to behave with respect in order to be treated with respect. In time we may come to know whether this effort is as productive of peace as we hope, but in Ireland we have already tried the alternative and it brought us some hundreds of years of misery.

At a recent psychoanalytical conference held close to Ground Zero in New York, one of the organizers, Dr Joe Cancelmo, made reference to some reassuring words spoken by an American airline captain to his nervous passengers at the start of a flight, shortly after the events of September 11th. He tried to give them a sense of mutual support by declaring, "We are all family for the duration of the journey". Globalization, with its positive opportunities to address the needs of humanity and the dangers exemplified by September 11th, ensures that all—Protestants and Catholics in Northern Ireland, Israelis and Palestinians in the Middle East, Blacks and Whites in South Africa, East and West, North and South, rich and poor—all of us on this single planet hurtling through space, are "family for the duration". Psychoanalysts know that "being family" is not always a comforting reassurance, but it does imply that understanding is possible if we can find the time, the space and the language to look for it. I hope that this book helps us a little further on the journey.

TERRORISM

Introduction

Coline Covington

"The mere prospect of a bombardment will cause a huge panic to break out in New York"

These prescient words were not written last year, but last century: in March 1899 as part of Kaiser Wilhelm's strategy to overcome the United States' resistance to his goal of establishing colonies and military bases around the world. His plan of attack was quite specifically to throw New Yorkers and their fellow Americans so off guard that they could neither think nor defend themselves effectively. This destabilization through fear is certainly one of the central aims and consequences of terrorism, whether it is on a political level or between individuals.

In this opening section of the book, we start with the sheer impact of terrorism as witnessed in the attacks on the World Trade Centre on 11th September 2001. Justin Beal, a young architect, living across the street from the WTC, walked out of his apartment for a meeting on the morning of 11th September only to be stunned by the force and what he described as "the awesome beauty" of the first dreadful attack. His photographs record those moments: such visual brilliance of massive destruction makes for disturbing viewing. His commentaries, both immediately following the attacks and his reflections a month later, give us a first hand sense of the traumatic nature of his and many others' experience.

Following the attacks of 11th September, one of the resounding questions asked was, "What would make anyone do such a thing?" The psychological mentality of the suicidal terrorist left a gaping hole in people's understanding. Ron Britton's paper, "The 11th of September massacre", addresses this question by viewing it in terms of an urge to an exalted death or the sacrifice to a higher ideal which must be made as a way of maintaining an idealized parental image. The individual profile of terrorism is broadened in Phil Ringstrom's paper, "Thoughts on 11th September", and linked to the cultural clashes between Modernity and Fundamentalism. Using concepts from psychoanalysis and information systems theory, Ringstrom analyses these cultural perspectives as open and closed systems respectively, resulting in strikingly different mentalities that are in conflict with each other.

With Aleksander Vucho's paper, "Beyond bombs and sanctions", we see the devastating effects of this kind of splitting within the borders of the former Yugoslavia and witness how the "other" is turned into an enemy, how a terrorist regime takes over individuals and groups, how it destroys the ability to think or differentiate, and how it even invades the confines of personal analysis. The impact of terrorism within the therapeutic setting is explored in Dvora Miller-Florsheim's paper, "From containment to leakage, from the collective to the unique: therapist and patient in shared national trauma". Written at the time of the terrorist attacks under the El-Aqsa Intifada in Israel, Miller-Florsheim addresses the central question of how the therapeutic process can continue in the face of overwhelming external threat and how we can help each other to go on living in the wake of collective trauma.

The societal and individual components of terrorism are analysed in Salman Akhtar's concise paper, "The psychodynamic dimension of terrorism". Akhtar makes the important point that terrorism necessarily entails an element of covert masochism and self-destructiveness. This means that the stated aim of terrorism must, paradoxically, never succeed because, as Akhtar argues, "if the group were to succeed, it would no longer be needed. Its projectively buttressed identity would collapse and the pain of its own suffering would insist on being recognized and psychically metabolized. Because the terrorist leader cannot tolerate such a depressive crisis, he unconsciously aims for the impossible." On an individual level, Akhtar identifies four factors that lead the way out of this sado–masochistic dynamic and towards forgiveness. These factors are: repetition, revenge, reparation, and reconsideration. When the need to repeat traumatic memories and to seek some degree of revenge for the hurt that was done can be acknowledged, reparation and reconsideration can take place.

The final paper by Stuart Twemlow and Frank Sacco, "Reflections on the making of a terrorist", outlines the "life history" of terrorism by locating the nascent terrorist within a particular social context in which it is incubated, either by virtue of denial or collusion. Twemlow and Sacco conclude on a positive and hopeful note with some theoretical suggestions, rooted in psychoanalysis, for an "antidote" to terrorism. While it can be argued that the aim of psychoanalysis is to preserve freedom of thought, in this call to arms by Twemlow and Sacco we are left not only to reflect upon the underlying causes, both in the outside world and in the individual psyche, of terrorism but also to consider ways of actively combating these whether it is in the consulting room, the class room, the community centre or the wider political arena.

CHAPTER ONE

Thoughts and photographs, World Trade Centre: 11th September 2001

Justin Beal

Here is the first thing I wrote after my experience of the morning of September 11th:

I got up around 8:30, earlier than usual, because I was going to talk to Rafi and I wanted to have a cup of coffee and look over my portfolio first. I put all the relevant work in my portfolio and put it, along with some dirty clothes (for airbrushing) and my cell phone in my bag. Because of the huge HVAC unit across the street, almost no outside noise came into our apartment. I took a shower around 8:45 and when I got out Annie was sitting by the window smoking a cigarette. Annie didn't have a job yet, and that made her nervous so she was usually up as soon as anyone else got up. She was sitting on one of the benches we had made together in the spring looking out the window and she said there was a lot of smoke in the air or something and I remember responding, as I pulled my shoes on, "maybe the world trade centre is on fire?" Annie said she was going up to the roof to see what was going on. I grabbed my camera as I walked out the door because I thought the smoke might create an effect similar to the one in the fog photographs I had taken in August from the street below our apartment. I thought Gina had

23

already gone to work, but she had actually gotten into the shower while I was getting dressed and somehow we hadn't seen each other. Brennan and Andrew were already up and out of the apartment. It was now 8:55. I walked out onto the street and immediately took the first photograph as I walked up Greenwich. The sky was full of 8½ by 11 sheets of paper floating to the ground like snow. There was an aspect of magical realism to it all ... I was discovering that the largest office building in the world had exploded and the only visible evidence is copier paper. The thousands of papers in the sky kept me from looking at the carnage underfoot. They floated to the ground like confetti ... all the heavy stuff fell instantly, but the paper drifted in the sky for a long time afterwards. I remember stopping in front of the fire station at the corner of Liberty (where I had taken my fog photographs). From that corner the view was particularly powerful because the perspective was so extreme and the height of the building always evoked that classic feeling of sky-scraper vertigo. For weeks later, I would have nightmares about standing below tall buildings and looking up at them ... a fear of heights from the ground. A truck came out of the station behind my right shoulder as I was taking photographs. I walked by that fire station every day ... I remember Heather talking before she left for Barcelona about how hot the firemen were. I was not sure what was going on, but I was taking photographs with my right hand and trying to call Annie with my left ... the network was already swamped, so nobody's cell phones worked. The street was crowded with commuters, but no-one seemed to know what was going on. From where I was standing, it looked like there was a fire on the far side of the south tower (my view of the north tower was obstructed by the south tower, so I could not see the extent of the damage).

I was trying to recreate the composition of the fog photograph from the week before. I was holding the camera in front of my face and I was zooming in on the top of the south tower when the second plane hit from the opposite side. I saw the impact through the lens and closed the shutter. I remember looking down at my camera to make sure I had taken a photograph before turning to run away. I had. I felt the explosion in my stomach, I felt the heat on my face, but because I was already looking through the camera, the image that I saw was bound by the rectangular viewfinder and only lasted for 1/250th of a second. Nobody had any idea what was going on, but by now rumours of planes were circulating everywhere. It was pretty frantic for a few seconds right after the impact, but once the initial blaze of the explosion died down, people just stood around looking. The fire department had blocked off Greenwich and it didn't look like I could get back to the apartment the way I had come, so I kept trying to get Annie on the phone. I remember worrying about her being the only person other than me stupid enough to stand under a burning building and take photographs. Though, it's worth mentioning that it never even occurred to me that the buildings might fall over.

As things settled, I looked at my watch and realized I still had some time before I had to meet Rafi. I began walking up Broadway and I stopped near J&R to buy another roll of film. When the man charged me $6 I thanked him for not charging me $60 because I would have bought it anyway. Everyone was saying that a plane had hit the Pentagon and Fort Knox. I nearly got my film developed at a 20 minute processing place on Broadway right below canal. I went to get a cup of coffee on that block near the Pearl Paint frame store. I found the Lifeform office and buzzed up. I got upstairs and they told me Rafi had left as soon as the first plane hit. "He's Israeli", a woman at the desk remarked (i.e. anyone who is accustomed to terrorism runs away from it instead of running towards it). I asked if I could use the phone while I was there. I couldn't get a call through to Essex, so I called Clelia (who, mind you, had only arrived home the night before). She started crying when I said hello. I was standing on a fire escape with a portable phone, next to some computer guy who shared the office with Rafi. I had just left a message for Sophie when the south tower collapsed. The smoke made it hard to see it fall, but it was obvious when it was no longer there ... the plume of dust from the collapse cast a shadow all the way down Broadway, so the whole street looked like a badly lit movie set. I started walking up town and my shoes (the one's Mila bought me for my 21st birthday that never fit me) were killing my feet so I walked in my socks. I was on a cobbled street (just below Claire's apartment) when the second tower fell down. I continued up through Washington Square park. I was walking past the public library (was Brennan there?) when I finally got a hold of Annie and Gina at Rachel's apartment. That was the first time I thought of the studio Annie and I had applied for. I stopped on 6th Avenue and got $600 out of two different ATM machines, just in case. Next I stopped at Pete's to make some phone calls (and get a new pair of shoes ... I still had 30 blocks to Clelia's and I had begun the morning two blocks from the bottom of Manhattan). I called Pete at work, I called the Kuntz's. Pete came home and walked me up to 86th street. Somehow, Bunting got through on the cell phone as I passed the Museum of Natural History.

21 October 2001

I was holding the camera in front of my face and I was zooming in on the top of the south tower when the second plane hit from the opposite side. I saw the impact through the lens and closed the shutter. I remember looking down at my camera to make sure I had taken a photograph before turning to run away. I had. I felt the explosion in my stomach and heat on my face, but because I was already looking through the camera, the image that I saw was bound by the rectangular viewfinder and only lasted for 1/250th of a second. It was strange to have such a visceral experience mitigated by a lens: it means, among other things, that the photograph that remains is the same as the memory I have. What I remember most vividly was a feeling of excitement. This may sound perverse, but it was the most beautiful thing I have ever seen. The sky that morning was bluer and clearer than I had seen it before and the explosion was a brilliant cadmium orange; two fields of colour—spectral opposites—interrupted by the hard metallic verticals of the building. The composition of the visual image coupled with the sound, vibration, smell, and heat was an overwhelmingly sensual experience. It was precisely the terror/ecstasy phenomenon that Burke and Kant employed to explain the sublime. It was sublime in the sense of Burke's definition ... "the experience of the sublime is so overwhelming it makes reasoning impossible."

Burke said, "there is something so overruling in whatever inspires us with awe, in all things that belong ever so remotely to terror, that nothing can stand in their presence." He describes this awe as "a pleasure that turns on pain. Those things in nature that cause terror by their association with potential danger are sources of the sublime ... these things are capable of producing delight, not pleasure, but a sort of delightful horror" (taken from *A Philosophical Enquiry into the Origin of our Ideas of the Sublime and Beautiful*). I was personally so scared and so confused that I was overcome by a sensation of ecstasy; it felt exciting—the "delightful horror" Burke describes.

I realize much more now how my experience of that morning was changed because I had the camera with me. From the moment I stepped out of my door, I was looking for an interesting image ... and though this may seem incidental, I think it gave me a certain predisposition that affected my relationship to the ensuing situation enormously. Understanding the situation "through a lens" gave me a comfortable distance from what was actually going on. Eventually, that distance was coupled with a sense of urgency ... I did not understand what was going on, but I knew that it was important that I document it. The urgency, in turn, gave me a role in the situation, made me feel like an active participant (perhaps more so than a victim). The role as documentor also meant that I was focused on the "significance" of the event before I had fathomed or apprehended what had actually happened ... I was more aware of other people's reactions than my own. It was "beautiful" and "significant", but it was not "real" (in many respects it remains "unreal" today). I remember my hands shaking and my heart racing, but I don't remember any impulse to flee. I was excited and intrigued and terrified, but not afraid that something would happen to me. I wonder now how much of this had to do with the camera?

I found myself thinking of the way the camera let me engage with the situation, but also allowed for a certain detachment. I've been looking at the work of Robert Capa whose photographs are characterized by a fearlessness that can only be a consequence of that feeling of detachment. His famous photograph Soldier at the Moment of Death, Spanish Civil War (1936) is remarkable because it tells the story not only of a soldier dying, but also of Capa's role as a witness to that death. Volumes have been written on the influence of the camera on the way we understand war and Capa himself once stated, "if your pictures aren't good enough, you aren't close enough" (from David Mellor's essay, "Scenes of conflict"). Whether this proximity is a measure of time or distance, what makes every photograph that anyone took that September 11th morning so remarkable is the fact that no one understood what it was they were documenting.

The fifteen-minute pause between impacts meant that the attack on the World Trade Centre was the most well documented act of terrorism in history. There are thousands of photographs just like mine, but what makes each one of them fascinating is the implied presence of the photographer in the face of something utterly incomprehensible and traumatizing. Each photograph locates, with horrifying precision, the "sublime" moment. As one example, I might refer to the closely-cropped photograph I took at the moment of impact. I could see this precise image perfectly in my mind before the film had even been developed. The memory was "processed" as the film was "processed" and the strange coincidence of witnessing the impact through the camera lens meant that the image that would return to me constantly for the next few days came in the form of a neatly cropped rectangle.

Recently, I have been reflecting on the connection between the processes of photography and memory. The cliché of a media-dependent society is that we take photographs so we can see what we are looking at. There is so much in my photographs I did not see until they were developed. The details—the passport on the street, the people leaning out of windows, the carnage underfoot. The symbols—the American flag at the foot of the towers in one image, the faint crescent moon against the blue sky in several others. The number of photographs I have seen from that morning make it easy for me (or anyone) to appropriate images as part of my own memory... to "remember" things I know happened, but I did not see at the time (one of the deceptive characteristics of photography).

On one level, I was a witness to the terror that happened as I stood at the foot of the building, but on another, I was unaware of what I was seeing. Kafka said, "we photograph things in order to drive them out of our minds." (cf. Barthes; *Camera Lucida*) For the most part he is correct, but what such a statement fails to take into account is the force with which photographs, after the fact, can drive these things back into our minds.

The other detail curiously absent from many media photographs were the thousands of pieces of office paper in the sky. Perhaps it didn't even last that long, but from where I was standing at the foot of the building they filled the sky like snow. Each piece drifted to the ground as if in a world totally separate from the frenzy that was consuming the street below. It was beautiful. There is a certain Marquez-ian logic to the idea that when these massive buildings

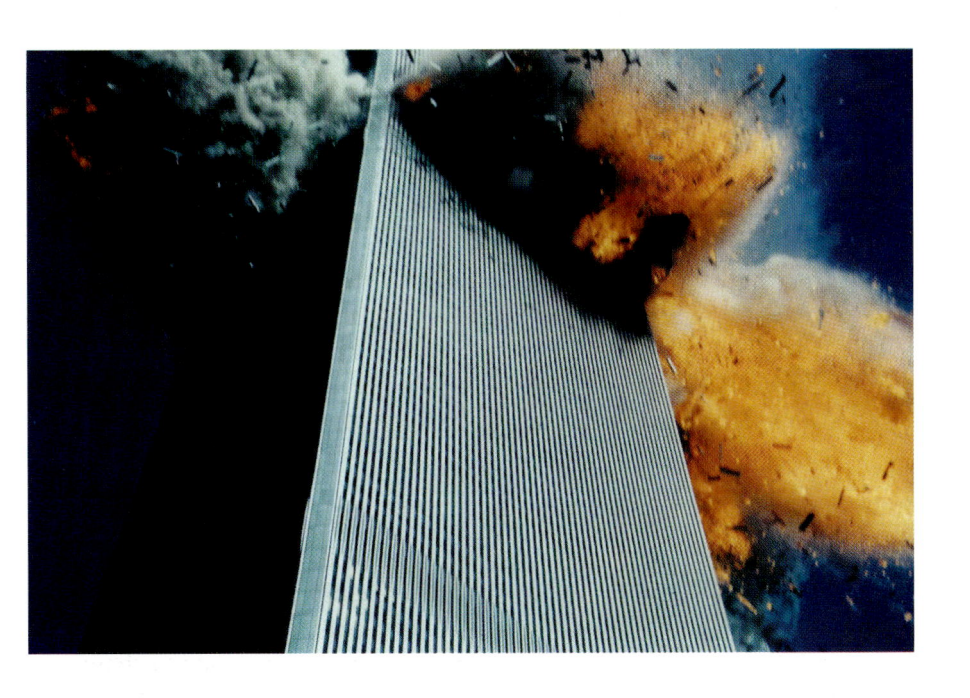

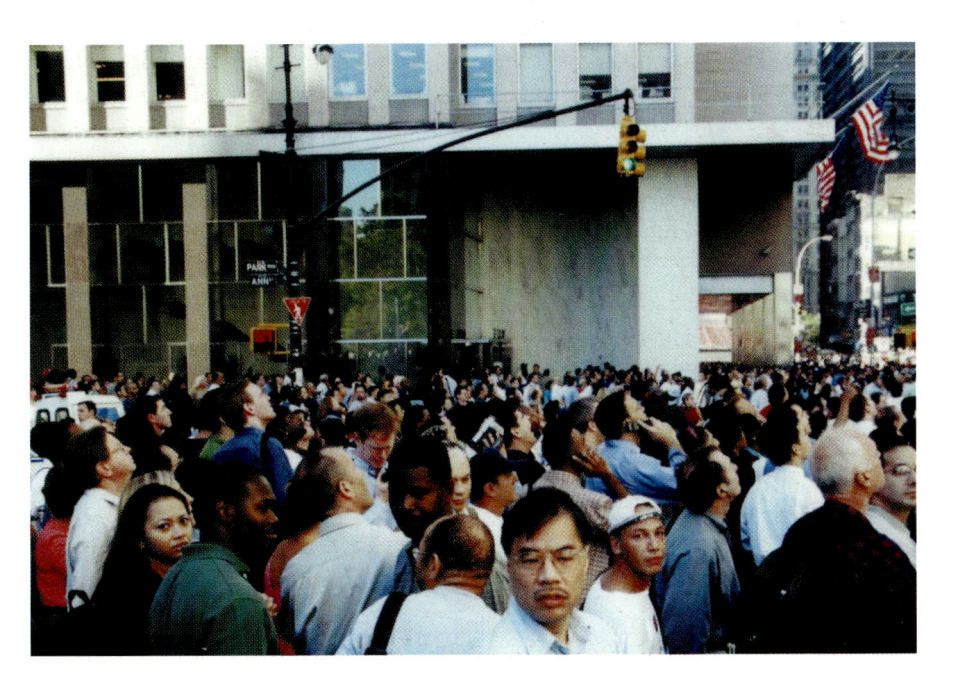

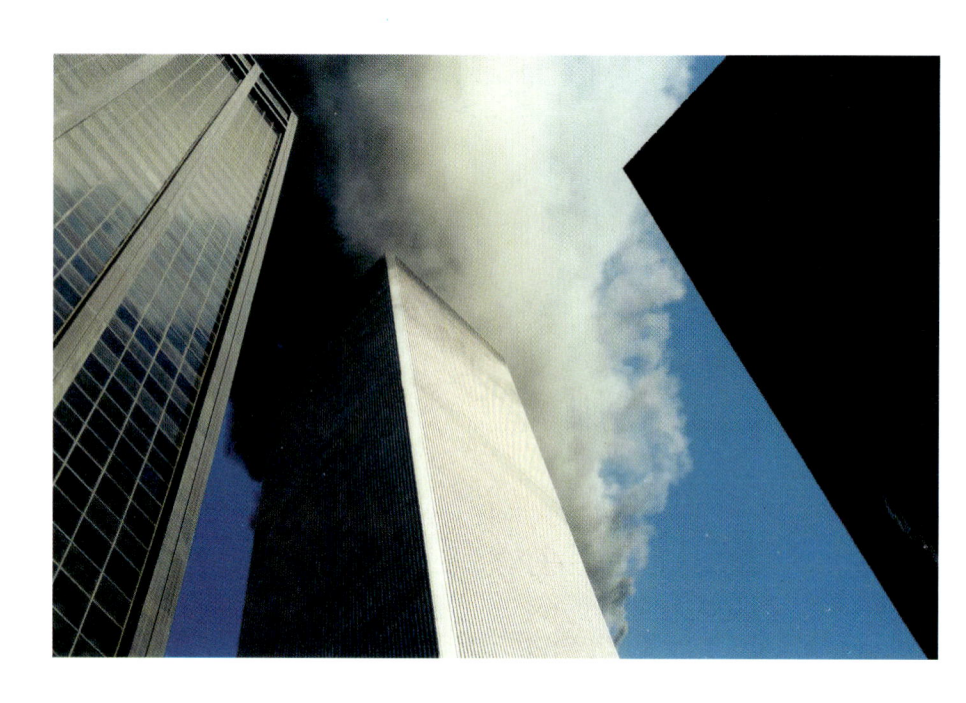

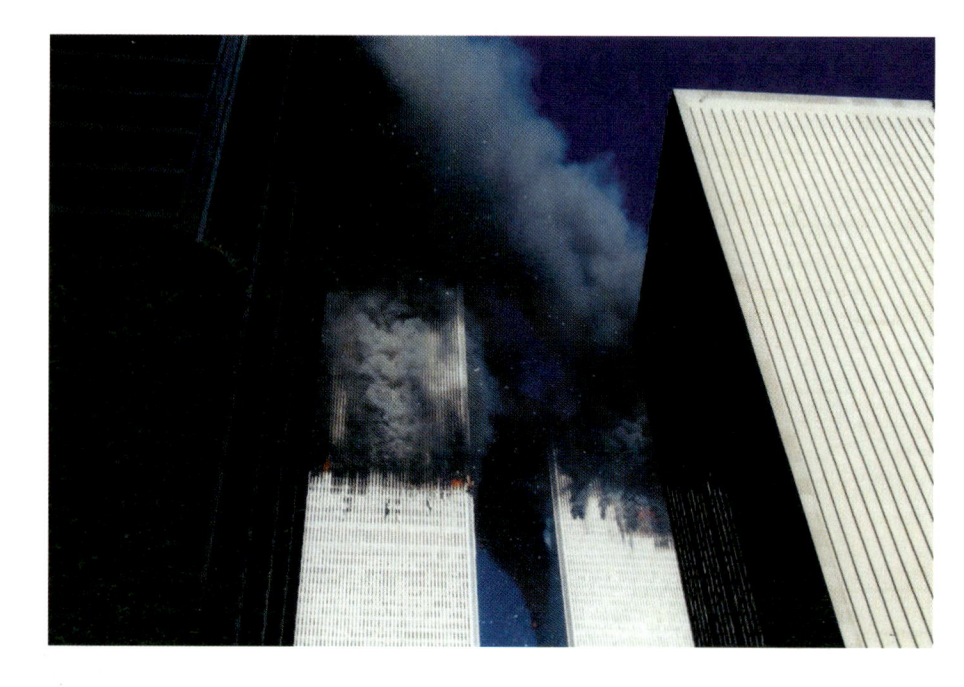

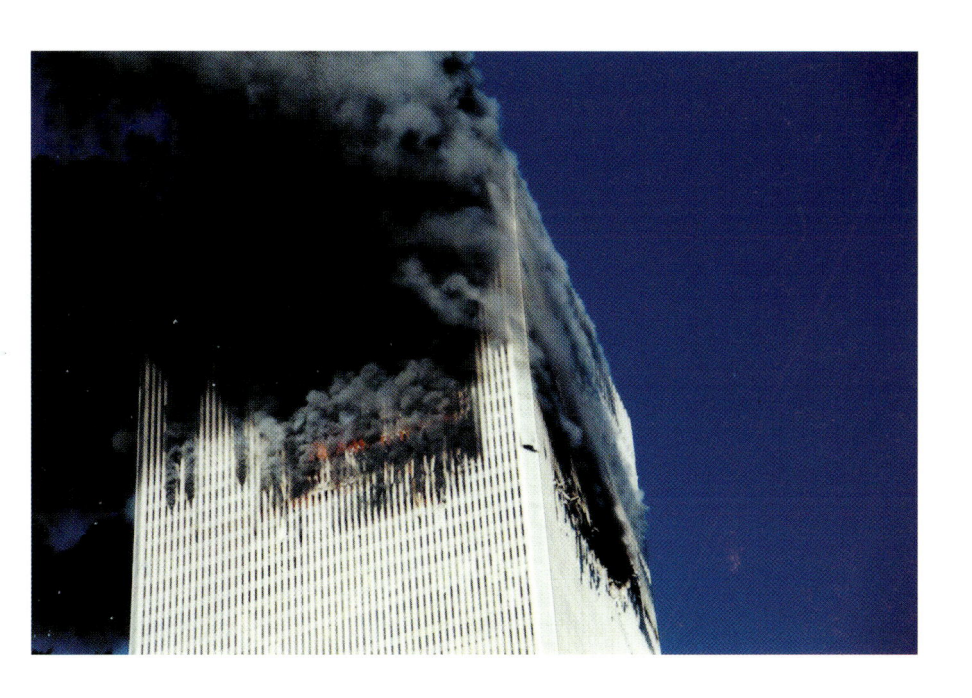

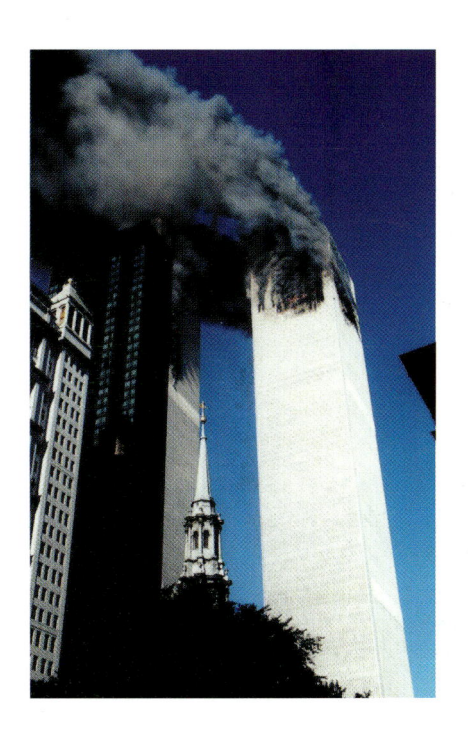

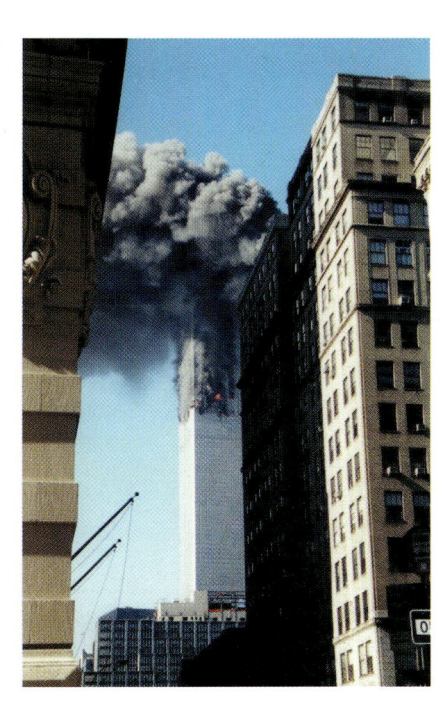

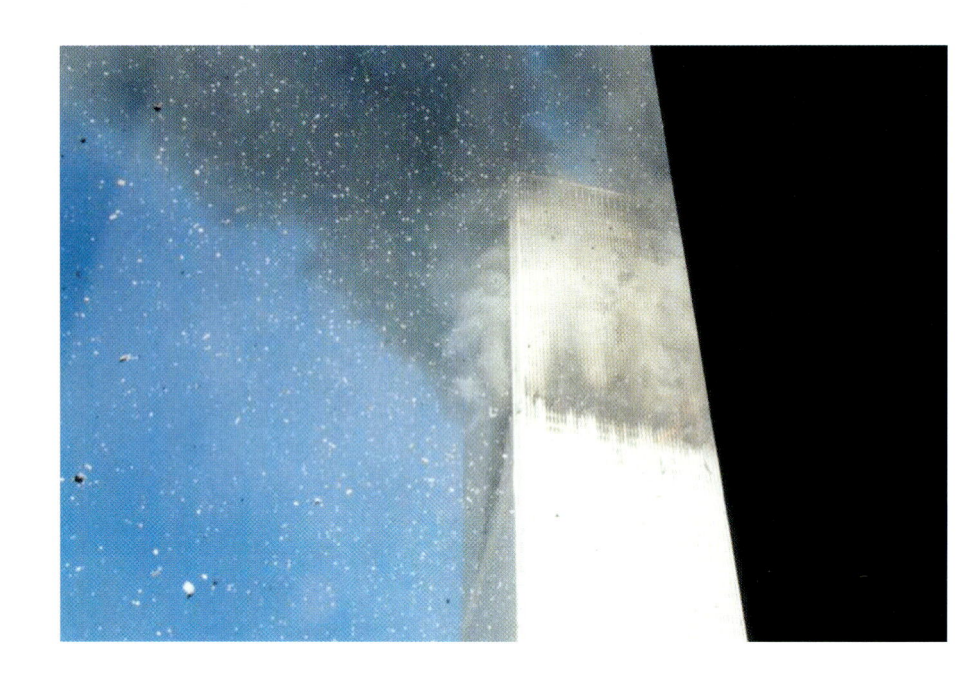

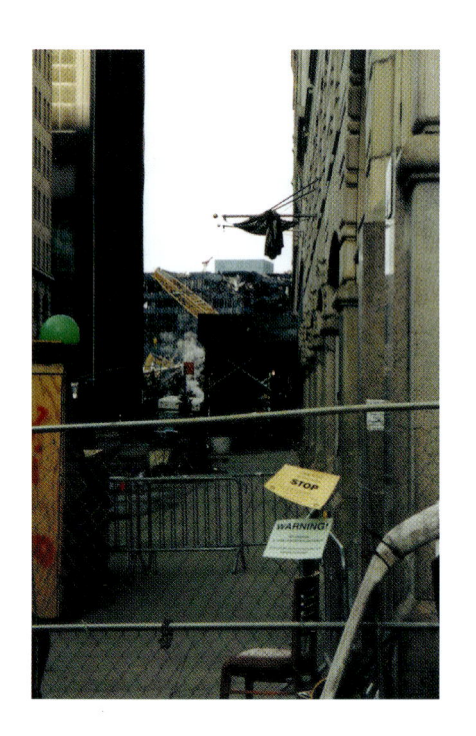

exploded, the sky wasn't full of blood or steel or glass, just paper. When I finally got back into my apartment weeks later there were pieces of this paper on my bed ... I still have several of them—a half-burnt invoice for some contracting work, fragments of a photocopied stock portfolio—that found their way in through the open window across the apartment and onto my bed.

CHAPTER TWO

The eleventh of September massacre

Ron Britton

> "The storm of airplanes will not stop, and there are thousands of young people who look forward to death like the Americans look forward to living"
>
> Osama bin Laden

Having read several excellent accounts on the religious, political and social background to the 11th September massacre, when asked to contribute something I asked myself what as a psychoanalyst can I usefully add. I wrote a paper on 'Fundamentalism' some years ago (1992) but I do not want to repeat that. So as I was already writing a paper on 'Sex, death and psychoanalysis', I thought I might offer a few thoughts on the suicidal act as a means of gaining divine approval and self-glorification.

A love affair with death

Those who died in the god's service, undergoing a violent death either by battle or by sacrifice, had entry into his realm ... the hero will be welcomed with feasting and hospitality because he died fearlessly. [Ellis Davidson, 1964, p. 149]

This is from the myths of the ninth century Norsemen of Europe, not from the creed of al-Qaeda. But Osama bin Laden in his *fatwa* of 1996 used almost the same words, describing how his 'young men' knew they would go directly to Paradise after sacrificing themselves in destroying the enemy.

I was reading these Nordic myths this summer when violent action based on such beliefs still seemed to be comfortably located in the remote past. My reason for doing so was that I was writing a paper on sex and death in hysteria, and exploring the ideas of Sabina Spielrein who was the first analyst to write on a 'destructive drive'. In her paper (1912) Spielrein, unlike Freud, locates "the destructive drive" *within* the "reproductive drive" (Spielrein, 1994, p. 184). I suggest in my paper that this location of the death drive is characteristic of a particular pathological organisation (Steiner, 1979) rather than its being a normal constituent of the sexual drive. In this system death is believed to produce eternal union rather than loss, whereas continued life is felt to cause separation.

In her paper, Spielrein brings Nietzsche to bear on the topic, "Loving and dying have gone together from eternity. The Will to Love: that is to be willing to die" (*ibid.*, p. 168), and she leans heavily on Wagner. "In Wagner, longing for death is often desire for dying in love" (*ibid.*, p. 177). She instances *The Flying Dutchman, Tristan and Isolde,* and most of all Siegfried and Brunhilde in *The Ring of the Nibelung*: Wagner's sources were the Nordic myths so this took me to reading them. As Nordic mythology, infatuation with Wagner's operas and a bad reading of Nietzsche all contributed to Hitler's idealism, the link made between Nazism and al-Qaeda in President Bush's speech to Congress may have some merit. Women had a place in Valhalla as the maids of Odin, serving pork, mead and sex to the warriors. Otherwise they could only enter "if they suffered a sacrificial death. They could be strangled and stabbed and burned after death in the name of the god" (Ellis Davidson, 1963, p. 150). Should they be burned on the hero's pyre their reward would be a marriage in the afterlife that they could not have in this one.

These ideas are not confined to Nordic paganism and Muslim fundamentalism. Christianity also has this theme of transfiguration through death and usually contains it in the person of Christ symbolically expressed in the 'Sacrifice of the Mass'. Less contained forms do appear in fundamentalist Christian sects from time to time and there have been examples in these of mass suicidal sacrifice.

In the individual, as psychoanalysts, we can posit explanations for this urge to an exalted death. Spielrein expressed this in these words,

> Their passion ... finds peace only with complete annihilation, with death of the personality. The strong fixation of libido on the parents makes transference to the external world impossible; no object completely resembles the parents ... I am dead means I have attained the desired regression to the parent and am disappearing there. [Spielrein, 1994, p. 173]

To this I would add that the fixation is to the infantile imago of an idealised parent who is more likely to be represented as God than as a human being.

I leave it to others to suggest how such individual psychopathology, if it is relevant, could be mirrored in group beliefs and behaviour. That it can history has repeatedly demonstrated, never more so than on the tragic day of 11th September 2001. The event itself still looms so large, and casts such a shadow on so many lives that it seems presumptuous to speculate on it as a psychological phenomenon. Similarly when hearing the news that a young man one knew well as a child has killed his father with an axe, saying to oneself 'how oedipal' seems unfitting to the shocking tragedy of the occasion. And yet it is what psychoanalysis can contribute.

CHAPTER THREE

Thoughts on September 11th, 2001

Philip A. Ringstrom

As none of us will forget, on September 11th, 2001 the unimaginable occurred when Muslim Extremist terrorists turned passenger airplanes into human-guided missiles targeting the Twin Trade Towers of New York City, the Pentagon, and an uncertain other failed target, perhaps the Capitol Building or White House. Shortly after this event, I took my ten-year-old daughter to our favourite Japanese restaurant. I asked her what she was learning in school about the events surrounding the September 11th attack. She was unclear, but wondered why on earth some people would do such a thing; what could they have against America, and what had we done to incur their hatred? As best I could, I tried to describe how we were witnessing a terrible clash of cultures. Islamic Fundamentalism was finding itself threatened by our culture, which embodies elements of modernity that we in the West take for granted. To elaborate in terms she could understand I spoke of the treatment of girls and of women in an extremist Fundamentalist culture such as Taliban society. They are prohibited from engaging in all the things she expects to be able to do; to be educated, to choose a life of her own, a career and to have a family, to move about as she pleases, to dress as she sees fit and to live with the understanding and burden that she will have to develop a mind of her own and be responsible for the choices she makes. When I described the fate of women in Islamic Fundamentalist culture she was powerfully affected. She was incapable of conceiving of what I was describing, asking incredulously, "Why don't they just leave? Why don't they just come to America?" Her naive inquiry conveyed a simplicity of thought that is so humanly natural yet is soon dispelled by the vicissitudes of maturity.

A war of cultures is what we face, and, as psychoanalysts, we recognize that this war is also a clash of differing attitudes to what must be loosely described as clashing states of minds or mental sets. In this light, it is critical for psychoanalysts to participate in conceptualizing what we see going on in order to preserve the freedom of mind that we aver, and to provide insight that may contribute to socio-political analysis. We need to contend with extremist Fundamentalist forces that are in conflict with our modernity. Modernity is exemplified and defended by what must be the most powerful evolutionary statement of western civilization —the Constitution of the United States of America. This document guarantees freedom of thought, freedom of faith, and most importantly freedom of expression of both. As this social contract openly embraces a range of beliefs, including those of Fundamentalists of both religious and secular systems, those who pose a threat to the psycho/social/political context the Constitution defends must be taken seriously. We need to be able to understand the prevailing clash between Fundamentalism and Modernity; to examine how that clash can lead to the type of terrorist assault that has finally awakened America from its isolationist, dogmatic slumbers, and pressed it into a role reflecting its Constitution—not only for its sake, but for the preservation of freedom as defined by its Constitution.

Fundamentalism in extremis

Fundamentalism, it should be noted, has been a social fact throughout history, and the reigns of terror associated with it were seldom found to be more ferocious than in the conduct of Christianity. While Andrew Sullivan (2001) noted that the Western world has grown up and learned from its egregious past, we still witness occasions within cells of Christian fundamentalism of perverse thinking such as Reverent Jerry Falwell's pronouncement that September 11th was God's way of punishing secularist America for straying from a moralistic path. Falwell's comments, targeting gays and liberals in particular, were withdrawn under an onslaught of outrage, but not soon enough to mark his form of fundamentalism as a curious bed-fellow of the Islamic fundamentalism that led to the September 11th assault.

With Farwell's version of Christianity more the exception than the rule, we may look to the history of Western culture as having spawned Modernist thought. The roots of modernity, cultivated four hundred years ago by John Locke and others, represent a tradition that relies on personal choice in faith. The tradition argues that there can be no true faith without this freedom. This choice is burdensome to the individual believer (or non-believer) and often leaves its communities ill at ease in the uncertainties that they must tolerate in order to live this way. Modernity lacks the assuredness of Fundamentalism and tends to vex us with doubt. This is the tradition of mind that Freud grew up in, and that allowed him to address a question that Fundamentalists find difficult to contemplate. What is this thing, this mind of man's, that is capable of so deceiving itself? It is only in this study, the examination of the unconscious as Freud delineated, that we are remotely free to exercise what might be termed "choice". This position refines Socrates' admonition that the unexamined life is not worth living, while inadvertently perhaps moves us in the direction of hermeneutics: in other words, the text is always interpreted by the interpreter. Or, as applied to psychoanalytic work, reality is understood to be an "interpretative text", so to speak, interpreted through the personal narratives and unconscious (psychic) realities of both analyst and patient. What elevates modernity above solipsistic relativism is the agreement that where multiple interpreters are free to argue their views, ever evolving dialogical truths are likely to prevail (Cavell, 1998; Gabbard, 1997; Orange et al., 1997; Renik, 1998). These principles are unacceptable to the Fundamentalist and constitute a threat to Fundamentalist Islam and above all to it most extremist outcroppings such as Taliban, Al Qaeda, and the forces led by charismatic leaders such as Osama Bin Laden.

In the Fundamentalist tradition, the text is viewed as *objet fixe*; a literal translation only is permissible and deviation constitutes heresy, sometimes punishable by death. Christianity once also suffered from this but must have learned something along the way. I am unaware, for example, of any current version of Christian faith or nation state that embodies the principles of Christianity that would threaten to execute humanitarian aid workers for introducing their faith as did the Taliban to eight Western workers convicted of having committed the crime of proselytizing.

The principal difficulty with Fundamentalism is that there is no place for difference and we know that where such contexts proliferate we find interpersonal strife characterized by dominance and submission. Sullivan points out that all that is not in accordance with the Fundamentalist's beliefs must be eradicated, lest the Fundamentalist lapse into capitulation with the heretical and thereby threaten his faith, his community, and its well being. Jessica Benjamin (1999) referred to these attitudes as complementary relational structures of dominance and submission. They cultivate a type of cultural projective identification wherein the West readily buys into asymmetrical dominance–submission gambits. Some of this became evident in the White House's rhetorical riposte, post-September 11th, against "evil" and "evildoers" who must be eradicated. It even led, lamentably, to the use of the term "crusade" against terrorism. This blunder colluded with the language structure of extreme Islamic Fundamentalists and was exploited as evidence of the "West's" intent to eliminate Islam, when in fact it was a reaction to Islamic terrorists' pledge to eliminate the West. If this were the end point of the discussion we would be engaging in little more than a kind of mimicry where each party takes the position of victim self-righteously fighting the evil other. But the projective identificatory link goes further. Mark Twain's novel the *The Mysterious Stranger* captured how each side in a war ironically invokes God as theirs and that He will, "God willing", save our side from that of the infidels. Comparably, the transcript of a videotape of Osama Bin Laden along with several leaders of the Al Qaeda movement showed them invoking "Allah Be Praised", and Allah was interspersed in virtually every sentence, whilst at the same time President Bush completed all of his speeches with "God Bless America". (See verbatim transcript of the video reported in the *Los Angeles Times* newspaper, December 14, 2001.)

The contribution of information theory

Ideas from the information sciences have influenced the evolution of certain ideas in contemporary psychoanalysis. The concern I shall focus on in this paper, pertains to conflictual differences between one culture founded on principles of Fundamentalism and another entrenched in Modernity. The Fundamentalism I am discussing is not only religious but also secular, as has been discussed by Robert Young (2001). The introduction of information science thinking (in particular semiotics—the study of signs) poses a challenge to the traditional dual drive theory of psychoanalysis. Information systems create links between the biological, the cultural, the intrapsychic, and the intersubjective in permutations from dyad to triad to family and community. They provide ways of conceptualizing that are meaningful in a cultural debate about principles of freedom versus principles of rigidified constraint. David Olds' article "A semiotic model of mind" (2000) is informative in this respect. Semiotics, a branch of information theory, addresses the cultural usage of signs to represent reality and provides a model of mind and of "mentalization" (cf. Fonagy & Target, 1996) that corresponds with recognition and interpretation of signs, signals, icons, and symbols. Semiotics asserts that reality is not directly knowable, but is constructed in the verbal and non-verbal language of culture. Employing information theory and semiotics provides a framework from which to construct a theory of mind that captures cultural conflict. In information terms, Fundamentalism posits and enforces systems of signs, signals, and symbols that strictly and literally rule-in what is good and rule-out what is bad. That which is ruled-out as evil *must* be eliminated while that which is good *must* be followed. From an avowed position of certainty, Fundamentalism proscribes that which cannot be viewed as contending points of view. There is power in this form of certainty in that ideologues may gather masses of the uncertain and lost around them.

In contrast to such closed system thinking, modernity, with all its faults, embodies information processing principles central to its cultural Weltanschauung that call upon and perpetually create greater and vastly more complex information systems. These are prone to processes of chaos (not necessarily randomness) that make things less certain, less predictable, and by virtue of this, more liberal, with all the complications that ensue. It is precisely this context of modernity that antagonises fundamentalists. The Reverent Falwell's Moral Majority, Nazi Germany, and the Taliban's response to this "heresy". One sees that the more complex thinking systems become, the more disturbing they are for those who find solace and security in the *diktats* of Fundamentalism.

We currently find ourselves in America akin to the psychoanalyst who is at times engulfed by transference attributions. Virtually everything he or she does may come to be perceived in terms of the patient's projections. For example, historically the USA in particular and the West in general, operating out of an information culture based on a considerable degree of social freedom, have had no overt interest in eliminating Islam. We have been interested in the oil that lies within many Islamic states in order to keep our particular lifestyle going. How responsible this objective is must, for reasons of space, remain another debate! The United States has also had a stake in preserving Israel, in part as a territorial imperative, both compensating for the atrocities Jews suffered during World War II, as well as insuring Jews their 3000 year old homeland. Devoid of an intentional design to eliminate Islam, the United States and much of the West struggles to comprehend the attributions made by Fundamentalists. However, Western Culture, with its porous boundaries and expansionist tendencies, exposes Fundamentalist Islamic countries (and others) to a cornucopia of popular western cultural temptations. Cultures that wash away semblances of class hierarchy, authority and dogma and promote an "anyone can have a shot at making it" message have been effective in diluting obvious class divisions, particularly in the USA. In the absence of any direct intent to eliminate Islam or control it beyond protecting and promoting Western national interests (in itself a powerful source of provocation), Bin Laden's and Al Qaeda's transference accusations could be understood as, at least to some degree, a projection of their own disavowed intentions. This is reflected in Bin Laden's call for the West's exodus from any involvement in the Middle East, discontinuation of our support for Israel and the entire Infidel world's conversion to the Muslim faith.

The outlook required for allegiance to a fundamentalist culture as depicted here may share certain characteristics with those patients who suffer a failure to imagine beyond their core constraining premises, as to do so threatens the fundamentals of their mental organizing criteria, i.e. their "invariant organizing principles". Considered in information terms this threat risks potential fragmentation at the level of the self-state and possibly at the level of the nation-state given that there exists a degree of identification between selfhood, group identity, and statehood in such societies.

What generations of psychoanalysts have attempted to learn from their clinical experiences is that to grasp the appeal of certainty we must find ourselves falling prey to re-enacting it. Hate in the countertransference is the vehicle for understanding hate in the transference. We have learned not to retaliate but to try to understand the nature of our patients' hatred and to respond not in kind but with emotional intelligence that may transform primitive, persecuting affects into food for thought.

Kleinian concepts; concern for the other

One way of thinking about this, from a psychoanalytic perspective, is to consider Klein's views on the depressive position.[1] Among the most compelling of Klein's ideas is that of the "epistemophilic instinct", or need to know what we as humans are about, starting from the centre of our own experience. This achievement materializes out of the capacity to reflect upon our motivations and not solely to react to them. It is linked to our ability to feel remorse and to recognize that there is more than one way to think about a subject and that things are seldom entirely good or entirely evil. Each of us is an admixture of positive and negative features in relation to others and we are prone to enact these unless we become able to reflect upon this personal truth about our condition. It lends itself to the developmental achievement of intersubjectivity: subject to subject relating wherein the other is recognized in terms of their subjectivity (Benjamin, 1988; Stern, 1985) and is no longer seen merely in terms of an object that either nurtures or persecutes.

Individuals and groups whose histories of trauma, individual and collective pathology or sense of injustice leave them fixated in the bifurcated position of paranoid/schizoid experience are left with little capacity to engage in the complex, variant expressions of intrapsychic and interpersonal concern for others that is constitutive of the depressive position. No individual, or group for that matter, is above slipping into the paranoid/schizoid position even if they have managed to develop beyond it—the relationship between P–S and D is probably one of lifelong flux. How do we infuse a closed system, frozen in a black and white mental process, with a way of thinking beyond an axis of pathological projection–introjection towards more reflective functioning? This remains our task whether we are faced with a borderline patient, a terrorist cell, or simply reactionary Americans who think only of bombing a country back into the dark ages, although the means we may employ in each of these situations will vary. Another way of considering this problem is to think in terms of variance and invariance of our capacity to think, feel, and act. How, developmentally, can we achieve multiple, fluidly organized perspectives rather than fixed, deterministic ones? Variance allows for measured, considered responses in the face of threat and is critical in the context of the terrorist's attempt to usurp "mentalization" (Fonagy & Target, 1996). Perhaps there was evidence of this in Western governments' responses in the aftermath of the September 11th assault. However imperfect or tainted by President Bush's rather simplistic rhetoric, the West exhibited restraint and reflection in framing its responses. It attempted to be deliberate in addressing as directly as possible those who vow to do it harm. At the same time it committed us to doing so in a manner that separates the terrorists (and those who wilfully harbour them) from the innocents that surround them and to do as little harm to the innocents as is technically possible. How practical this turns out to be is another question.

When examined from the perspective of modernity, the logic that supports terrorist acts cannot fail to embody elements of pathology, notwithstanding the necessary geopolitical explanations that help us understand from whence it arises. By paying careful, analytic attention to the pathological aspect, without demonizing it, it can assist us in avoiding lapses into our own potential for paranoid/schizoid thinking and reactionary retaliation. The psychological task is to recognize the primitive impulse and undertake a certain amount of mental work to metabolize the hated projection long enough to understand its source. We may then be more able to respond not only to a source of harm to the world, but to a sick organism, be it a region in particular or the globe at large, and one that requires care as much as surgery.

This way of thinking about terrorism, as a source of coercion, intimidation, and mind control when Fundamentalism becomes threatened by too much diversity, can help us to grasp why the extreme radicalization of the Fundamentalist's perspective lends itself to a shift away from its potentially more containing and socially organizing elements to something akin to nihilism. Karen Armstrong, who writes on the history of Islam as well as other forms of religious fundamentalism, underscored precisely this point when she commented that the terrorists' actions seemed more in accordance with nihilism than Fundamentalism. No true Fundamentalist, she added, would face Allah in Heaven with vodka on his breath or with having become involved with non-Muslim women as some of the terrorists had—in other words, having "succumbed" to western values. So whilst there may be a clear connection to Fundamentalism, it is important to recognize that a movement such as Al Qaeda has an additional purpose beyond Fundamentalism, expressed as destruction that is unamenable to reason or dialogue. Armstrong suggests that this additional purpose is characterized by an Armageddon quality in which destruction is conceived of and framed according to the premise "to save mankind, you must first destroy it" and that this must be expedited in biblical proportions.

When individuals or groups arrogate to themselves, in the manner outlined above, a position of absolute cultural authority, any form of coercion may be employed to protect what is at stake. Terrorism can be both highly economical and effective in this respect. According to *Webster's Dictionary*, terrorism is "the systematic use of terror especially as a means of coercion." It achieves this by inducing trauma, which elsewhere I have suggested involves the "visitation of the unimaginable" (Ringstrom, 1999). The coercion that terrorism imposes is less about physical trauma (notwithstanding the tremendous damage to New York City and Washington, DC) than it is about psychological oppression. Physical destruction of persons or property is a means to an end: the terrorists' wider goal is to impair and if possible immobilize its victims' ability to "mentalize" (Fonagy & Target, *ibid.*). This pathological objective aims to remove the ability to consider situations in their complexity; to eradicate a symbolic level of functioning that allows for reflection and revision of ideas in the face of new data; and in place of more complex ways of thinking to introduce ideas as equivalent to icons or concrete objects ("things" as opposed to "words") that are beyond question or examination and which bear comparison to "symbol equations" (cf. Segal, 1964). The casualty of the victims' impaired thinking is a mutual inability to relate. The extension of this casualty is an impairment of the capacity to recognize the other in terms of his or her subjective experience and only as a frightening object who will dominate them (if they are unable to dominate him). The terrorist's goal is to draw the other into paranoid–schizoid conflict that treats peace not as an objective (a developmental outlook being precluded) but as an obstacle to a more frightening agenda of domination, submission, and annihilation.

The traumatized mind that the terrorist seeks to induce is also likely to be a reflection of his own mental state: terrorism is driven in part by a type of malignant projective identification. It includes a perverse form of empathy, requiring first some ability to "enter the mind" of its potential victim, to best know how to cause havoc. Kohut noted this in his discussion of the way the Germans used the V-2 "buzzbomb" in the Battle of Britain. The weapon was strategically poor insofar as it was a relatively direction-less, target-less bomb that simply fell out of the sky when its fuel was spent. Psychologically, however, it was worth its weight in gold to the oppressor. Terror descended on those below when they heard its engine stop. The Al Qaeda terrorists in the present campaign are exercising a similar ingenuity, using to advantage the fruits of western modernization by identifying and capitalizing on our passion for freedom, privacy, and technology. All three of these are being marshalled against our democratically constituted society, with the object of inducing us to forsake more and more of these rights and to employ constraints more associated with Fundamentalist societies.

The traumatized mind of the terrorist's victim is required to function a-historically insofar as the past is collapsed into the present through the annulment of the capacity to feel and grasp a distinction between the two. Centuries-old wounds remain alive and are reactivated instantly by any actions that echo from the past. Vigilance is high, ambiguity intolerable and any situation must be codified as either safe or not, and since there is no room for error in judging safety, judgement is readily forsaken for the more seemingly foolproof paranoid position. This position can even call for pre-emptive strikes if moments of doubt intrude sufficiently. It is this state of mind that the terrorist hopes to inculcate in the West and it is certainly a responsibility of the psychoanalytic community to contribute our experience in whatever ways are necessary to illuminate and obstruct their objective. The traumatized mind the terrorists seek to create is prone to collapse into rigid dominant–submissive complementary structures, as noted by Benjamin (1998). Through these means, terrorists ensure that there is no room for dialogue, no place for peace and no condition for creating representative government. Note how every peace initiative in the Israeli–Palestinian conflict is punctuated by an act of extremist terrorism. War at any cost is the terrorist's mission.

Terrorist cells have little difficulty finding recruits in the tumultuous Middle East where it is common for young men to live with little sense of hope for the future. Often they have suffered personal losses of property, family, and friends. Despite such losses, the greatest loss to these impassioned youths must be their capacity to "mentalize". They resort to binary thinking which makes kinship to fundamentalists possible, though not inevitable. Right and wrong are proscribed by and enforced in terms of a literal (anti-hermeneutic) reading of religious or secular texts. The need to be told what is good and what is evil renders them submissive to the authority of their ideological leaders. The phrase, "having a mind of one's own" is antithetical, if not incomprehensible. Because the code of right and wrong is *a priori* dictated in a climate that supports no open debate of multiple perspectives, the appeal of collective certainty and imposed notions of "truth" in the face of complexity is compelling.[2]

As psychoanalysts, our theory and practice rests on the premise of freeing ourselves and our patients to think—to have our own minds. While we have conflicting points of view given our differing theories, we generally do not allow political analysis to temper our voice on the importance of preserving freedom of thought. We need to remain opposed to terrorism of all sorts and be vigilant against acts of our own in the West that risk engaging with them. Most of all, we need to support policies that serve to open up the capacity for broadened perspectives by creating potential or "transitional" space beyond the splitting and projective identification into which terrorists draw their victims. Our task is to examine the conditions under which minds are likely to be traumatized and under which they are more likely to be integrated. It may be of interest that a West Point graduate with eight subsequent years of humanitarian relief efforts was interviewed on the U.S. "Fresh Air" programme cited earlier. This former cadet commented that the current enlightened military perspective is that humanitarian aid may well become an important military strategy in the long-term, since every enemy you convert, as well as every enemy you do not create, is one less enemy that you will one day have to fight. This does not obviate the fact that we must be prepared to fight enemies such as the Al Qaeda terrorists, but we also need to provide damaged minds and starving bodies with food of different kinds.[3]

Macro to micro; cultural to personal

I want to shift from a macro lens perspective very briefly to the micro lens of dealing with the trauma of loss that the September 11th event forced upon us as individuals. Trauma, Grotstein (1997) suggests, arises when we are assaulted by an inability to imagine the events that overwhelm us. In effect, we have not been able to "create" the trauma in our mind prior to its occurrence. In fact, I believe the primary factor that differentiates the same event from being immobilizingly traumatic to some but less so to others is that the former have no chance (or perhaps the capacity) to imagine the event in advance. Bromberg (1998) notes that it literally shocks them. Furthermore, we are all the more devastated in circumstances when we are assaulted by the very thing our unconsciously omnipotent fantasies led us to feel we were impervious to.

Stolorow (1999) has written that in trauma, there is an experience of "estrangement and isolation" that lends itself to a "psychic partition" between those described by one of his patients as "normals" and the "traumatized ones". This partition is such, his patient informed him, "That there is no possibility for a normal to ever grasp the experience of a traumatised one." Though there are clear problems in reifying conceptually a partition analogy, there is a sense in which severely traumatized people undergo experiences which, by definition, the majority cannot grasp. Knowledge of this fact in the analyst or therapist and, if possible, recognition of it and working through it, can make a great difference to the patient's sense of unique, un-understandable separation from others.

In conclusion, the tragic events of September 11th bring to the attention of psychoanalysts around the world with great force a spectrum of issues from the macro to the micro. By understanding clashes in culture (between, for example, modernity and fundamentalism) we can become better equipped to understand how culture can operate to free the human spirit or to shackle it. By employing ideas from information systems theory and semiotics we can draw some parallels between the informational constraints of culture and those of the human psyche.

With regard to the micro or personal dimension it is important to remember how in trauma, the assault of the unimaginable preys on the trauma victim's subsequent imaginings. Perhaps more aptly, the assault can effect a failure to imagine, wherein the trauma robs those most directly affected of the ability to have controlled it in advance via some form of cognitive preparation. Such victims often become haunted by the task of trying to imagine—often obsessively —what was heretofore unimaginable. Helping the trauma victim with a failure to imagine with re-ignition of imagination as part of a less restrained mental capacity is fundamental to analytic work.

Notes

1. Those unfamiliar with Klein's taxonomy may be confused by the term "depressive position" which simply relates the intrapsychic experience of integration. That is, to a state of reconciliation of the loved and the hated rather than, for example, the hated being projected out and attributed to the other, this latter example reminiscent of the "splitting and projection" of the paranoid/schizoid positions. It appears that Klein chose the term depressive because of the sadness and remorse

that often accompanies the cognitive realizations of the depressive position.

2. Professor M. A. Muqtedar Khan, in his memo to American Muslims provides a compelling example when he beseeches his fellow American Muslims to examine their own cognitive impairment:

> While we loudly and consistently condemn Israel for its ill treatment of Palestinians, we are silent when Muslim regimes abuse the rights of Muslims and slaughter thousands of them. Remember Saddam Hussein and his use of chemical weapons against Muslims (Kurds)? Remember the Pakistani army's excesses against Muslims (Bengalis)? Remember the mujahideen of Afghanistan and their mutual slaughter? Have we ever condemned them for their excesses? Have we demanded international intervention or retribution against them? Do you know how the Saudis treat their minority Shiis? Have we protested the violation of their rights? But we all are eager to condemn Israel; not because we care for the rights and lives of the Palestinians; we don't. We condemn Israel because we hate "them."

He then adds,

> The biggest victims of hate-filled politics as embodied in the actions of several Muslim militias all over the world are Muslims themselves. Hate is the extreme form of intolerance and when individuals and groups succumb to it they can do nothing constructive. Militias like the Taliban have allowed their hate for the West to override their obligation to pursue the welfare of their people and as a result of their actions not only have thousands of innocent people died in America, but thousands of people will die in the Muslim world.

As evidence, he writes,

> Already, half a million Afghans have had to leave their homes and their country. It will only get worse as the war escalates. Hamas and Islamic Jihad may kill a few Jews, women and children included, with their suicide bombs and temporarily satisfy their lust for Jewish blood, but thousands of Palestinians then pay the price for their actions.

3. An American Muslim interviewed on NPR today spoke with great pride about America. He noted that with the exception of a few extremists (which he compared to Bin Laden incidentally) there have been very few attacks on Muslims in this country, and in fact a widespread outpouring of support. I think this is emblematic of a nation-state that has evidenced increasing multicultural maturity that represents a quality of life incomprehensible to a Middle Eastern world

vexed in far more collapsed and constrained beliefs that are not even allowed to be challenged. Those conditions are anathema to what we as analysts believe in and we should not hesitate to preserve and expand what we have in this country. The choice to live a life as a fundamentalist should be just that, a choice. It cannot be so in an environment that has no tolerance of difference.

CHAPTER FOUR

Beyond bombs and sanctions

Aleksander Vucho

I consider nationalism in terms of a malignant form of national identity based on the hate of those who do not belong to one's own nationality. Since identity is established on similarities and differences, the chances for intolerance of members of other nationalities are great. Few are those that have never felt hostility towards someone just because he/she belongs to another group. The form of this hostility may be benign as, for example, when we return from a trip abroad and do not exactly ascribe the best characteristics to the members of that nation. We see them through stereotypes, or broadly generalize the positive or negative traits of individuals to the entire nation. Sporting competitions between two nations usually lead to passionate reactions which are, generally, spent in front of television, but sometimes may become malevolent in the field. We may be suspicious or distant to members of other nations or, in multi-ethnic environments, we may vote for a member of our own nation just because s/he is a member, not seeing his/her aggression and willingness to provoke inter-ethnic conflict. Therefore we meet with an omnipresent phenomenon, existing in each of us and hence, as a group phenomenon, it represents a phenomenon requiring careful treatment. In order to flourish in its full and tragic force, nationalism requires a mass (Freud, 1921). Once the spirit of nationalism is released it is impossible to control it and return to the individual where it can be handled more easily.

Nationalism is, above all, a group phenomenon. Nevertheless, in its vehemence it exceeds other phenomena that may be related to groups of similar sizes, such as patriotism, for example. It is said that there is no war as hideous as the war between nations sharing the same territory. By the speed of its development, barbarity, the extended time necessary to find a peaceful solution to the differences which have arisen between the quarrelling nations, this clash resembles family conflicts. The quarrelling family members, who until that moment had been living seemingly peacefully, suddenly quarrel, break off all ties, accuse each other of disloyalty, betrayal, and of having been robbed by them. An outside observer will see all of this either as absurd or easily resolved, since he/she is not acquainted with the passions hidden behind the misunderstanding. It seems to an outside observer that the quarrelling parties may easily be reconciled since the conflict itself is insignificant, that it is simple to determine by rational methods who is right, or if all fails, the quarrelling parties can easily separate. In the case of former Yugoslavia, as we all unfortunately know, none of this has happened. The quarrelling parties got into a bloody fight, the parties who speak the same language, whether they like it or not. The other two nations, not sharing the same language, have more or less escaped the slaughter. Furthermore, the parties of war behaved like the three super states from Orwell's *1984*, continuously uniting forces against the third. So once again, we come to the family phenomenon—the closer they are the more they hate each other.

I belong to a generation born in the early fifties that has been taught throughout its entire schooling that brotherhood and unity are the most precious values. Yet I learnt as well, through the history of the Middle Ages, that sons, brothers, or relatives in conflict had destroyed large states (Serbia, Croatia, and Bosnia) and made them easy prey to various external enemies. When nationalism in Serbia gained momentum in 1987 I again had a chance to read that, for us, unity is most important, and somewhat later, that we must protect our brothers. We see what became of our unity, and of how we protected our brothers.

The social and political situation in former Yugoslavia was

fertile ground for the emergence of nationalist movements. The former Yugoslavia consisted of six republics, two autonomous provinces with six nations and many national minorities. The situation was rendered more complicated by the presence of Christianity and Islam: the Christians were mainly divided into Orthodox and Catholic with the presence of the majority of large Christian sects. About 80% of the population were of Slavic origin, 10% Albanians and some 10% of others. Approximately a quarter of all marriages were multi-ethnic, and in the areas where conflict was the most violent there were over 30% of multi-ethnic marriages. The line dividing the area with a predominantly Catholic population from the area with predominantly Orthodox population corresponded with the border between the west and east Roman Empire. The three Slavic languages and Albanian prevailed in the country. The Moslem population consisted of a Slavic population converted to Islam during the Turkish occupation.

Within the territories of the former Yugoslavia there had essentially been no democratic tradition. The western parts, which at one time had belonged to the Austro–Hungarian Empire, could not align themselves with democracy (like the Empire they once belonged to). In confirmation of this thesis are the histories of those countries which, with the exception of the Czech Republic, have all experienced dictatorial regimes. The ideology of the Communist regime was based on "not thinking". In addition to various repressive measures, the most repressive one in mental terms, skilfully spread by propaganda, was that we had no hope if we did not listen to the daily ideology. This provided the only route to surviving all the difficulties we were in, or the evils our neighbours wished to wreak on us. Thus, during the forty-year history of Communist Yugoslavia, threats from outside alternated with periodical purges following the left/right turns of the Party policy. In this manner the majority of the population was continuously afraid of the evil that the supreme wisdom could conquer. It is my impression that in everyday life the majority was concerned with the fact that it is possible to live in such a leisurely manner with so little work. The propaganda had constantly insisted on our uniqueness and that the laws applying to others did not apply to us. Any attempt to question the correctness or incorrectness of certain Party decisions was met by a severe response from the Party: the doubters were declared enemies and were often marked as destroyers of brotherhood and of the unity of the nation, of their sacred inheritance. So any idea of democracy was frustrated. Since democracy is a society where conflicts are always present but tend to be solved by dialogue, this kind of thinking was impossible for the whole group. What was left for the majority was a national alternative. Therefore, events from the previous war, with bloody inter-ethnic fights, were learned within the family through stories told by parents or by their parents. The horrors they were talking about created hostile feelings towards the members of other nations. This was further corroborated by the fact that the events had happened to close relatives, and the authority of the storyteller itself left no room to question why those events had taken place at all. Thus, black and white images were created by facilitating the idea that the happiness of a group constitutes the life of one nation on a particular territory.

In short, at times when the government was unable to provide satisfactory solutions to difficulties not created by the external enemy, the psychological situation of the group was that the solution would only be found through nationalist groupings, and that other nations were responsible for one's own troubles. The ruling oligarchy had passed the standard course of all communist societies from cosmopolitanism to nationalism. From the moment of Tito's death the ruling national communist oligarchies had misused, as some say (I am more inclined to think that they did not know how to think differently), inter-ethnic relations which had never been resolved. To talk about crimes that had taken place at inter-ethnic level was strictly forbidden during the communist regime. The system of thinking within a regime that presented the world as black and white was unable to cope with situations which consisted of various shades of grey. Moreover, talk about victims would inevitably bring to attention the victims of the regime as well. Thus, in the end, we did not even know the number of victims of the previous war. This situation gave various national leaders a huge arena for perverse manipulations. The ruling oligarchies started first by raising the question of who is supporting whom, and who is stealing from whom—hence, energy supplies were being stolen from the Serbs and they, in turn, were selling inferior quality cars to everyone at high prices. Later they moved onto counting the victims, and after that, to openly prompting inter-ethnic conflicts.

The conflict, in essence, took place among three nations sharing the same language but different religions.

Along with the similarities, the differences between former Yugoslavia and other East European countries were significant. The standards of living were closer to the standards of Western Europe until the mid-eighties. Travelling abroad was possible for all Yugoslav citizens and there were no visas required for the majority of countries. Citizens were inclined to sneer at the regime, while at the same time they lived well since their standard of living was just a bit lower than in the developed countries, in addition they had social security and worked considerably less than in the West. The crisis that began in the eighties, along with the incompetence of the ruling oligarch to change the socialist system peacefully, resulted in an accumulation of anger in the general population. A situation where there is an economic crisis and the ruling class does not know how, does not care, or does not want to offer a solution, causes feelings of fear and helplessness amongst the members of any group. This is when the group starts to pursue a solution to the situation in which it finds itself. The group begins to show the symptom of "gathering around a tent" (Volcan, 1997): since it consisted of various nations, each of the nations began to gather around its "national tent".

The second phenomenon of a group in crisis is that the group elects the "craziest" to be its leader (Bion, 1961). The leader is the craziest because he/she offers a simple and quick solution to the crisis. This phenomenon has appeared among the two largest nations of the former Yugoslavia, the Croats and the Serbs. Their leaders stressed the greatness of their respective nations, their uniqueness, and simultaneously indicated their oppressed status in Yugoslavia. The solution lay in the recognition of the supremacy of these two nations. The leaders of both the Croatians and the Serbs themselves have an unpleasant similarity within their own family histories—violent deaths of both parents.

Narcissism of minor differences

It is well-known that violence among individuals usually occurs between those who are acquainted, and the closer the ties, the greater the possibility for violence. It is likewise with violence between two nations: the closer they are, the greater the possibilities of violence. In his paper, "Civilisation and its Discontents" (1930), Freud believed that characteristic rituals of certain civilizations developed as a need to place aggressive and sexual impulses under control. Thus a group, through a ritual, symbolically represents certain forbidden acts. Freud also mentioned the relations between two different groups intolerant to each other's traditions and customs, and described these as the "narcissism of minor differences". He did not analyse the term further. We may assume that any ritual imposed by a society, and I do not mean only the standard rituals but also social rules, produces resistance in each individual. Rituals evoke our narcissism by offering a symbol instead of the real thing, and thus offend our omnipotence, making us feel unconsciously frustrated and helpless. When we travel as tourists in other countries we are prepared to disdain or admire their habits and customs. This attitude is usually ambivalent, filled with praise or criticism. The customs that are most frequently disdained are related to the food and hygiene of the nation concerned. Their cuisine either smells or is marvellous, the people are either clean or dirty, or dirty and perfumed. They are either cold or warm.

Rituals themselves, regardless of the civilization they belong to, are frequently concerned with food. There are forbidden animals, or days when certain rules impose what is allowed or forbidden to be eaten. These rules cause much astonishment, and in tense situations, anger and resentment. If we have two nations living side by side, having different rituals, they will usually mock the rituals of the other. They will describe them as stupid, as people who don't know a good thing when they see it, and are unaware that at the same time they also have their own rituals which limit them. Observing rituals of others causes in us feelings of helplessness with respect to our own rituals, which show us that we are not omnipotent. The rituals of others are similar enough to cause, in the majority, a sense of helplessness, yet not so similar as to allow consideration of our own limitations. Thus, all bad feelings are transferred to others; they are stupid, smell of their own food which they must eat due to their strange customs. Therefore, they are primitive, stupid, and evil. In our territories Moslems smell of tallow and Christians of lard. The division of the "good and bad breast" becomes obvious in the other, the neighbouring nation.

The second set of customs is related to hygiene habits, especially defecation. In that field there is a firm, positive evaluation of one's own rituals and firm repulsion towards those of others. Let us remind ourselves that one of the biggest humiliations we experience is toilet training. Therefore all habits of others, although little different from ours, seem dirty and make these people seem insufficiently clean: the humiliation we felt during the painstaking acquiring of hygiene habits is passed onto them. One of the stories about the hard life in the army was a story about the disgust with bottles of water which the Moslems kept in the army toilets. I assume that Moslems were similarly nauseated by toilet paper. Only second in rank was the story of the state of toilets in that institution, and the absence of privacy. It seems that all the humiliation and disgust had been transferred to the others, and, of all things, related to personal hygiene. To a certain degree the last ten years of the former Yugoslavia resembled the situation in an army lavatory. The nations derided each other without being aware of living in contaminated environments that were becoming dirtier and dirtier with each passing day.

The third area where the customs of people are kept in sight is the sexual behaviour of particular nations. Although we know from our personal experience that the sexual behaviour of nations living in the same locality is, above all, an individual concern, an account of sexual morality of a particular nation resembles a description of a group of clones. Thus, the Croats were fags, Moslems both potent and fags. I do not know what fantasy was related to the Serbs. I consider that this area of human relations is best suited for the phenomenon appearing in nationalism and relating to the total exclusion of personal experience in contact with other nations while thinking of a nation as a group. This perception of members of another race or nation is quite familiar and present among highly educated people, even those in the psychotherapeutic profession. I remember a case when at a professional meeting held at my clinic, for who knows what reason, a discussion began as to who is sexually more potent—the blacks or the whites—and subsequently moved to the length of the penis. One of my colleagues said that blacks are certainly more potent and have a longer penis because they are black and they are closer to animals. My colleague, a woman of experience, said, "I have tried; it has nothing to do with colour, it has to do with a person". This voice of common sense broke off the discussion (unfortunately such common sense was not evident among the politicians in former Yugoslavia). The attitude of men towards women of other nations is coloured by the perception of a woman as a type of prey. They are women who either openly love sex or just pretend not to. Therefore, being with a woman against her own will is not such a great sin. This attitude is also noticeable in former Yugoslavia. By all indications, rape of members of another nation was widely spread during the war. It ingrained an additional malevolence: the raped women would give birth to a member of the nation that had raped her.

I have specified three areas to which ritual is attached: food, toilet training, and sexual life. In all of them we experience frustrations, our omnipotence is limited and we feel undervalued and helpless. Watching rituals of another nation provokes in us ancient helplessness and we project this upon the members of other nations, evaluating them as a unique group and not as a set of individuals. Powerlessness prevents us from exercising our personal judgement so that our own group appears to be powerful and others do not. This mechanism of thinking becomes the same as the one in perversion. In order to feel powerful someone else must be humiliated and his/her procreative values must be annihilated (sadism, homosexuality, fetishism, etc.).

Dehumanization of others—a form of perversion of thinking

In this paper, I have compared the metamorphosis of the thinking of people overwhelmed by national fervour with the thinking of perverts. Perverse people, in every form of perversion, deny that a parental pair was necessary for their conception. In nationalist fervour we generally see an attack on members of other nations as inferior and more primitive or, if they are at a higher level of civilization, they are seen as being dehumanized by their own indifference. Therefore, only a member of a particular nation is the one that has a true measure of humanity. Noble but with feelings, aggressive but honourable. Another feature appearing in nationalist fervour is that either the particular nation is of special origin or, when this is difficult to maintain, then at least of the oldest origin.

It is characteristic that in nationalist fervour there exist two parallel tendencies. The first one is that the neighbour nations have originated from the chosen nation, but with time have accepted another religion due to their being corrupt and evil, or having renounced their noble origin. The second tendency is to proclaim some mysterious origin (noble of course) and to accuse other nations of having concealed that origin. Hence, there is a Serbian book, *Serbs, The Oldest Nation* that was very popular before the war. Even serious and educated people have elaborated all sorts of absurdities, of which the most notable was that the Serbian language is the foundation of other languages, and that it has somewhat obscure ties with Sanskrit, except it is unclear which is the older. Croats, in turn, have ascribed to themselves obscure Aryan–Iranian origins. All of these theories aim to establish a special origin which is noble and in that manner to reduce the damage emerging from the awareness that they have come into being by simple sexual intercourse between their parents. This way everyone becomes noble regardless of the reality of everyday life. We have, thus, two explanations expressing the pain of coming into being in the usual way. We have a situation very similar to the one in childhood when children deal emotionally with the fact that they came into being from their mother and father by inventing all sorts of romantic theories known to us as family romance. The chosen nation is noble, having come into being from noble parents, whereas the others have a semi-animal origin. I consider that this mechanism is the cause of numerous atrocities in the war. One of the historic examples is that crusaders ate the roasted flesh of Arabs in order to prove that they were not human (Rustin, 1991). Destruction of this opinion of oneself lies in aggrandizing one's own omnipotence, both through one's own greatness and through the lowliness of the others. To be of noble origin, or of the oldest nation, establishes a feeling of closeness among its members. As we are the oldest, the time difference between ancestors is wiped out. All members of a nation, both alive and dead, are thus alive. So, we can easily identify ourselves with mythical heroes of the past, but also with the victims of the past. What was done five hundred years ago feels as though it is happening now, not to our ancestors, but to us. Almost twenty years ago I had a patient, an intellectual who was born in an area where dreadful inter-ethnic conflicts had taken place during the

Second World War. The patient was neurotic and strongly attached to his mother whose family was killed during those conflicts. He often dreamed that he was going to war with his friends in order to avenge his ancestors.

Torture and fantasies of family relations

Unfortunately, events that had happened during the last war confirm the following thesis: that it seems that all three sides reported cases, not altogether rare, of forcing prisoners into homosexual, homosexual incestuous and heterosexual incestuous contacts. It seems as though the members of a chosen nation saw in the others a personification of their own perverse and incestuous fantasies, and therefore enjoyed both their humiliation and horror, and the transformation of fantasies into reality. It was as if members of the chosen nation had acted out, through non-humans, their own fantasies related to their relationships with loved ones—father, mother, sister, and brothers. This behaviour shows a similarity with disturbed family relations or fantasies related to family life. Incestuous bans, which are a humiliation, always tend to be overcome. Forcing others to do what we fantasize humiliates them and elevates us. The fact that the same language had bound all, and that they had yet all wished to be far apart, reminds one of the stories in every family that there are poor relatives who are miserable, evil, dirty, and have doubtful interrelations.

Atrocious tortures occurring during the war were widespread in the terrain outside the usual institutions (police), as usually happens in wars. Those tortures in their treatment were similar to children taking dolls apart or torturing domestic animals, and their only aim was the satisfaction derived by the torturers experiencing their own divine omnipotence. The events resembled the novels of the Marquis de Sade (Chassguet-Smirgel, 1990) which have elements of childish brutality, but in contrast to the works of the respected Marquis—where the tortured revive in order to be tortured again, and the lucky ones escape—there was none of this here. The events also reminded one of the tortures to which small children are exposed by disturbed parents. All this was done by recent neighbours and friends, one to another. Thus the events acquired the characteristics of family violence where murders often happen to be brutal.

It was observed that guards allowed their friends to enter the prison camps in order to participate in atrocities. It is a known fact that in Srebrenica soldiers who were executing prisoners were forcing truck and bus drivers to participate personally in the executions under the threat of being executed themselves. The shame for a committed act sometimes has strange ways of nullification. I would not defend people who did this, but I have an impression that they wanted to share their own evil with others in order to sully those few normal people among them who did not participate in the crime. In any event, the simultaneous existence of omnipotence and guilt did not bring about any good in this case either.

Campfire stories

After the Second World War the Yugoslav institutions were unable to start the process of public debate on inter-ethnic events that had taken place during the war. History was mainly presented as the fight against the Germans and domestic traitors. The propaganda itself was about the resistance of partisans against Germans, while domestic opponents of partisans were mentioned from time to time without any profound explanations. This policy of the Yugoslav authorities is understandable to some degree, since there was, at this time, a parallel ideological war which also sought adherents. The partisans were presented as absolutely good, noble towards the enemy and justly harsh towards themselves. Each murder attempt among the natives would also bring to the surface ideologically founded murders. This situation has remained unresolved to this day; hence the number of victims in the territory of Yugoslavia during World War II is still unknown. During World War II, on Yugoslavian territory, bloody inter-ethnic clashes occurred between Serbs, Croats, and Moslems. The parties had been in different positions. Croats had a state that institutionalized terror over the members of other nations, yet the other two parties, although without their own states and institutionalized terror, had not remained beholden.

The official party had tried to keep secret the entire problem of war trauma by propaganda about strong ties between the nations, the unbreakable brotherhood. All of this seemed a complete denial of cruel events that had occurred. On the other hand, power itself was divided not only in ideological but also in national principle. Cadres who had fought in the war came to power, and they originated from the areas where the most horrific inter-ethnic events took place. According to a traditional custom which some call the "old boy's network" and others call the "Mafia style", cadres who came to power later also originated mostly from the same areas. This means that the latter had been told about the events during the war, but had not experienced the pain that would make them able to observe people around them as individuals and not as members of a national "herd".

The process of elaborating fantasies connected to parents' trauma took place at the same sites where the original trauma had happened; accounts of events were handed down from parents or other ancestors. The children passing the scenic clearings and hills on their way to school, and from the stories told by their parents, knew that at these same spots members of their nation had been brutally killed. Most often children going to school belonged to different nations, and each of them had their "secret graves". At school they were learning about brotherhood, but in the evenings, sitting by the fire, they listened to emotional stories about others in their neighbourhood. Children heard stories about slaughters with an underlying message of the parents' impotence in the face of the pursuing evil. The parents' impotence had a devastating effect on the self-respect of the children, who were left vulnerable in the face of the external evil of their stories, but essentially vulnerable before their own internal aggressive impulses. The second message of the storyteller was: never trust a neighbour and always be prepared for anything. To a child nationalist hatred may be an attempt to avenge the parents' impotence. A child strives to retain the omnipotent picture of his/her parent, the power and strength he/she simultaneously adores and fears. This is how revenge becomes an important part of the child's identity. The child tries to overcome the traumatizing effects of the parents' trauma, combining both his father's strength with the aggressor's hatred which are then directed against the members of other nations. The hitherto safe world, offering protection from all evil either outside or inside, fell apart in the evening when these fireside stories describe the truth of the ancestors' fate. As long as the regime was successful in maintaining a tolerable harmony, it had sufficient followers. The moment citizens observed national antagonism on the part of the leadership, the protective strength of the regime burst like a bubble. The only thing left was to pick up arms, at first for protection, and later on for revenge.

Fighting against recent friends

A person advancing against a member of another nation is in a complex position. The members of the other nation are usually neighbours, school friends, friends from work, people the person grew up, and kept company with. Stories from our war are similar to all previous stories of ethnic cleansing which happened in other places at other times. People who came from outside, usually people with dubious histories whose services had been offered to each of the three warring parties, mostly started the genocide itself. I would like to stress that each police force of the warring parties had maintained the *modus operandi* as was usual in the Yugoslav police service. The Yugoslav police had a strong tradition of the KGB which, of course, had accepted Stalin's statement about criminals: "These people are socially close to us." Such people start a blood bath which is gradually joined by the local residents. The unresolved war traumas of ancestors facilitated vengeance and made this process much easier. I say "easier" because multi-ethnic conflicts have a mutual dimension in any war: fear for one's life makes picking up arms and attacking others easier. It is a heavy burden on our conscience to fight against those we know, and therefore the enemy must be additionally dehumanized in order to tolerably justify our own aggression.

This is again behaviour similar to that displayed in family conflicts. The quarrelling parties disown each other, demand a change of family name, and disinherit each other. Paradoxically, this additional dehumanization of a member of another nation is necessary because of the mutual proximity. They need to be made evil or inhuman so that war against them could be possible. Total detachment from one's own experience of positive emotions towards former friends was necessary to enable shooting at them. Thus a terrible war was started where there was no surrender possible, since surrendering usually implied torture and horrible death.

Immediately after the war between the Serbs and the Croats it was not permitted for each to listen to the music of the other. Now, almost ten years later, both in Croatia and Serbia the music of the other may be heard. In Serbia, the music broadcast on the radio is mostly from the pre-war period originating from Croatia and Bosnia. Authorities of both countries (unwillingly) allow guest performances of musicians of the opposite camp. At these rare concerts attendance is enormous, and members of the audience frequently sing with the performers. The Yugo-nostalgia phenomenon is increasingly present, resembling the pain felt after sufficient time had elapsed after a family quarrel.

Communism and nationalism

The strength of nationalism lies in the group. I will not be adding anything new if I state that a person within a group feels protected no matter what he/she does. Protection is based on a group identity that is experienced as powerful, indestructible and mighty, those qualities being incarnated in the leader of the group, who represents its condensed strength. The leader is the omnipotent self-object (Kohut, 1972) with all the traits of a "Mafia gang leader" (Rosenfeld, 1988). The leader and the group are interdependent because the group projects its desires upon the leader, who must realize them in order to achieve the group's admiration and submission. The leader receives the strength and worship from the group if he follows it's desires, and members of the group have the strength and admiration of their leader if they follow him. Undoubtedly, this relationship does not leave much room for contemplating one's actions. Language, ideology, origin, and culture are strong cohesive factors in a large group. The Communist Party was the strongest group in former Yugoslavia. When communism as an ideology was in crisis it suffered the destiny of large systems unable to solve the crisis in which they find themselves. It behaved as a courtier in the tale, "The Emperor's New Suit" and destroyed any idea which might bring about a solution to the crisis.

The system reacted nervously to the development of any alternative organization. One of the characteristics of communism was to destroy any type of professionalism and to subjugate it to ideology. One of the directors of the clinic where I was working, who was also a police colonel, had defended psychoanalysis when it came under attack during a meeting of the Serbian Medical Association. He said: "I don't care that Freud's ideology is unlike Marxism. It heals people, and if I heal people I develop socialism." The Party and the government strictly controlled intellectual professions. University education had alternately been a place of purgatory for the unfit—a sort of ivory tower, or a battlefield of ideological fights where the defeated party would leave the university and seek employment in institutions which exerted no influence on society. Therefore it was not possible to develop a sense of belonging to a legitimate professional group. The education system did not develop the ability to think critically. The prevailing, indeed the only possible way of acquiring knowledge was ex-cathedra. Consequently, the quality of knowledge of degree holders was poor, and this created an additional barrier to the development of an intellectual as an individual capable of an independent life. As communism grew weaker and weaker, nationalism grew stronger and stronger. The sense of belonging to a particular people, language, and culture was something that communism was unable to destroy. Furthermore, communists and nationalists understood each other well. Both systems function according to a black and white principle; both systems can survive only by permanently discovering outside enemies, and if this enemy does not exist (which is most often the case) it must be invented. Both systems do not allow dogma to be questioned—dogma that is the same for communism and for nationalism, but with different names. In one, the system is that which is the best and the most humane in the world, and in the other, it is the people who are the most intelligent, the most hospitable and the most honourable in the world. Danilo Kish, our well-known writer, said that he ceased to believe in national distinctions as he went to elementary schools in both Hungary and Yugoslavia. At both schools he learned that the Hungarians, i.e. the Serbs were the most intelligent, the most hospitable and the most honourable people in the world. Both systems easily invented enemies who were green with envy of the other's marvellous qualities and wealth—thus the enemy was motivated to take this treasure away. Subsequently, regime propaganda stated that Yugoslavia was the only country in Europe fighting against the new colonization and that its allies were Iraq, India and China. Earlier, the ally had been Belorussia as well, but this alliance had vanished.

It is no wonder that the most obsessed communists so easily change sides and leave communism for nationalism. I will quote a quite detestable character, Joseph Goebbels (Brown, 1963): "Give me a communist and I will easily make a national socialist out of him. I will never succeed with a citizen." A mixture of crisis and lack of democracy had led to the election of a leader in the manner described by Bion (1961): "A group in crisis always elects the craziest among themselves as the leader." It seems that it was necessary to elect leaders capable of announcing that other nations were guilty for the crisis and subsequently to offer the shortest and the most violent ways of getting out of it. Simple and quick solutions are always the most cruel ones, at first against the opposing group and later on, when they are spent, against the group within which these ideas have developed. At the beginning people had the right to change their nationality—under humiliating conditions, of course (in the former Yugoslavia this affected the language, culture, and the type of script used—Cyrillic or Latin). This solution has a double effect. "Other people" resist the assimilation, whereas the "first people" become paranoid—they are afraid of traitors amongst themselves and despise those "other people" who have adopted their conditions. The "first people" become angry towards the "other people" because they have rejected their generous conditions. It is interesting to note that in the former Yugoslavia all leaders had offered such conditions to the others. What followed after these offers was a call to arms to defend one's own flesh and blood and territories. A territory shared by the peoples would overnight become a territory of only one nation which subsequently expanded day-by-day. Illustrative was the saying in Serbia, half-joke and half-slogan: "Serbia up to Tokyo". The consequence, of course, not mentioned by propaganda, was the destruction or relocation of the "others". Through propaganda the time and space condensed and thus each group was promised that they were on the verge of Plato's Golden Age, in an era where people originate from gods. An era with promises that we will all love each other, live like brothers with no differences, as all will be good, intelligent, and honourable. There will be no envy in this new society and everybody will be happy. Thus the Serbs became a celestial nation. The unconscious message of the propaganda was that there would be no tensions, no hate among the members of the chosen group. It is only necessary to move and destroy those who do not love us, who envy our values which we have lost but will now recover. Thus, some of the ecclesiastical dignitaries and politicians calculated how many victims it was necessary to have in order to achieve the goal of a life of eternal happiness. For the majority of its members the nation, hence, became a symbol of divine time, space and a life of which we consciously have no experience. The only test of reality was a pleasant fantasy which, no matter how pleasant, is not the best means for testing. The idea of life in a society without tensions and envy resembles the fantasy of life in the mother's womb, or a life in heaven before picking the fruit from the Tree of Knowledge. This idyllic situation represents a powerful defence against the aggressive fantasies towards the mother's womb that carries the threat of other babies. As all babies are mono-ethnic there is no need to worry about which is loved more. All babies receive the same quantity of love, warmth, and food. So everyone has the same quantity of everything and there is no need for envy. That way, both communism and nationalism achieve the mutual goal.

Sanctions, Kosovo and bombing

I will repeat that former Yugoslavia had been, since the mid-sixties, an open country in the sense that entry visas were not required and citizens also did not need visas to travel to the West. The goods from the West were readily available on the Yugoslav market, together with cult products such as Coca-Cola and chewing gum. Western culture flowed freely into Yugoslavia. Therefore the sanctions imposed in 1992 had a most painful impact on the very layer of the population which was closest to the West by its upbringing and culture. A well-known group phenomena appeared: when a group feels deprived it turns against the group which it holds responsible for that deprivation. Still greater gathering around the regime occurred because everyone felt threatened and this newly-created situation suited the regime well. Through its propaganda it presented the West as the major culprit for the war and for other life misfortunes. Instead of weakening the Milosevic regime the sanctions strengthened it. Hundreds and hundreds of thousands of young people left the country in search of a better life. Most of them were opponents of the regime. Those who kept their contact with the West cursed the bad telephone lines and eight-hour drives by mini-bus to Budapest, the nearest airport. I do not know who was cursed more—the regime, or those who had imposed the sanctions.

During the past years much has been said about Kosovo. For the last ten years Kosovo has been a place where the relations between the Albanian and non-Albanian populations were organized along the principles of apartheid, although the system, of course, was not called by that name. Instead of giving a historical presentation of the situation in Kosovo which finally led to an armed conflict between the Serbs and Albanians, I will try to illustrate the history of this situation through a group experience. Seven years ago, a project was started for giving help to the traumatized, financed by the Soros Foundation for psycho-traumatized in Pristina. Within this project I ran a multi-ethnic education–experiential group consisting of psychiatrists and psychologists. After approximately three months' work, members of the group began to talk about interethnic relations. Both Serbs and Albanians participated in discussions in an atmosphere which I experienced as a constructive one. Towards the end of the discussion a Turkish woman spoke, saying that in Kosovo when Serbs are in power they mistreat Albanians and when Albanians are in power they mistreat Serbs, but both of these nations mistreat Turks. With shy smiles both Serbs and Albanians agreed with her. Then I considered what she had said as a starting point from which Serbs and Albanians have a chance to perceive their own behaviour. A group consisting of people who were not captivated by nationalism was able to use her words. Unfortunately, many of those who lived in Kosovo were not. A desire for vengeance was too strong.

During the bombing of Kosovo, this issue also arose in the therapy of one of my clients. Unfortunately I was not able to keep to protocol during the bombing, and therefore the material presented will be insufficient both on account of the bombing and for the protection of the client.

The client is an Albanian, born and brought up in Belgrade where he completely fitted into the life of his peer group. Among them he never had any problems related to his origin. Needless to say, that group was not exactly typical in Yugoslav territories. It is interesting that his best friend is an ardent Serbian nationalist, but the relationship had survived until now, with fiery discussion of course. As the client is a person with separation problems, his enduring difficulty was not the bombing, but the fact that after the end of a session he was left without my protection and he was very angry that my children had my protection while he was deprived of it. After about a month of bombing he came to the session very upset because while at the home of relatives in Pec (a town on the southwest of Kosovo) he encountered not his relatives, but an unknown person saying that everybody had left. In this situation, it was very difficult for me to continue to interpret my patient's material in an analytic way, so the sessions became places where he was able to talk about his fears of persecution and his fears about what may happen at work, as well as his fears for his parents and sister. A week later he telephoned me to tell me that something terrible had happened and that he did not know if he would be able to come to the session. He could not say any more over the phone. I told him that I would wait for him. He came and informed me that his brother-in-law had disappeared on his way home from the flat of my patient's parents. He told me he did not understand where his brother-in-law might have been because he went out with little money. My reaction was completely unanalytical. I told him that as his brother-in-law was a journalist it was likely that he had been kidnapped by the secret police, and until his release after discussions with them, he (the patient) would probably be unable to contact him. I directed him to a friend of mine who is running the Centre for Human Rights and who held out bravely during the war. I also told him that he should make a lot of fuss about the disappearance, as his brother-in-law would be safer then. Three days later the relatives phoned from Montenegro to say that the brother-in-law had come back. The war roared on and in the therapy, my patient resumed being able to speak of his fears and to receive adequate support. There was a change in the patient's attitude towards me.

Having been the most hated person in the world, I became the most loved one in the world. It was true that when the war ended and normal psychoanalytical work resumed, I again became the person who was hearing only how awful the parents were.

My origin is multi-ethnic, and I think that from my paper you will get the impression that nationalistic ideas do not rank highly in my value system. Nevertheless, during the sessions with this young man I felt ashamed of all the things that were happening to him. I was constantly examining myself about whether there was something more I could have done to help prevent the development of such a bloody conflict.

Sometimes, sitting talking with patients about their problems struck me as completely useless and insane while nearby or three-hundred kilometres away, people were disappearing or being killed simply because they belonged to another nation. From time to time I felt entirely unprotected, not from the NATO bombing, but from the madness boiling amongst the members of the warring nations. However, the fact that my patients had endured the bombing and other misfortunes better than "normal" people helped me to continue with my work. Subsequent months and years will show whether I have been mistaken in staying with the hope that I will be able to protect those I love.

CHAPTER FIVE

From containment to leakage, from the collective to the unique: therapist and patient in shared national trauma

Dvora Miller-Florsheim

"I wasn't one of the six million who died in the Shoah, I wasn't even among the survivors. And I wasn't one of the six hundred thousand who went out of Egypt. I came to the Promised Land by sea. No, I was not in that number, though I still have the fire and the smoke within me, pillars of fire and pillars of smoke that guide me by night and by day. I still have inside me the mad search for emergency exit, for soft places, for the nakedness of the land, for the escape into weakness and hope ... Afterwards, silence. No questions, no answers. Jewish history and world history grind me between them like two grindstones, sometimes to a powder ... Sometimes I fall into the gap between to hide, or sink the way down"

Yehuda Amichai, 2000

Introduction

The first version of this article was written in March 1996, following the upheaval caused by the assassination of Prime Minister Yitzhak Rabin—architect of the peace process—

and the wave of terrorist attacks that came in its wake. It was originally presented as a paper in New York, where American psychoanalysts made an effort to connect what was presented to their own world and cited examples, mainly of victims of personal trauma: robbery and rape.

After several quiet years, the obviously naive and fanciful thought crossed my mind that I could file away the article because it was no longer relevant. But the events of these past two years of the El-Aqsa Intifada and its terrible terrorists attacks, have revived, with even greater intensity, a painful feeling we have been carrying with us throughout history: the feeling of helplessness and rage in the face of the loss of life, the dangers lurking in every corner, and the growing uncertainty. The hope, perhaps the false hope, that this is a temporary situation and soon, very soon, the path to peace will be found—or at least the path to some kind of agreement or even a few days' respite—is fading, and the knowledge that any of us could be a victim in one way or another has seeped into our consciousness.

Then, when the updated version of this article was being prepared, the terrible event of September 11th occurred in the US, an event that instantaneously transformed the entire world into an unsafe place. Shavit writes (2001):

> The defining moment of our generation, with all of its horrifying images, resonates in all of us ... but we are left unable to truly decipher it, unable to clarify for ourselves its full meaning. For Israelis, the change is less dramatic than for citizens of other Western nations. In fact, a claim could be made that if, in the wake of September 2000 (the outbreak of the present Intifada), many Israelis lost their faith that the peace process would free them from the Israeli situation and give them the sort of life Americans live, then in the wake of September 2001, they learned that American life is taking on some of the features that characterize the Israeli situation.

While many books and articles have been written in the mental health field about traumatic stress reactions, research and articles on the psychotherapist's in such situations are still in their infancy. Limentani (1989) for example, noted an amazing contrast between "the buoyancy of the scientific life" in the British Psychoanalytic Society and the fact that there is almost no publication about the experience of being an analyst in wartime Britain.

Noy (2000), in his comprehensive volume on therapy in traumatic stress situations, published in Israel, devotes only one page to an item he calls "Dangers to the Therapist's Mental Health". These dangers, he writes, exist because therapists, in response to trauma, do not merely observe, they are involved in the process.

At a time when therapeutic methods used in treating Holocaust survivors were being discussed (twenty to thirty years after the war), isolated examples could be found of the avoidance and denial that characterized the way mental health professionals in Israel were dealing with "those who had returned from death". In discussing their own reluctance to face the Holocaust, Williams & Kestenberg (1974) wrote on the latency period that had to be traversed before one could give up the denial and repression of the unspeakable terror. Moses (1987) spoke of having been, with others, "a partner to the denial of the impact", not only of the Holocaust but also of several wars that threatened the State of Israel. It has been assumed that the patients, along with the society to which they belonged, were attempting to avoid personal confrontation with "the extreme" and with hidden feelings of mourning, rage, shame, and fear of death, experienced by both the therapist and the survivor (Davidson, 1980). Keinan-Kon (1998) pointed to a similar phenomenon which occurred during the Gulf War. Her paper (written seven years after the Gulf War) is one of few exceptions (Berman, 1991; Molad, 1991; Stern, 1992) that dare to raise the question: "When analyst and patient alike are threatened by the same traumatizing reality, is it possible to bring back to the common symmetrical factual reality, the asymmetry necessary for the therapeutic space?" (*ibid.*, p. 440).

Nonetheless, Lifton (1978) and Lindy (1989), who worked with Vietnam veterans, believe that without an awareness of countertransference and its power, it is impossible to engage in meaningful therapy with survivors and comprehend their unexpressed pain; nor is it possible to arrive at a meaningful understanding of the unique forms of evil in our times. Therapists must be willing to reconsider social and scientific values they have believed in. For us, this means confronting our fears and our hopes about our own death and survival, including our professional survival. (Lifton, *ibid*.)

The question arises as to whether, in our tumultuous reality, deprived of objective distance, we will have the ability to observe a process? Should we be speaking not about trauma victims and their therapists, but about *all of us* living in the shadow of trauma? Or is it perhaps, precisely because of this, that we avoid discussing the difficult questions and dilemmas the situation imposes upon us?

The hypothesis of this article is that the therapist's identity is formed in a cultural context, and therefore, the collective narrative and the associations connected with it will be an inseparable part of this context. In Israel one of the fundamental themes that comprise the national narrative is war and coping with it. Therapists are not just neutral objects but rather subjects sharing in collective, cumulative, traumatic experience. Apparently this shared destiny has many implications on whatever happens in psychotherapy, especially during a period when the difference between the home front and the battle front is blurred, and so is the boundary between therapist and patient.

Conscious and unconscious collective identity

Loewenberg (1995) as well as Volkan & Itzkowitz (2000), revise Erikson's (1950) statement on identity and note that nations are "born" differently. Shared realistic or fantasized perceptions of the past and the manner in which a large group's identity was established, influence common attitudes and actions within a given society.

The sociologist Ben-David (1962) believes that, particularly during the formative years of Israel, there was "a nearly perfect harmony between individual values and the needs of the collective" (*ibid.*, p. 408). Though remembrance of persecution is rooted deeply in Jewish tradition, the trauma of the Holocaust stamped itself indelibly on the national psychology of the New Society (Davidson, 1985; Eilon, 1981) and the memory of the inferno permeated all levels of society. Yet, Holocaust survivors were expected to remain silent with no way of mourning their unmetabolized loss. Gampel (2000) introduces the concept of "radioactivity" to describe how massive trauma does not only nestle itself within in the victims' inner world: it is transmitted within the family and across to future generations, a process Robben (2000) suggests labelling as "transgenerational indigestible trauma".

The dream that the new homeland will supply a "background of safety" (Sandler, 1960) soon turned into a nightmare, becoming Freud's *"unheimliich"* or the "background of the uncanny", as Gampel (2000) uses the concept. This contradiction is an integral component of our attitude towards the Israeli army: at the collective level the army serves to provide the "background of safety". However, at the individual level it has come to be the "background of the uncanny".

The Israel Defence Forces can be considered a civilian army, so that almost every family has a member serving in compulsory or reserved duty. Developmental issues such as separation–individuation, adolescence and the formation of masculine identity are firmly linked to the military service. This is an ambivalent developmental stage, both significant and threatening, from the time a child is born. Israel is a small country with a "Jewish" mentality, a country in which everyone knows everyone else—and if you don't actually know the victim, then one of your acquaintances surely does. Klein (1973) emphasizes that Israel, as a society, provides an environment where unresolved mourning can be worked through. On Israel's annual days of commemoration the community mourns together. The term "Family of Bereavement" reflects the importance the Israeli society accords to the death of its young people.

Paradoxically, intertwined with remembering and mourning is a most prominent dominant desire to forget, to "clean up" the evidence of destruction, to be reborn into normal life. Though denial helps us to go on living, on an unconscious level, there is a high price to cumulative trauma (Khan, 1981; Berman, 1991).

It can be hypothesized that in Israel the "radioactivity" of trauma also leaks into the intimacy and safety zone of the analyst's consulting room and that the anguish becomes intermingled within the inner worlds of both patients and therapists.

Denial, disavowal or escape to normality?

Observing daily life in Israel over the years creates the impression of a normal existence disguising the terrible price of cumulative trauma. Undoubtedly, the external reality of inherent historical threat forces us to use denial to keep our sanity. To an outside observer we might even be seen as indifferent, obtuse or alienated. This kind of defence mechanism marks all sorts of strange "defensible borders". When katyushas missiles fell in the northern part of the country, some two hundred and fifty kilometres from our home, the danger could be denied. When a bus is blown up in Jerusalem, some sixty kilometres from our home, denial still works. But when the explosion takes place on the corner of the street our children cross every day, denial is much more difficult. Nevertheless, it seems that such threats can and actually are denied when entering the psychotherapy room.

It is always astonishing when patients come into the room and begin speaking, with the utmost naturalness, about the emotional agonies of their inner world without saying a word about the external reality, without the need for even a transitional comment. More than once, the question arises of how to respect patients' choice, without wondering about their coping or alternatively, without pathologizing projected guilt and anxiety. This ability may actually be evidence of positive developments in t80
he therapeutic process and of the ability to work things through in the inner theatre of the mind rather than in the dramatic arena outside.

And what about the therapists? We can assume that they are also not immune to denial. How will therapists' denial affect the space left for patients to deal with what is troubling them? After all, it is well known how much unconscious power and influence therapists have on patients.

> A psychotherapy group is meeting in a city where many terrorist attacks have occurred. In a supervision session, the group leaders are surprised to realize the extent to which content related to external reality is absent from the group's discussions, and they wonder about its meaning and their part in it. In one session, as they are discussing self-actualization of femininity and masculinity, the air quivers with the frighteningly powerful booming sounds of planes breaking the sound barrier. One of the participant's attempts to draw the group's attention to the sounds coming from outside are interpreted as an effort to run away from the explosive sounds and drives inside her and move far away to what is happening in the sky. Only through supervision does one of the group leaders

become aware of the sense of dread also threatening to overwhelm her at hearing the noise, and perhaps of the urgent need to summon up denial in the face of such a complex reality, even if that means limiting her perception.

Freud (1938a,b) tentatively distinguished between repression and disavowal which is directed against external reality. Freud related to disavowal as a split in the ego, and as defining circumstances where an individual proves adept at keeping two apparently contradictory ideas in mind, without feeling the obligation to reconcile the two. Unable to assimilate the traumatic reality, the person splits his ego, disavowing his perception of this reality.

Kubler-Ross (1969) describes the response of terminal patients that suddenly hint they can no longer continue looking at reality as it is, and temporarily cling to denial. At an even later stage patients use splitting instead of denial. They can talk about their health and their illness, about their life and their death, as if these were twin entities entitled to exist side by side. In this way, they can confront death and still keep hoping. Spiro (1987) formulated the concept of a "culturally constituted defence mechanism". This concept is crucial for understanding the subtleties of the use of defence mechanisms where the content is heavily drawn from collective representations.

Are we—patients and therapists—taking part in a "conspiracy of silence" so typical of Holocaust survivors? Do we choose to ignore reality because we feel caught in an impasse? Is this nothing more than a healthy process, the only option possible, preserving the inner continuation of the self in terms of "going on being" (Winnicott, 1949)?

Leakage or overlapping worlds?

When patient and analyst are both exposed to the same traumatic external circumstances, they share a common external reality and their worlds overlap. On Commemoration Days, at the sound of the two minutes' siren, both therapist and patient will unquestioningly get up and stand at attention. However, this unique experience concretely exposes the leakage. Comparably, the recent presence of mobile telephones in the therapeutic hour introduces new challenges. The shared anxiety concerning children's safety and the need to be constantly in touch, poses dilemmas such as: does the turned-on phone protect the therapeutic potential space or violate it? What about symmetry? Even experienced therapists and analysts, usually careful to preserve the boundaries of therapy, find themselves crossing the lines, seduced into acting as rescuers, affected by the heavy pressures of traumatic transference and countertransference.

Keinan-Kon (1998) describes how she bought a second gas mask for a patient who refused to bring his to psychotherapy, because she could not bear the possibility enacted in the situation of a forced-choice decision along the lines "one to life, one to death".

The following example demonstrates the extent to which subjects raised during therapy relate to major, almost sacred issues in Israeli life, where social and personal identities are liable to cause therapists to side with society against the patient. Dasberg (1987) even suggests the concept of "social counter-transference" to describe such a process.

> A patient of mine created a fictitious medical record for her son that would lower his medical profile and prevent his being assigned to a combat unit. I am flooded with emotion thinking of my son. I doubt that I can do that with my own son who is approaching draft age. I am aware of the patient's discomfort—a combination of shame, guilt and the intense desire to save her son. Perhaps the words of Benyamin Galai's poem, "Sarah's Life", were going through my mind: Sarah, wife of Abraham the Patriarch, had died emotionally many years before she was laid to rest in the ground. Her coffin was the memory of the logs her husband had split to make an altar for the sacrifice of their son, Isaac.
>
> In the end, I pull myself together and choose to say something like: "In a place where we are again and again being put to the test of 'the Sacrifice of Isaac', who knows what the right thing to do is?"

Approaching the zone of the unspeakable and unthinkable

Apfel & Simon (2000) argue that we, analysts, are not accustomed to analysing our political positions and political "countertransference" and hence rationalize our insecurities by a kind of phobic avoidance. Even when victims of violence have been analysed, they have tended to protect the analyst from the full onslaught of their terrible experiences (*ibid*.).

The political and social situation in Israel makes it impossible to remain a neutral observer and we are constantly required to touch the boundaries of our tolerance. There are many "others" in Israeli reality: idealistic settlers and ordinary people in search of better life across the "green line"; the ultra-orthodox who do not serve in the army, but do the sacred work of collecting the pieces of the dead victims in order to bring them to proper burial; secular people, left-wing urban sophisticates; new immigrants; Israeli Arabs and, of course, Palestinians.

In Israel political discussion focuses on the country's survival and the feeling is that what for one side is a background of safety represents for the other side the uncanny. Can such a complex reality not threaten to intrude the psychotherapy room, when just a moment before we started the session, we heard horrifying, painful, infuriating or bewildering news? We become enraged, anxious and hateful, unable to sympathize with those who are, at this moment, a terrible enemy, but whose children are being killed in the hopeless poverty and cesspool of their lives. All in a state of extraordinary agitation. "Unthinkable thoughts" come to our mind—vengeful, murderous, unethical thoughts. Then, how can we help our patients and ourselves cope with evil? Where does one draw the strength and resiliency of spirit to contain the divisiveness and complexity of the situation, with no resolution in sight? I think that not only do we find it difficult to observe the Jewish edict "Love Thy Brother as Thyself", but find it difficult to keep in mind the fundamental law that "Man is Created in God's Image".

> An annual conference of psychologists. It is taking place in December, some two months after the outbreak of the Al-Aqsa Intifida, at a time when the settlers in the territories feel that they are sitting ducks for terrorist attacks, and after the October riots, when twelve Israeli Arab citizens were killed by the police. Naomi is the only participant who lives in the settlements. Something in her appearance projects a mixture of aloofness and serenity, a kind of stoicism. She talks about how her participation in the group had

merely solidified the feeling that she arrived with—being isolated, rejected and demonized by the group, a feeling which represents the way most settlers feel. Something has been disrupted and distorted in this Intifada, she says. The settlers are hated, abandoned to their fate, and "when I look back I don't see my nation standing behind me". Being marked as an obstacle to peace, there are even people who gloat at their suffering. In a matter of minutes, the members are actually reproducing the attitudes she has described. Alona, the only child of Holocaust survivors, is very angry that her son, a soldier, is serving in the territories and endangering his life guarding the settlers. Rachel, who had lost her husband and father in a terrorist attack many years ago, is outraged by Naomi presenting herself as the only victim. Galia is sure that emotions cannot be separated from the political debate. She grew up in a kibbutz, and who knows better than her, how much a part of structure ideology is.

As the leader, I feel torn, but mostly paralysed, like a parent whose secrets are divulged, whose weakness and confusion have been exposed. The split between left and right exists in my extended family. We avoid visiting our relatives in the settlements, abstain from heart to heart talks. My thoughts wander to a patient of mine who became clinically depressed when she moved to a settlement, a move which opened ideological, emotional and existential chasms in her. I recalled her childhood fantasy in which she was marching at the head of a group of children who would make peace with the Arabs. I return to Naomi, feeling angry that she limits herself to restraint and rationality, finding it difficult to empathize with her pain and anxiety. The session ends in emotional chaos.

During the lunch break I try to empty my mind and heart of all the noise, and I feel that, at the beginning of the next session, I want to say to Naomi: "Don't tell me something big and important, just tell me something small and idiotic". And that's what I do. The intervention seems artificial, but she agrees and chooses to talk about a children's story she is reading. This is the turning point. A part of the fortress wall is breached; Naomi begins talking about her fear that her children will be orphaned, about her wishes and hopes. The others in the group can now show empathy and not leave her in isolation, and can bear the complexity.

This example indicates how easily mutual, collective, apocalyptic fears can penetrate a group and threaten its integrity, where both the group and the leader find it difficult to maintain a psychological stance. Group leaders must undergo an internal process if they are to find, in all that chaos, an empathetic, human approach towards the small things in life that we all share.

The exhausting session ends. All the psychologists are invited to a dialogue with our Arab colleagues, who speak fervently about their identity dilemmas, ongoing discrimination, and feelings of humiliation. They couldn't understand how their Jewish colleagues did not even call them while they were coping with the emergency situation in their schools. Once again, I am emotionally torn. I try to balance the voices, to contain them inside me, by identifying on a certain level with all the various sides, but in fact, not with any of them. I doubt, that it is possible, at this particular point in time, to do something beyond trying to listen and perhaps pray only to the "God of Small Things" (Roy, 1997).

From collective to unique experiences

Traumatic situations, by their very nature, contain dramatic, overwhelming, and painful elements, which can make it difficult to make the vital switch from the real to the symbolic aspects that contain the therapeutic potential. Freud (1912) referred to the therapist's ability to become carried away, by projection, into the patient's contents. Besides self-analysis, he suggested "evenly suspended or poised attention" as a technical solution, aimed at helping the therapist to get beyond the wall of the recounted story to its hidden meanings. Listening to the concealed story enables us to understand what makes our world unique within the collective bond. In order for the therapeutic process to take place, extra care must be exercised in establishing the difference between each side's subjective reality. In the following example one may ask how the specific therapeutic session contributed to the transformation from fragmentation to coherence, from despair to hope, from death to life.

> A patient, second generation Holocaust survivor, born in Israel, the mother of grown children, has been living for years in a border kibbutz. She came to therapy because of inexplicable catastrophic

anxieties and feelings of insecurity. Many times in the past, she has expressed concern about terrorist attacks with relation to her children, who live in large cities. These days, she does not go to work along the same route she always did, because of the terrorist attacks that have occurred on it. She is preoccupied with the dominance of her mother and sister, who continue to treat her like a child, and with her supposedly ancient guilt about other people's catastrophes, of which she had been spared.

Not too long ago, this patient, who is a psychotherapist, was called upon to intervene in the post-traumatic situation of an entire community. In our therapy, I feel that she is becoming over-burdened. A short time later, while she is in session with a patient, terrorists begin shooting at people in the street. She hears the shots but the patient continues talking. Later, the psychotherapist receives phone calls: a patient suffering from post-traumatic stress refuses to come to his session with his children; another asks for her sessions to be moved to a different location because she will not set foot in that "marked city". The therapist calms her down and suggests she waits a week, when they would reconsider and discuss the matter. A third patient asks her directly, "Are you afraid?" And she replies, "Of course, but we have to go on living", although she herself is not convinced.

She is depressed and frightened in our session, two days later, reliving those fearful moments with her patients, looking at me for an answer. It seems strange to her that she is frightened for herself and not for her children. She says, smiling a bittersweet smile, "Maybe it's a good sign that, because of therapy, I've started thinking more about myself". She recalls that when her son was a baby, she would cover his bed, which was opposite the door, so that if terrorists broke in, they would not realize that a baby was lying in it. At this stage, I too feel unfocused. My mind drifts to the dreadful memories as well as communal memories Israelis have of Smadar Haran, whose house was invaded by terrorists and to the death of her two children, suffocated in her effort to keep them quiet. I am thinking about the Holocaust and similar impossible parental dilemmas.

Should I tell the patient about my associations? Would that be of any benefit? I feel the need to say something natural, something about my own fears on that day, when every news broadcast mentioned that the police were searching the area I live in, to avert terrorist attacks. I wanted to say, as my patient had said to her own patient directly, humanly: "Yes, I'm afraid too and I don't have an answer either". My patient continues, "I'd like to *get rid* of the 'baggage' by leaving it with you, but I feel that it's harder to *separate* from the 'baggage' because it's attached to my body like a lichen".

Maybe, she says, she only needs "a day off" from the events, and I add, "Maybe a week", exactly the same advice she offered to her own patient. She smiles.

In my mind, I try to connect the contents of this session with the previous ones, when she had been full of life, looking elegant, wearing jewellery she had recently bought for herself. Finally, I say something about the intermediate stage, when she can no longer protect her grown children and separate from them, when she is no longer her mother's little child. But now that she is the one facing danger and death, she can use her own vitality and vigour. I detect a sense of relief. And she says, "That's interesting, do we have time left? Because that's exactly what I wanted to talk about, about how I can maintain a relationship with my mother and sister, but be free of them too".

My patient leaves and I am left troubled, musing, definitely feeling what she has projected onto me, thus relieving herself. I try to clarify for myself the function I fulfilled for this patient. Did I provide her with a "day off", a resting place where she could set aside the madness, where she could experience the "illusory moments" (Winnicott, 1959), that would enable her to move into this dangerous reality? The next week, she begins our session by saying, "Those things that happened *seem far away*, and each of those three words is meaningful". After all, both of us are aware enough to know that concrete reality has not changed, but for a brief while, we could ostensibly push it out of our internal reality. Perhaps, beyond containing, what enabled the transformation from fragmentation to coherence was the interpretation which separated the collective from the personal, and separated her from her past. Only against such a background could her own vitality emerge.

Prologue

In Amos Gitai's internationally known film—*Kippur*—about the

Yom Kippur War (1973), Gitai intends, whether consciously or unconsciously, to free individual recollections from bonds of collective identifications. He tries to do the impossible: to present a war without relating to the national and cultural narrative. A kind of war that could happen in any place and time but leads nowhere. Most of the film takes place in a protected and protecting place: in a helicopter where the crew rescues and treats the injured. A violent event strikes the supposedly safe zone, when the helicopter is shot down and crashes. At another dreadful moment, the frightened doctor speaks of his mother who survived the horrors of the Holocaust. And so, contrary to the original intention of the film, the national narrative leaks into the personal and becomes powerfully present. Only in the end, does the film return to the point of the beginning, a colourful intimate love-making scene, where the main character is able to reattach himself to life.

One of Bion's (a First World War post-traumatic survivor), most controversial recommendations was that the analyst should approach the session without "memory and desire" (1970). Can we accept this suggestion when it becomes increasingly clear that in the psychotherapy room there are two frightened subjects with fresh collective memories?

In this paper, I have attempted to open a window to the collective Israeli narrative that analysts and patients share, the radioactivity of cumulative trauma that leaks into psychotherapy and the effort needed in order to provide psychotherapeutic help and to go on living. Obviously, more intense feelings of counter-transference are aroused, and therapists are confronted by moral and humanistic questions they usually avoid in order to maintain analytic stance. Many questions arise with no answers. Nevertheless, it is my belief that the psychotherapy room must be kept as a containing, protecting space, neither exposed nor sealed off, thus enabling us to return safely to our inner intimate selves like Gitai's hero.

Moreover, as Buber (1965) says, in a reality where both therapist and patient share a common *interhuman* sphere, therapists must connect with their own humanity, in an "I and Thou" encounter with their patients. This means that therapists—without burdening patients with their own personal problems—should not be afraid to be present as subjects, with their own associations, experiences and feelings, which are an inseparable part of the therapeutic dialogue. They must posses a kind of serenity that will allow them not to rush into interpretations or to cover up pain, rifts, and helplessness with supposed "understanding".

In one of the dramatic moments in Hebrew literature, Izhar, in a story called *Prisoner of War* (1949), writes about an Israeli soldier who is torn between the obligation to obey orders and his conscience. A splendid scenery is used by the author as a place of refuge for the soldier, when his dilemma reaches its peak. While writing this article I felt like the soldier who in the midst of the terrible turmoil stopped and used the splendid scenery to pause and reflect on the inner scenery. Such a pause is the only possible way to survive creatively.

When Primo Levi was asked once how he managed to survive Auschwitz, he sardonically replied: "Apart from my knowledge of German and sheer luck—I never stopped looking curiously and passionately at the world around me".

CHAPTER SIX

The psychodynamic dimension of terrorism

Salman Akhtar

Like a psychosocial smallpox, eruptions of terrorism are scattered all over the skin of today's world. These range from the chronic violent strife between Catholics and Protestants in Ireland to the sudden shock of the World Trade Centre bombing in New York City; from the continuing Israeli–Arab bloodshed in the Middle East to the horror of the explosion at Oklahoma's Murrah Federal Building, and from the religiously sanctified suicide bombings by the Lebanese Hezbollah to the violent tactics of the Basque liberation organisation, Euzkadi Ta Azkatasura. The complexities underlying these phenomena are profound. Understanding them would necessitate a multidisciplinary approach with contributions from the perspectives of history, political science, economics, religion, social anthropology, and psychology. Although it is acknowledged that multilayered socio-economic factors contribute to the emergence of terrorism, this article focuses on the psychological dimension of terrorism.

This article begins by taking up the difficulties that lie in the path of defining the term 'terrorism'. Once an operational definition is arrived at, the psychodynamic characteristics of terrorist leaders and their followers are delineated, using concepts from both individual and group psychology. Following this, a brief digression is made into the clinical realm and some parallels between the terrorist violence against peace-seeking forces and certain patients' destructive attacks on the psychotherapeutic process are demonstrated. In conclusion, comments are made regarding the dynamics of overcoming hate and achieving the psychic stance of forgiveness.

The problem of definition

Although terms such as terrorism and terrorist have become a part of our sociopolitical lexicon, their definition remains far from clear. Many factors contribute to this conceptual murkiness.

First and foremost, when the word terrorism was introduced in 1795, it denoted the acts of intimidation of civilians by their government (Volkan, 1997). Such "terrorism from above" has indeed far exceeded, in the sheer number of its victims, any act of "terrorism from below" (i.e. certain people's attempt to rebel against, disrupt, or overthrow an established government). Yet the term terrorism is largely employed today for the latter phenomena, excusing from its denotative jurisdiction the concentration camps of the Holocaust, the Gulags of Stalin, the killing fields of the Pol Pot regime, the torture chambers of Pinochet, and the recent Serbian massacre of ethnic Albanians. A deeply ensconced, large organisation with a well-oiled machinery and a powerful means of mass destruction is referred to as a totalitarian or fascist regime and a small, poorly organised zealous group with haphazardly collected ammunition is termed a terrorist organisation.

Second, the label terrorist is invariably applied to an individual or a group by others and is not a self-assigned designation. As a result, the same individual might be declared a terrorist by the group targeted by his assault and a hero by those whose interests he represents. For instance, during India's struggle for independence from British rule, the fiery Sikh leader, Bhagat Singh, was deemed a terrorist by the British, and a shaheed (literally, a glorious martyr) by the Indians. The same contradictory diagnosis applies to Sheik Yasin, leader of the militant Palestinian group, Hamas, which is responsible for violent attacks against innocent Israeli citizens. Viewed as an evil terrorist by the Israelis, Yasin is revered by the fundamentalist Palestinians. Of course, there are many more examples of this.

Third, because the term terrorism is context based, it becomes inextricably bound with the passage of time. Yesterday's terrorist might well be tomorrow's hero. In his Irgun days, Manachem Begin often recoursed to organised violence in the struggle against the British political order and was deemed a terrorist by his oppressors. Today he is revered in Israel. Yasir Arafat's transformation from leader of the Palestine Liberation Organisation (PLO), to Nobel laureate for world peace is another instance of the temporally vulnerable nature of terminology in this realm.

Finally, defining who is a terrorist is also complicated by the fact that destructive acts perpetrated by loners, even if ethnopolitically motivated, are often exempt from the scope of the term terrorism. Thus, Baruch Goldstein's showering of Palestinian Muslims praying in a mosque and Ted Kaczynski's (the Unabomber) stealthy campaign against technologic modernity are viewed as symptoms of deranged minds and not as terrorist acts. In all fairness, it should be acknowledged that Timothy McVeigh might be an exception here.

When such denotative pitfalls are taken into consideration, one is led to conclude that the term terrorism refers to the violent expression of a political agenda by an organised group of individuals who operate in a clandestine manner and who are bound to each other by hatred of a common enemy and love of a common political, ethnic, or ideological goal. Terrorists need to be distinguished from two other groups with overlapping characteristics—cultists and members of street gangs. The latter two groups also consist of individuals herding around a charismatic leader, idealising themselves, devaluing the rest of the society, and leading a socially marginal, if not clandestine, existence.

The differences between a terrorist organisation on the one hand and cults and gangs on the other hand involve the degree, overtness, and direction of violence and the underlying agenda that holds these groups together. Violence is the chief means of expression in terrorism. Gangs too are often violent toward non-members. Cults, although overtly decrying violence, can break out in grotesque acts of self-destructiveness. The mass suicides of Reverend Jones' Guyana and, more recently, of the Heaven's Gate in California are two vivid examples. The second difference among terrorist organisations, cults and street gangs resides in their overt agendas being political, spiritual, and materialistic, respectively.

Multifactorial dynamics

The terrorism-prone individual

Although psychological studies of terrorists are few, evidence does exist that most major players in a terrorist organisation are, themselves, deeply traumatised individuals (Volkan, 1997). As children they suffered chronic physical abuse and profound emotional humiliation. The "safety feeling" (Sandler, 1987) which is necessary for healthy psychic growth, was thus violated. They grew up mistrusting others, loathing passivity, and dreading the recurrence of a violation of their psychophysical boundaries. "At the base, this intense anxiety over future loss is driven by the semiconscious inner knowledge that passivity ensures victimisation" (Volkan, 1997). To eliminate this fear, such individuals feel the need to "kill off" their view of themselves as victims. One way to accomplish this is to turn passivity into activity, masochism into sadism, and victimhood into victimising others. Hatred and violent tendencies toward others thus develop. Devaluing others buttresses fragile self-esteem. The resulting "malignant narcissism" (Kernberg, 1984) renders mute the voice of reason and morality. Sociopathic behaviour and outright cruelty are thus justified. The narrowed cognition characteristic of paranoid mentality (Akhtar, 1992; Bollas, 1992; Shapiro, 1965), along with a thin patina of political rationalisation, gives a gloss of logic to the entire psychic organisation.

Social triggers

A terrorism-prone individual is pushed over the edge by a trigger from the environment. An unexpected wave of economic deprivation, territorial disenfranchisement, curtailment of civil liberties, or outright state-sanctioned violence are among the factors that shake up the vulnerable individual's self-esteem, mobilise his "narcissistic rage" (Kohut, 1972) and propel him toward establishing or joining a terrorist organisation.

The terrorist organisation

Like most groups, a terrorist organisation consists of a leader and his followers. The leader is usually a traumatised but charismatic individual who is capable of exerting a powerful fascinating effect on others (Olden, 1941). The followers are usually single, sexually inhibited young men, equally traumatised themselves and struggling to achieve a sense of selfhood and a cohesive identity. Through his fiery oratory and bold actions, the leader appeals to the group members' infantile hunger for love and acceptance. He evokes "chosen glories" (Volkan, 1988) through exaggerated accounts of past achievements of the group. He offers a new family, as it were, placing himself in the father's role. He forcefully reminds the group of their "chosen trauma" (*ibid*.) through exaggerated accounts of past injustices against the group by their enemies. He thus helps his followers shift their aggression toward those outside the group. This enhances group cohesion, which, in turn, furthers the leader's grip on the members. He comes to exert a hypnotic influence on his followers. He can diminish their shame and guilt, increase their narcissism, and help project their felt inferiority onto others. The "destructive pied piper" (Blum, 1995) thus promotes prejudice, hatred, and violence toward debased outsiders. At the same time, once the terrorist leader begins accepting overt or covert political and financial backing from established nations, he himself becomes subject to large group processes.

Two cardinal features of group psychology (Freud, 1921), namely intensified affect and diminished intellectual acumen, contribute to the regression set in motion by the group leader. Individual members lose their previous sense of right and wrong, surrendering their personal values on the altar of group approval. Under the influence of an inciting social trigger and the mesmerising power of a leader, the group regresses further. Feeling itself to be a victim, the group begins to victimise others in an act of externalisation. The oppressed of yesterday become the oppressors of today. Individual acts of terrorism (e.g. bombing, hijacking planes, or hostage taking), although largely chosen for their destructive potential and shock value, also contain unconscious enactments of childhood abuse by the parents, with a reversal of the roles of perpetrator and victim. Such violent medleys provide the discharge of repressed sexual impulses as well and prepare the psychosocial floor for an "inevitable dance with death" (Neubauer, 1995).

The secondary role of the other

The cohesion of a terrorist group is furthered by the overt or covert financial aid and praise for its activities from agencies supportive of its cause. The shock and horror of the victims also, paradoxically, fuels the narcissism of the terrorist; this dynamic is akin to the satisfaction a sexual exhibitionist draws from his onlooker's startled response. Notoriety achieved through public media services a similar mirroring function.

The covert factor of masochism and self-destructiveness

Because the terrorist organisation is established on the principle of externalisation of one's own victimhood in search of an exalted and conflict-free identity, it inherently cannot afford to succeed in its surface agenda. If the group were to succeed, it would no longer be needed. Its projectively buttressed identity would collapse and the pain of its own suffering would insist on being recognised and psychically metabolised. Because the terrorist leader cannot tolerate such a depressive crisis, he unconsciously aims for the impossible (Volkan, 1997; Post, 1990). The resulting failure to achieve the officially stated goal is unconsciously desired because it facilitates the continued externalisation of the victimised aspects of the individual and group self. Such self-destructiveness also gratifies the remnant capacity for unconscious guilt regarding the cruelty perpetrated against others.

An intrapsychic terrorist organisation

Like a terrorist organisation that seeks an impossible and ideal goal, some patients reveal an unconscious striving for totally undoing the effects of their childhood traumas or even erasing their occurrence in the first place. The terrorist organisation seeks omnipotence and has no concern for the opponent's rights. It even attacks those within its own ranks who seek peace with the 'enemy'. Similarly, the patient, who suffers from pathological hope and harbours a malignant "someday" fantasy (Akhtar, 1996), strives to obtain absolute satisfaction from the therapist without any concern for the latter. He demands that the therapist provide such things as exquisite empathy, love, sex, treatment for reduced fees, access to his or her home, sessions on demand, and encounters at all kinds of hours. If the patient finds the therapist to be lacking in any of these regards, he berates him or her as useless, unloving, and even cruel. In a fashion akin to a terrorist organisation, the patient thus attacks not only the therapist's concern and devotion, but also those parts of his own personality that seem aligned with the therapist and can see the inconsolable nature of his own hunger. It is as if the patient has an internal terrorist organisation that seeks to assassinate his observing ego because it is collaborating with the therapist and seems willing to give up the search for the lost, dimly remembered, and retrospectively idealised 'all-good' days of early infancy in favour of milder but more realistic satisfactions in the current life.

Also, like the terrorist organisation that seduces its members into overlooking their current misery and setting their eyes on the glorious future promised by their struggle, this internal destructive agency renders the patient enormously stoic. Recourse to infantile omnipotence makes any amount of waiting bearable (Potamianou, 1992). For such individuals, the present has only secondary importance. They can tolerate any current suffering in the hope that future rewards will make it all worthwhile. The promise of receiving the love of *hoors* (celestial maidens) in the heaven made to the Hezbollah suicide bombers (Volkan, 1997) is akin to these patients' insistence that all the self-induced suffering is acceptable because "someday" (Akhtar, 1996) their childhood traumas will be completely reversed.

Toward forgiveness

The Rabin–Arafat handshake at the 1995 peace accord between Israelis and Palestinians at The White House is emblematic of a psychological state of reconciliation between fierce opponents, letting go of grudges, making compromises, renouncing omnipotent claims, and settling for less than ideal handouts from life. In Kleinian terms (Klein, 1948a), this is a move from the "paranoid" position to the "depressive" position. In the paranoid position, "goodness" is claimed for oneself and "badness" is totally externalised. The world is viewed in black and white terms. The self is regarded as a victim and the other as an oppressor. Mistrust, fear, rage, greed, and ruthlessness predominate. In the depressive position, it is acknowledged that the self is not "all good" and the other not "all bad". Capacity for empathy appears on the horizon. There also emerge feelings of gratitude for what one has indeed received, guilt and sadness for having hurt others, and reparative longings to redress the damage done. Reality testing improves and the capacity for reciprocal relationships develops. Four factors seem to be of importance in making such an advance possible.

Repetition

With the attack–revenge–counter-revenge cycle repeating itself over and over with little actual benefit, it becomes difficult to deny that such bloody warfare is futile. The informative potential of repetition gradually accumulates. True to old wisdom then, the passage of time does facilitate a move toward forgiveness. Like the diminution of rage in an ageing borderline individual, the destructive energies of a terrorist organisation also gradually run out. Non-hostile exchanges between the group it represents and its opponents accrue over time and begin to have psychostructural presence. External realities surrounding the warring factions also change and affect what is going on within the dyad.

Revenge

Although 'politically incorrect', some revenge is actually good for the victim. It puts the victim's ego in an active rather than a passive position. This imparts a sense of mastery and autonomy that makes further destructiveness a matter of choice rather than of an inner demonic mandate. Having taken some revenge and tasted the pleasure of sadism also changes the libido–aggression balance in the self-object relationship. The victim no longer remains innocent and the perpetrator is no longer the sole cruel party. Both now seem to have been hurt and to have caused hurt. This shift lays the groundwork for empathy and reduces hatred. Forgiveness is the next step.

Reparation

Acknowledgement by the perpetrator that he has indeed harmed the victim is an important factor in the latter's recovery from the trauma (Akhtar, 1995, 1999). It undoes the profoundly deleterious effects of "gaslighting" (i.e. denying that anything destructive is being done to someone). To harm someone and then to question his or her perception of it is a double jeopardy, tantamount to "soul murder" (Shengold, 1989). Note in this connection the pain those who deny the Holocaust cause Jews and, in a clinical parallel, the anguish induced in a sexually abused child whose 'non-abusive' parent refused to believe the occurrence of such an event. Recognising the Holocaust and the sexual abuse, in contrast, improves reality testing and facilitates mourning. Such a move is given further impetus if the perpetrator shows signs of remorse, apologises, and offers emotional reparation, material reparation, or both. This testifies to the verity of one's grievance and functions as a graft over one's psychic wounds. A secondary increase in self-esteem follows that permits further mourning. A dialectic relationship gradually develops between such enhanced healthy narcissism and the emerging capacity to let go of the grief.

Reconsideration

Together, the experiential knowledge derived from the passage of time, the libido–aggression shift as a result of taking some revenge, and the rectified perceptual and narcissistic economy as a consequence of receiving reparation result in the capacity for better reality testing. This makes it possible to reconsider the 'memories' of one's traumas. Kafka's (Kafka, 1992) view that we repeat not what we have repressed but what we remember in a particular rigid way is pertinent in this context. Its implication for the clinical as well as the social situation is that to let go of grudges we do not need to recall what has been forgotten, but an amplification, elaboration, and revision of what indeed is remembered.

In tandem, these four factors (repetition, revenge, reparation, and reconsideration) improve reality testing, facilitate mourning of earlier injustices, enhance ownership of one's own destructiveness, permit the capacity for concern for the opponent, and allow forgiveness to emerge and consolidate. To return to the metaphor invoked at the beginning of this section, the Rabin–Arafat handshake seems to have been a product of such dynamics. In the clinical situation, too, repetition (a long duration of treatment), revenge (sadistic assaults on the therapist), reparation (the therapist's lasting empathy and devotion), and reconsideration (re-contextualisation and revision of childhood memories) gradually facilitate the letting go of chronic anguish and omnipotent hope emanating from severe childhood traumas and deprivations. Pathological optimism gives way to realistic hope, which paves the way to a peaceful existence.

Conclusion

The social evil of terrorism has multiple determinants, ranging from political and economic factors to the role played by the deeply traumatised childhoods of the participants in such activities. Elaborating on the complex interplay of these variables, this article portrays the terrorist as a sociopolitical Ahab: grievously injured, possessed by the lust of revenge, unmindful of reality, boundless in his demonic hope, ruthless and cruel toward others, and, ultimately, not even good for his own self. This article further suggests that a combination of repetition, the opportunity to take some revenge, reparation from the perpetrator, and reconsideration of the psychic and external reality helps the traumatised–vengeful individual (whether a terrorist on the social scene or a malignantly sadomasochistic patient in treatment) gradually let go of the searing pain that fuels his destructive hope. Lessening of pain causes a diminution of pathological optimism. Hope for realistic compromises thus becomes possible, leading to a peaceful life.

CHAPTER SEVEN

Reflections on the making of a terrorist

Stuart W. Twemlow and Frank C. Sacco

"Listen children, your father is dead. From his old coats I will make you little jackets. I'll make you little trousers from his old pants. There'll be in his pockets, things he used to put there. Keys and pennies covered with tobacco. Dan shall have the pennies to save in his bank. Ann shall have the keys to make a pretty noise with. Life must go on and the dead be forgotten. Life must go on, though good men die. Ann eat your breakfast, Dan take your medicine. Life must go on. I forgot just why."

"Lament", by Edna St. Vincent Millay

Introduction

Keeping life going on somehow preoccupies the minds of virtually every American since September 11th, when more people died in a single incident than in any other non-wartime period in U.S. history and still countless others continue to lament the loss of loved ones. In this paper, we will outline an approach to an evolving understanding of social activism, fanaticism, and its potential progression to martyrdom and terrorism. In the necessary painful self-examination that is being undertaken by Americans, we offer some thoughts on social context as a crucible for the making of a terrorist.

What is obvious from a review of the scholarly literature is that not a lot is known about terrorists as individuals but there are many theories. One can speculate that particular social factors are important to the incubation of the nascent terrorist. This paper will outline a tentative "life history" of terrorism in a way that suggests how all of us can become more aware of how we unwittingly encourage terrorism, and can instead make other choices which offer a theoretical direction toward an "antidote".

We begin with observations that we Americans have been impaired by the trauma of September 11th with damage to our collective self-esteem and narcissism like that of Goliath brought to his knees by a tiny, almost invisible, human being with a well placed slingshot made from Goliath's loincloth. In the chapter we examine a few, certainly not all, of the irrational reactions to this serious narcissistic injury to a powerful nation, including the decision to "declare war" on Osama bin Laden.

More specifically, we wish to focus on how terrorism develops in its social context. Our view is that often terrorists began their idealism during adolescent years since adolescents experience a normative crisis in which all aspects of their being and values are questioned. We hypothesize that while some adolescents align themselves with the mores of what Spiro Agnew called the "silent majority", others may become committed social activists. A culture such as America's, with its democratic freedoms protected through the Constitution, is a potential breeding ground for terrorism if certain conditions are not met. Our speculation is that if a culture does not accept, or more actively rejects, the ideals of the committed social activist, then a nascent fanatic could emerge. The issue is how social aggression is directed, controlled, and modulated. This chapter gives an example of the social impact of committed social activists who are not marginalized and do find a place within their culture.

The primary energy that drives the terrorist and fanatic is aggression; we refer in a later section of this paper to work we have done with homicidal children in school settings in the USA with analogous fanatical and terrorist mindsets and actions. In these instances, the coercive power dynamics that seem to motivate such killers seem to be mainly a product of a social context in which human relationships have become devalued. Such dynamics involve a complicated dialectical relationship between the victim of coercion, the victimizer, and the audience of bystanders, resulting in collusive murderousness.

We finish with a tentative antidote for terrorism; a set of suggestions for a social context that will enable a committed social activist to collaborate with the existing system to create a safe, caring, and responsive social context within which people can actualize their wishes, goals, and desires without infringing upon the freedoms of others. Such a proposal if successful, could answer Aristotle's fear that in a democracy the workers could suffer from an excess of freedom and elect a tyrant as leader who would act out their vengeful fantasies against preceding oligarchs and monarchs. Could such an antidote possibly work?

Shattered mindsets: people process September 11th

Immediately after the attack on the World Trade Centre and the Pentagon, there was outrage. Irrational fears, rituals, and poorly thought through reactions became rampant. Americans became afraid of travelling, of investing, and of strangers; to name only three major and obvious fears in our culture. A memo distributed in October, 2001, by the administration of Stuyvesant High School in New York City to students, parents, and staff exemplified these responses in stark terms. This school is located a few blocks from the World Trade Centre.[1]

Q: Why do we need to wear ID cards in school?
A: Because every fanatic and every nut in North America has seen/heard/read about Stuyvesant since the WTC attack. We are THE high-profile school in America. We need to be able to identify who does not belong here at a glance.
Q: But we are students. We don't look like terrorists. Why do you have to wear ID cards in school?
A: All terrorists do not look like Osama bin Laden. Let me repeat, every nut and fanatic has heard of Stuyvesant. Everyone who didn't make the cut-off on the test, everyone who is angry at his

teacher, everyone who hates. Everyone. There are about a quarter of a billion people in this country alone. [Comment: so now every angry rebel fits into the category of potential terrorist.]

Q: You fascist pigs with your Big Brother mentality are just trying to scare us. There's no real danger.

A: Are you for real? There are bad people out there who believe that they will spend all eternity in heaven with seventy-two virgins if they can kill some of us while killing themselves. They really believe that. There are nuts who see Satan, there are an infinite variety of other kinds of nuts and wackos, and you think that you are above wearing an ID card while in school? We are in a war and this is a potential front.

This outraged sarcasm and defensive–aggressive posturing contrasts with the helpful efforts of many psychoanalytically trained individuals in the immediate New York area who volunteered their services free of charge, initially, to all citizens and then, specifically, to fire and police department personnel who had suffered a high loss of life during rescue attempts. A number of national associations of psychoanalysts, psychologists, and psychiatrists created volunteer service organizations, which were also joined by professionals from all over the country who travelled to New York City, some closing their practices to volunteer their services to the needy. It became apparent in working with survivors and rescuers that, along with the individual reactions to trauma and loss, there was a destruction of the invulnerable, omnipotent American cultural identity that was felt as a pervasive "existential" depression difficult to process. It became clear that the experience of September 11th had been a major narcissistic injury to the U.S. "cultural identity".

Social activists, fanatics, martyrs, and terrorists: a progression

Scholars like Haynal (2001), Haldane (1995), and Haynal *et al.* (1983) take a historical perspective on fanaticism and its role in human cultures. It certainly has not always been a pejorative term: the soothsayers in ancient Rome were called fanatics, a word derived from "fanum"; a temple where the oracles were pronounced. The mystical and more gentle, and committed qualities of fanaticism do not linger as clearly today. Over the centuries since the age of enlightenment, fanatics became distinguishable from the reasonable man, soothsayer, and priest by their destructiveness, although some (Haynal et al., p. 243) note that the fanatic's refusal of "what is" in society, by no means always implies illness or immaturity, but can stem from an individual's stand against the inadmissible perversion of a whole society.

It is our observation that the emergence of the "fanatical man" is the potential outcome of any intensely held human belief and that there is a continuum from normal intense conviction to highly destructive fanaticism. It is also our opinion that social pathologizing of fanaticism results from a failure to recognize the potential for such behaviour in all human beings, and especially, for the responsibility of all of us for the social context and conditions, which we suggest, can sometimes convert intense social commitment into martyrdom and destructive terrorism. Writers like Colvard (2002), suggest similarly that terrorists are not inherently violent, but are victims of a network of psychological and ideological legitimacy.

The Greek root *Martyrs* defines a martyr as a witness, perhaps related to the Greek gk; "mermera", which means a thoughtful witness who voluntarily suffers death as the penalty for knowing (*Websters*, 1993; The Barnhardt Dictionary of Etymology, 1988). Further, to be martyred means to renounce one's religion, tenet, practice or principle, extended later to one's sacrifice of a life station or what is of great value for the sake of a principle or to sustain a cause. This more idealistic definition has evolved in the twentieth century to include one who adopts "a specious air of suffering or deprivation, especially as a means of attracting sympathy or attention." Terrorism, the systematic use of terror as a means of coercion, has been adapted by a number including Corrado (1982) to include activities with an exhibitionistic quality used for political objectives with "publicity as a goal" (p. 294).

From this social perspective, there is a continuum that ranges from fanaticism, primarily an internal state, to martyrdom, where there is a willingness to sacrifice oneself for a cause, and finally to terrorism, where the rage is more homicidally directed towards others in the name of a cause. This can be destruction by an individual like Jim Jones or political, like the suicide bombers being trained by the Hamas group in Palestine.[2] This destructiveness seems based on a build-up of aggressive impulses in a variety of social contexts ranging from dismissive houses/schools (school shooter), to oppressed or closed cultures or groups (suicide bomber).

In summary, fanaticism is characterized by:

1. A coercive narcissism: where the fanatic is intolerant of differences from his or her opinions and in which there is a denial of personhood with cause taking precedence over person. Envy is prominent since what belongs to others is felt to be "mine".
2. Pathological certainty: impervious to reason and for which there is irrational zeal and commitment, thought by many to cover a deeper seated fear of annihilation.
3. Contempt for the enemy or for non-believers: with humiliation being used as the primary tool to coerce compliance.
4. Oversimplified theories and causal chains: the fanatical mindset leads to simplified cognitive processes and exaggerated cathexis of certain ideas. Often, religion creates a fertile medium for fanatical beliefs, with sometimes an implied fanatical adherence to a non-human entity, for example, Saint Augustine's suggestion that one should only love God. Simplified conditioning techniques used to train suicide bombers in Palestine included that there would be sexual and other favours in heaven as rewards. Thus, if the social context accepts and validates some elements of the nascent fanatic's belief, or rejects them, then distinctly different outcomes are possible. Table 1 lists these possible outcomes.

Although the transition from committed social activist to fanatic is not a straightforward one, the socially committed altruistic and politically tough and resilient activist can be a potent agent for social change. (Twemlow & Sacco, 1996; Twemlow, 2001). However, the social context must be receptive and respectful of the activist mission, at least in allowing its exploration and expression. Democracies like the USA, in theory provide an accepting, although sceptical, incubator for activist ideas. Social activists often emerge from adolescent identity diffusion, although true social activists consistently find outlets for their beliefs in their cultures and in their

Table 1.

Fanatical ideas integrated into the culture	Fanatical ideas not integrated into the culture
Purity of the believer	Sickness of the believer
	Insanity
Charisma	Satanic beliefs
	Judgement of the damned
God inspired wisdom	Omnipotent self-inflation
Vindication of the just	A hypocrite and criminal
Inspiring or revolutionary idea	Social isolation
Seen as honest and committed	
Social acceptance	

social mores over a lifetime. The cause usually becomes less narrowly political and more generally altruistic as the activist grows older.

In another context (Twemlow & Sacco, 1996, 1999), we have examined the attributes of committed social activists. Although our researches occurred in Jamaica, the colonial influences suggest some comparability with the USA. The attributes of a peacemaker were derived from a variety of psychological tests and self-report inventories as well as behavioural observation of the effectiveness of the peacemaker. These qualities included being:

1. More altruistic than egoistic;
2. Aware of and takes responsibility for community problems;
3. Willing to take physical risks for peace and not easily frightened;
4. Relationship-oriented and humanistic;
5. Self-motivated and a motivator of others;
6. Alert, strong, and positive;
7. Self-rewarding with low need for praise;
8. Personally well organized;
9. Advocate and protector of the vulnerable and disempowered;
10. Able to see potential in all people;
11. Low in sadism; and
12. An enthusiastic advocate, committed and understanding of the "cause".

A social case study also illustrates some of these principles.[3]

The Great Peace March for Global Nuclear Disarmament in 1986 (Folsom & Fledderjohan, 1988) was an example of the impact of the social context for the budding social activist—turned harmless fanatic. It began as PRO Peace; People Reaching Out For Peace with fundraising under the guidance of David Mixner, a public relations consultant and seventies peace activist with strong political connections. The march to Washington, DC, from California was a carefully planned affair with camping, medical assistance, food, and protection organized in meticulous detail along the route. Even before the march began, the venture bankrupted. By then, the followers were "socially committed". They marched anyway using what had been previously arranged and making do for the rest. Some four hundred people of all ages completed the course from March to November, finishing with a peace rally and march, which spawned others including a march in the Soviet Union.

However, integration of the fanatic's ideas into the culture does not ensure that he/she will become happy, grateful, and part of that culture. It partly depends on history and how that integration occurs. The French Revolution is an example of revolutionary ideas that created martyrs whose ideas were ultimately integrated into a political transformation for the culture. For example, Robespierre was a classic martyr/fanatic who, from his writings, seemed to enjoy and glorify in the role of victim. He insisted on spilling his blood for the good of the revolution saying: "We shall trace the road to immortality with our blood. Oh, sublime people! Receive the sacrifice of my entire being: happy is he who is born in your midst! Even happier is he who can die for your happiness!"[4] Undoubtedly, individual psychopathology can make a difference. Charisma, whose etymology means an immediate relationship with the divine without intermediary, may inspire an omnipotently disposed fanatic to behave like God, The Father. However, if the fanatic becomes a revered figure, there is always ambivalence. Jim Jones, responsible for the mass suicide of nine hundred individuals in Ghana, insisted that all followers call him "The Father". Any questioning of his judgement, he said, implied betrayal. In his long sermons he berated his followers in a contemptuous way (Peter Olsson, MD, 2001, personal communication). Some leaders, such as Robespierre, Churchill, and perhaps Ralph Nader, are eventually vindicated by history. Others, like Hitler and the Bolsheviks, are instead eternally damned, while yet others are held more ambivalently, like Napoleon.

Clearly, for an understanding of the complex interaction between the social activist, fanatic, martyr, terrorist, and the social context, whether individual psychopathology plays a part is an important issue. By its very nature, there are difficulties in answering this question, for even though valiant attempts have been made to collect information about fanatics and terrorists, often that information is scanty, grossly biased, and even if a psychiatrist has performed the examination, is fettered by the particular characteristics of the situation making the findings suspect. Shaw (1986) in a telling critique of the psychopathology model of political terrorism, summarizes the scant psychiatric literature, noting that terrorists have been regularly diagnosed with Antisocial Personality Disorder and Narcissistic Personality Disorder. He criticizes these pathologizing approaches as plagued with fundamental attribution errors, i.e. vilifying personalities we don't like. Although fanaticism may result in behaviours that are pathological, there is clearly no gross disorganization of the capacity to think nor personality distortions that make an individual incapable of perceiving a consensual reality and attempting to destroy that reality. Certain social traumata may be central. For example, Dr Eyad Sarraj, a psychiatrist and founder of the Palestinian Independent Commission for Citizen's Rights, reflects that:

> What propels (Palestinian) people into such action is a long history of humiliation and a desire for revenge that every Arab harbours. Since the establishment of Israel in 1948, and the resultant uprooting of Palestinians, a deep-seated feeling of shame has taken root in the Arab psyche, producing the feeling that one is unworthy to live. The honourable Arab is the one who refuses to suffer shame and dies in dignity. The thirty-five years of Israeli military occupation of the West Bank and the Gaza strip has served as a continuous reminder of Arab weakness. [Sarraj, 2002]

He points out that Palestinians feel that they are restoring their honour by fighting the aggressor and not just being helpless victims. Facing a well-equipped army with stones and suicide bombers, reinforces Palestinians' feelings of strength, courage, and defiance.[5]

Heatherton *et al.* (2000), in a landmark summary of the literature on stigma, provides a clue to some features of the social context from several research perspectives: Evidence suggests that stigma has three primary functions for the stigmatizer: the control of self-esteem, the establishment of control over others, and the buffering of anxiety. All can be seen as socially mediated mechanisms to control and stabilize the psyche of the stigmatizer.

In the social crucible for terrorism, the bystander role is also pivotal. What a community does with the fanatic's ideas has a critical impact on his/her psychopathology, especially if the social rejection from peer groups perceived as important is sufficiently disturbing. It is not always necessary for the bystanding social group to be external. By that we mean that a bystanding social group can be entertained in fantasy only, although the historical roots may have been in a real social group. The internet offers instant global access to bystanding groups around the world Our work with fanatical children (Twemlow *et al.*, in press,a) and in harassment and bullying in workplace settings (Twemlow, 1999) indicates that such social trauma can create a cast of characters in the field of internal objects that maintains a pressure to fantasize in dream-life, daydreams, and in hypnagogic and hypnopompic states.

Individuals and groups with linked interests can become clusters of bully bystanders (groups or individuals who vicariously enjoy victimization), thus gaining an advantage through projection of their own disavowed fantasies into the fanaticizer, while contributing to the pressure to fantasize and avoiding actual danger themselves. Several Australian colleagues commented that America often appears to take on the worries of the world, being more than willing to step into the rescuer role. Although it may well be that this role is appropriate and even necessary, group processes of this type can lead to serious misjudgements.

The absence of enemies

With the collapse of the Soviet Union in 1989 there has since been a frantic search for enemies. Biesel (1994), in an informative article, summarizes the media reaction to super power politics: the *New York Times* commented on March 4, 1990, "Democracy is winning, the arms race is over. Villains are friendly now ... the jackpot so long desired was America's. So then, why doesn't it feel better?" Psychoanalysts like Volkan (1999) have postulated the value of a familiar enemy in containing and holding disavowed self and object representations. He has pointed out the dangers when the enemy is no longer familiar; since there is less hope for diplomatic solutions. One reporter for *Newsweek* (Meg Greenfred) said, "Conducting this nation's business overseas has become more difficult with the disappearance of the unifying, clearly defined and universally understood threat (the Soviet Union). Whose side are we on? And how many sides are there?"—reflecting, somewhat nostalgically, that things were simpler during the cold war. A Paris intellectual, Bernard-Henri Levi, noted that the western world is having great trouble getting used to the death of communism, which another writer half jokingly called "Communostalgia!" Newscasters and politicians who have never been near a psychoanalytic couch seem to be missing the familiar enemy. As we make Osama bin Laden into a less familiar enemy, we are unconsciously more controlled by him and enactments abound. In 1994, *Newsweek* reported how the U.S. and the west were "building an Islamic enemy" and that there was a Muslim sect with a dirty agenda preparing for a holy war.[6]

In contrast with this demonic depiction of the unfamiliar enemy, Russell & Miller (1983) compiled a demographic profile of 350 known terrorists deriving information from many news sources. The profile of a terrorist is a single male, 22–24 years of age with a university education. Backgrounds include doctors, lawyers, journalists, and teachers except in the Middle East where technical training prevails. Terrorists generally have come from affluent middle to upper middle class families who have enjoyed social prestige. Osama bin Laden left his wealthy, politically influential family as a young man to fight against the Soviet invasion of Afghanistan with the assistance of the CIA and the blessing of several governments including those of Saudi Arabia and Pakistan. It was only after the Soviet withdrawal from Afghanistan that he turned against the U.S. and its allies. He never lost his revolutionary interests in spite of a brief attempt to return to the family construction business. His university and family background included early idealistic religious interests from when he was quite young.

School terrorists and suicide bombers

Young people are prone to fanatical beliefs. Adolescence with its social and physiological demands for unprecedented growth and separation from the "nuclear" family is a natural incubator for extremism, as many parents and therapists have experienced. International terrorism may also have its roots in separation/ individuation dynamics, since it is during adolescence that idealistic/altruistic/fanatical beliefs often first emerge. We speculate that an understanding of extremist children, exemplified in the "school shooters" in the U.S., may provide understanding both of a developmental perspective on terrorism, and the unique vulnerabilities of growing adolescents to unscrupulous military strategists, and extremism in all its forms. Even in the U.S., with arguably more freedoms than in any other democracy, this form of fanaticism usually emerges in its own closed peer-focused culture felt by the adolescent to be of prime importance, and preferable to any other social norms.

Eissler (2000) elegantly outlines a theory of hatred as a force for social change. The cause can be subjugated to destructive impulses and personal vendettas as is seen in school shooters, or personal motives and impulses can be suppressed and manipulated by the cause as in the case of Palestinian suicide bombers[7] and Japanese kamikaze pilots[8] (Taylor & Ryan, 1988), where the fanatic/terrorist is created and used by political forces in the name of a cause.

Terror, from the Latin *terrere*, to induce intense fear, apprehension, or dread, often renders the targets overwhelmed and under-prepared, such as were schools in the homicides in the U.S.A.[9] In Jonesboro, Arkansas, an eleven and a thirteen year-old team turned into snipers firing on students exiting a school building, killing and wounding children they did not know. The local community experienced this as a terrorist act against the school. There is a process propelling these children to act like extremists rather than to act out their adolescent angst in less violent ways. In some ways they are like suicide bombers who instead kill themselves at school as a symbolic act of revenge and retaliation for what is perceived as a source of great personal humiliation and shame. Unlike idealist Palestinian teens exploding themselves for a political cause, these young school shooters end their lives to end their psychological pain, in a megalomaniacal spree of revenge.[10]

Dylan Klebold, voDKa to his friends, a seventeen year-old boy who on April 20, 1999, with his eighteen year-old colleague and friend, Eric Harris, close to the anniversary of Adolf Hilter's birthday and that of the David Koresh cult shootout in Waco, Texas, actualized a carefully engineered, premeditated plot with the ultimate goal to destroy their high school as well as the community of Littleton, Colorado around it. There had been detailed planning for more than a year with maps and notes being made not only on weaponry used but also on strategies to maximize the kill. By chance, Stuart Twemlow happened to be treating a man whose son had gone to stay with his mother in Littleton and had spent some three months at Columbine High School, six months before the shootings occurred. Although the boy wanted to stay with his mother, he found the school climate intolerable, indicating that the bullying was overt; any children who were not sexually active and strong members of the athletic teams were overtly and regularly, physically bullied and sexually humiliated in front of girls. My patient's son would be classified as a nerd, an American idiom for children who are bookish, not gifted athletically, and who are somewhat sexually and socially shy.

The fanatical hatred of these two boys flourished in a strange dehumanized bond based on alienation and a common external enemy, revealed in their numerous notes and diaries. In one of them, Dylan Klebold, said simply, "The lonely man strikes with absolute rage". Although many of their writings and videotapes explaining their crimes are still not available to the general public, what is available reflects an uncontrolled chaotic hatred. On the tapes they spoke of how easy it was to make other people believe what they wanted them to, how evolved they felt, and how dying was something they looked forward to. Harris said, "I'm full of hate and I love it. God, I can't wait till they die. I can taste the blood now", calling themselves NBK's (natural born killers). "You know what I hate?" Klebold said, "Mankind. Kill everything. Kill everything". The fragments of their diaries are full of vitriol but it is not discriminatory; the railing is against almost every conceivable group. Harris said, "We hate Niggers, Spics, let's not forget you white POS (pieces of shit) also". Included also were: the rich, the white, the poor, all races and racism, and what Harris called "fitness fuckheads", martial arts experts, and people who try to impress others by bragging about their cars, Star Wars fans, people who mispronounce words, people who drive slow in a fast lane, along with several named television channels. Hatred was a common bond inspiring, energizing and invigorating these boys with the attendant mindset, making the world simple enough to cope with, and with an end in sight for their misery and alienation.

The school shooter unlike the political fanatic is not bred to be part of a larger political movement. Hamas begins training young Palestinian minds from pre-school and there is community and family involvement in the "growth" of a political fanatic. In contrast, the school shooter evolves in isolation from his family, although he goes through many of the same steps: he becomes zealous about personal grievances, while the political fanatic fights for a collective cause. He may be part of a cult, as was the case in Pearl, Mississippi, where the shooter was trained by a group of peers called "Kroth".[11] Retaliation is the school shooter's motive, whereas the political terrorist is sending somebody else's message about perceived collective oppression. The fantasy of future reward or vindication creates part of the necessary mindset to carry out the political act. Both the bombers and the shooters fantasize some relief for themselves or their culture after the completion of their lethal rampage with suicide. Klebold and Harris felt like revolutionaries fighting for the socially oppressed at Columbine High in the same way as a suicide bomber is engulfed in the promised reward of an afterlife full of status and sensual reward.

Adolescents, who are suicidal from other causes, experience a very similar transition in their mindsets before they take lethal actions. A key element of this self-destructive mindset is a narrowing of perspective creating a feeling of intolerable mental pressure and the need to act. The suicidal adolescent and the school shooter both despair that their existence of humiliation will ever change and that their future consists only of unendurable psychological pain. The suicide bomber in contrast is selected for a mission and thinks of being a religious hero. Both begin their lethal countdown isolated from the reality-based social supports that could offer another perspective on life.

A Secret Service study (Vossekuil *et al.*, 2000) found that in 75% of the thirty-seven school shooting incidents they studied, the children communicated their lethal plans indirectly, mostly to peers in the immediate seventy-two hours before the actual attack. In contrast, when Hamas chooses a young Palestinian martyr, they do not tell the parents or friends when the mission is to occur, they take the young person into seclusion.[12] The seventy-two-hour period before the school shooter attack is a critical point in this cycle for potential intervention. The targets of school shooters are selected based on a personal grievance, while the young martyrs' targets are selected for them for a strategic political purpose. Both school shooters and suicide bombers seek public places of significance for their lethal attacks. The school shooter's mindset shifts to a "ready" mode that sets the stage for the final act, while the suicide bombers see themselves as one in a series of chosen martyrs in a holy war.

There was clearly a copycat effect noticed by the FBI in school shootings;[13] many of the school shooters had a morbid fascination with prior school shootings. Both the school shooters and the suicide bombers appear to be looking at themselves as messengers seeking a form of redemption or justice. Whether the style is symbolic or political, there is a contagious element to these lethal acts. Suicide bombers are viewed as heroes in their oppressed and wounded cultures. School shooters are reviled and either commit suicide after the attack or spend their lives in prison, and the families of school shooters are often sued and viciously criticized.[14] In contrast, suicide bombers' families are often held in great esteem and are compensated financially after the attack.

The critical role of shame (Gilligan, 2001) for these young American school terrorists is cited by the FBI (O'Toole, 2000) and Secret Service (Vossekuil *et al.*, 2000) as being rooted in bullying or the repeated use of exclusion, rumours, and being the target of dirty tricks, and other language-based, social aggression. There are many opportunities for the world powers to be aware of social injustices leading to shame in various ethnic and religious groups. Just like school shooters who cannot refrain from telling their friends about their plan, fanatical groups also send signals to any containing authority that a group of people is being oppressed and on the road to terrorism. For example, it is reported in *Jane's Terrorism & Security Monitor* (September 17, 2001), that Abdel-Bari Atwan, editor of London's *al-Quds-al-Arabi* newspaper, told Reuters that bin Laden warned three weeks prior to September 11th, that he would attack American interests in an unprecedented way.

In summary, there are several clues that can perhaps inform prevention strategies; shaming and a dismissive home and social environment promote social isolation and disconnection from peer and community group objectives. As these factors percolate, the dialogue between the container (school or nation) and the oppressed (child or political factions) stops and fantasy takes over. Fantasy is made easier by modern technology. The anonymity of the Internet allows a violent retaliatory fantasy to be fuelled. Many of the school shooters attached themselves to cyber images masquerading as aggression containing father figures, e.g., Adolf Hitler and Stalin (Twemlow *et al.*, in press,b). The Internet provides information and connections to hate or similarly oppressed views, international news, and plans and ingredients for making destructive devices, together with oversimplified formulae for success that reinforces enraged grandiose fantasies. Ichimura *et al.* (2001) describes an excellent example: a young man who hijacked a plane, and then tried to fly the plane after years of practice on a homemade flight simulator designed from Internet information. He had failed in a competitive university and in spite of fanatical interest in flying planes, was never accepted for pilot training. In tape recordings of conversations in the cockpit of the plane with the captain, the cyber criminal found it quite perplexing that he was unable to really fly the plane, commenting that it surprised him since he was so good on his home flight simulator!

At home the school shooters were allowed a great deal of freedom to plan and to prepare attacks; this dismissive and permissive environment may have also been a fundamental ingredient in the evolution of this cycle of violence. None of the school shooters were ever stopped at the source (in their own homes or at school), since their containers of aggression were not functional. If a school container (teachers, administration, and peer group) dismisses the social pressure and pain experienced by the prospective school shooter, the young shooter is cut off from sources of acceptance and protection, and the psychological pain is no longer endurable. Adults in a dismissive social environment not only themselves dismiss human relationships as a viable means of problem solving, but are dismissed by the budding terrorist as being a source of support.

Antidotes to terrorism: I Lessons from the martial arts

The deeply held convictions of fanatics are frightening. Aside from the unconscious reasons for war, there are consequences of declaring war that can oversimplify both the enemy and the social context. When training blackbelts in his martial arts school, Stuart Twemlow would pose the following conundrum: "Who would win a fight between the reigning world heavyweight boxing champion and a homeless person in a street setting?" The intense commitment of someone with nothing to lose is clear for all to see in the war on Afghanistan. In one recent incident, half a dozen Taliban hospitalized prisoners held hundreds of other soldiers including American Special Forces at bay before finally being routed. It is a cliché of martial arts, and common sense, that one would never fight anyone with nothing to lose.

It is our hypothesis that before war is declared, the following issues should be considered:

1. Contempt fuels the enemy's outrage

For every fanatic destroyed there are a thousand waiting to take their place with the possibility of becoming martyrs. Bodansky (1999) in a detailed analysis of Osama bin Laden and his strategies states, "Perhaps the most important and lasting legacy of bin Laden is his impact on Muslim youth all over the world, for whom he is a source of inspiration" (p. 405). Bodansky reports that one Pakistani newspaper said, "No matter wherever he is and wherever he decides to live, the number of people who love him will never lessen", noting also that the giving of the name Osama to babies throughout the Muslim world has increased dramatically. A recent news release noted that Taliban prisoners incarcerated at the American base at Guatanamo Bay in Cuba cover many religions including Christianity with twenty-six countries represented.[15] While the last word has not been said about vicious propaganda, one effect of it is to stereotype and distort, thereby adding to the potential to underestimate the enemy in an effort to mobilize feeling against that enemy. A Japanese colleague of Stuart Twemlow who was a small child during World War II remembers his parents telling him that they had heard that American soldiers killed and ate their own children. We believe that belittling Osama bin Laden as "the evil one", and wanting him dead or alive as in Wild West posters, has hurt, not helped efforts to unite other nations against an otherwise highly supportable world-wide mission against terrorism.

2. Declaration of war inflates the status and grandiosity of the enemy, and the resulting corporatism degrades altruism

Sir Michael Howard[16] noted that America had made a "natural but terrible and irrevocable error" in declaring war on Al Qaeda. He points out that the British prefer to consider such situations not as war but the mobilization of valuable resources against dangerous antisocial activity. Such "situations" can never be entirely eliminated but can be reduced to and kept at a level that does not threaten social stability. These should instead be "emergencies" fought within civil authority in a peacetime framework using espionage and without interrupting the normal tenor of civilian life. If not dignified with the status of enemy, Howard declares, "Enemies instead become criminals whose lesser status makes them easier to fight". Benito Mussolini once said that fascism should be more properly called corporatism since it is the merger of state and corporate power; profitable wars encourage defensive narcissistic absorption when helping others becomes a secondary concern.

3. Declaration of war can lead to an oversimplified mindset to the enemy

Declaring a war in an atmosphere of contempt can lead to incorrect assumptions about the enemy, that the adversary is identifiable and containable and that the action will lead to decisive results. While the political impact of showing respect for the enemy may be undesirable, wars must be conducted with such respect. Expecting Osama bin Laden to be holed up in a cave waiting for martyrdom is clearly a gross underestimation. War should be concluded as quickly and decisively as possible, setting the scene after it for peace in a culture that has not been devastated physically or psychologically. After all, if genocide does occur, the conquering army has an expensive, time consuming, and very difficult task before it.

Since we have now elevated Osama bin Laden and his network

of Al Qaeda to the status of enemy, how then would it be possible to convert this war into one that could be won? Our point is that it is necessary to adopt a code of respectful conduct for a constructive outcome. One young Vietnam Veteran told me he had the job of digging up Vietnamese graveyards to bury ... American trash. The contempt implied in such actions is undoubtedly not consciously intended. It can be seen as part of a "war psychosis"; the outcome of the fantasy that the enemy can be defeated only if every last one is destroyed.

Victoriano Crillio, a famous Secoya Chief who Stuart Twemlow met while exploring in the upper Amazon Valley of Ecuador, was known for his gentleness, legendary strength, and agility. He represented six tribes of the upper Amazon Valley in the Ecuadorian Parliament. A quiet and gentle voice boomed from this man of immense power and strength. He responded to my question, "What are the qualities needed to be a chief and to win a war?" He felt there were three: the first is knowledge. Knowledge must be culturally relevant, based on experience, capable of being translated into common sense terms understandable to all, and useable with effective and predictable results, since in war, he said, the culture of both sides must be preserved at all costs. Second is diplomacy, which he dismissed with a twinkle in his eye as the ability to get along with people you don't like. Third, and finally, is the capacity to wield a big stick with a soft voice, pointing out that the softness of the voice tempers the destructiveness and perceived justness of the stick. The stick, he said, should only be used out of love (respect in our terms). Can the compassionate gentle philosophy of this powerful Amazon Chief whom Nietszche might have called, a "Roman Caesar with Christ's soul", teach us something? Only if the enemy is not dehumanized.

In a project to reduce violence in a Jamaican city (Twemlow & Sacco, 1996), after two lessons in the principles and philosophy of the martial arts, one police officer while on patrol, was attacked by a man wielding a machete. His usual practice would have been to shoot the individual. He remembered, however, what he had been taught and so instead disarmed the man and brought him under control utilizing talk down and joint locks. The officer discovered that the man had found his wife in bed with someone else and had begun to drink and run amok. The policeman was proud that he had not killed this man whom he did not consider a bad person, and instead, he had been able to be helpful to him in understanding his rage and jealousy. The policeman later became a natural helper in the community in which he lived, his work being very much facilitated both by his strength, his gentleness, and by then, this legendary act of benevolent compassion.

In our dojo *"there is no enemy"*, is a conundrum to be understood by all black belts. The enemy from this perspective is potentially understandable rather than a monstrous subhuman species created by propaganda and oversimplification. Once the possibility of human contact with the enemy is resurrected, negotiation can begin. The real object of war is no fighting embodied in the Kanji—Bushido, meaning both fighting (Bushi) and not fighting (do: the way). Paradoxically, the Bushido code of conduct for war was an integral part of the training of the Samurai during the several hundred years of war in Japan with not only the goal of teaching ethical behaviour and values to soldiers, but also as clever strategies to handle the enemy and win the war. This code includes "values" like: *respect, courtesy, honour, rectitude, benevolence, veracity, self-control, courage, and loyalty*. Table 2 is a summary of how these principles can be translated into fighting strategies.

In summary, from the point of view of martial arts, the role of victim and victimizer are psychological postures that necessitate a code or set of rules that involves deep knowing of your enemy and respect for the cause of the enemy. Thus, there is a mutual implied agreement with the enemy that the war is winnable and with minimal "collateral damage". Modern warfare, mainly fought at great distances with machines, has unfortunately enabled the human element and compassion to be largely dissociated from combat.

Antidotes to terrorism: II A framework for creating safe connected communities

It is our working hypothesis that for communities to become safe havens instead of breeding grounds for fanaticism and terrorism, several conditions must be met:[17]

Table 2. The Bushido Approach to Winning A War.

Principle	Lesson of the Martial Way (Do)	Value as a Battle Strategy
Respect	Consider all types of attackers as skilled masters	Better assessment and judgement of the enemy
Courtesy	"Even when you are quietly seated, not the roughest ruffian can dare make onset on your person" Ogasawara	Keeping a reserve of energy, maintaining strength, controlling fear and anger
Honour	Allowing the enemy to save face	Not provoking to the enemy
Rectitude (justice)	"To die when it is right to die, to strike when to strike is right" Courageously using good judgement	Conveying a sense of irresistible, intent and strength
Benevolence	"Bushi no Nasaki" the tenderness of a warrior	Paradoxical surprise of the enemy, avoiding a "nothing to lose" mentality
Veracity and loyalty	"Bushi-no-Ichi-gon" the word of the Samurai is guarantee of truthfulness	Allow preservation of strength and energy, courage, intense commitment of the fighter to the goal, avoidance of cognitive dissonance
Self-control	Absorbing the strike without complaint and with intelligence (giving way)	Stoicism, relentlessness
Courage	Endurance in the course of righteousness	Intense commitment to the battle, willing to die for the cause

- The presence of satisfying connections between people which in turn depend upon:
  - the quality of the leadership;
  - shared interests, experiences and values;
  - a relatively low level of unacknowledged conflict;
  - stable, non-threatening external conditions.
- Work connections between people depend on all of the above and a shared task considered to be worthwhile.
- A safe connected community recognizes the authority and responsibility of all as members of the community and draws upon the various strengths of community members.
- Within this space members can connect spontaneously according to their interests, but to accomplish a work task, this space must be structured into a forum for wide ranging discussion.
- Respectful, non-blaming discussion, which has a number of good outcomes:
  - people develop the capacity to see the other's point of view;
  - people develop their individual voices and learn about personal responsibility;
  - people learn about inter-dependence: that is, each member or sub-group can best achieve its goals by collaboration and helping to solve the problems of other individuals/sub-groups; and altruism and compassion develop hand in hand with enlightened self-interest.
- Dysfunctional communities tend to develop pathological power dynamics among individuals and sub-groups:
  - the phenomenon of "pseudospeciation", (Erikson, E., 1985, Erikson, K., 1996), or the tendency to view others as alien, inferior, and not-fully-human, licenses cruelty to others;
  - a community fragmented by pathological power dynamics does not develop a collective knowledge or spirit through which to address its problems;
  - unhealthy forms of escapism (drugs, perverse sexuality, etc.) occur.
- A working hypothesis about pathological power dynamics that can be applied to communities includes the following:

— Pathological power dynamics are reflected in communities through the living out of complex, dysfunctional Bully–Victim–Bystander roles. These three roles can be seen as representing a dissociative process; the Victim is dissociated from the community (as not-us) by the Bully on behalf of the bystanding community. The Bully–Victim relationship represents a dyadic structure and the Bystanders are an abdicating Third. The focus of work is with the Bystanders and the desired transformation is from Bystander to involved and committed community member/witness. The intervention aims at the recognition within the large group of the dissociated element (represented by the Victim) as a part of themselves about which they are anxious, and the recognition of the dissociative process (represented by the Bully), as a defensive action for which they are responsible.
— Connected people make safe communities. These connections are restored when the fragmenting effects of dissociative processes are interrupted by grasping the meaning of this action as an effort to deal with anxiety felt by all.
— Dissociation is a violent process and often produces violence. The goal is the transformation of brute power into passionate statement and respectful communication; this requires the survival of the container and of the task.

— In a larger sense, the cohesiveness of a community depends upon its "stabilizing systems". Each of these systems takes up a basic aspect of the community's developmental task (for example, health, learning, order, spirituality).
— Each stabilizing system represents a primary authorised role in the community. This opens the field to an examination of the community's relationship to authority and vice versa. The power dynamics within a subsystem (for example, the student body of a school) are greatly affected by the power dynamics of the larger system, which contain it (for example, the power dynamics among teachers and between teachers and students).
— Symptomatic behaviour within any sub-group system can be seen as a consultation-in-action to the authority structure of that stabilizing system. Symptomatic behaviour is not simply a

problem to be solved, but rather a dysfunctional solution, which keeps a larger, potentially more painful and more meaningful problem unseen.

Is it possible for strangers in a community to become connected in these ways? Indeed it is. Americans pulled together dramatically in response to September 11th. There was a 30% drop in crime rate in the Bronx, although within two to three months that had returned to "normal". People in New York City were and still are, more than usually helpful to each other and tolerant of other's mood swings and demandingness. Stories abound about the bravery of individuals and strangers who would help each other in self-sacrificing altruistic ways: *United We Stand, God Bless America* is still seen decorating many buildings, billboards and homes. The connected attitude of Americans is typified in an airline pilot's September 15th, 2001, pre-flight announcement for flight 564 bound from Denver, Colorado, to Washington, DC. He said:[18]

> First I want to thank you for being brave enough to fly today. The doors are now closed and we have no help from the outside for any problems that might occur inside this plane. As you could tell when you checked in, the government has made some changes to increase security in the airports. They have not, however, made any rules about what happens after those doors close. Until they do that, we have made our own rules and I want to share them with you ... Here is our plan and our rules. If someone or several people stand up and say they are hijacking this plane, I want you all to stand up together. Then take whatever you have available to you and throw it at them. Throw it at their faces and heads so they will have to raise their hands to protect themselves. The very best protection you have against knives are the pillows and blankets. Whoever is close to these people should then try to get a blanket over their heads. Then they won't be able to see. Once that is done, get them down and keep them there. Do not let them up. I will then land the plane at the closest place and we *will* take care of them. After all, there are usually only a few of them and we are two-hundred-plus strong. We will not allow them to take over this plane. I find it interesting that the U.S. Constitution begins with the words "We the people". That's who we are, the people, and we will not be defeated.

The passengers were then asked to turn and introduce themselves to any strangers around them. The pilot said "For today we will consider you family. We will treat you as such and ask that you do the same with us."

Safe communities require connected and tolerant people. Figure 1 summarizes the model.

Conclusions

If one accepts that the aetiology of fanaticism is primarily social and on a continuum with normality, we believe a deeper psychological and psychoanalytic understanding of fanaticism, the fear it produces, and the difficulties in controlling it become possible. Perhaps with the exception of killing that results primarily from internal motivation, violence is always dialectically determined. The fanaticized–fanaticizer relationships are co-created roles always embedded in a participating bystanding social context, i.e. fanaticism as we have hypothesized it, is a state of consciousness, the

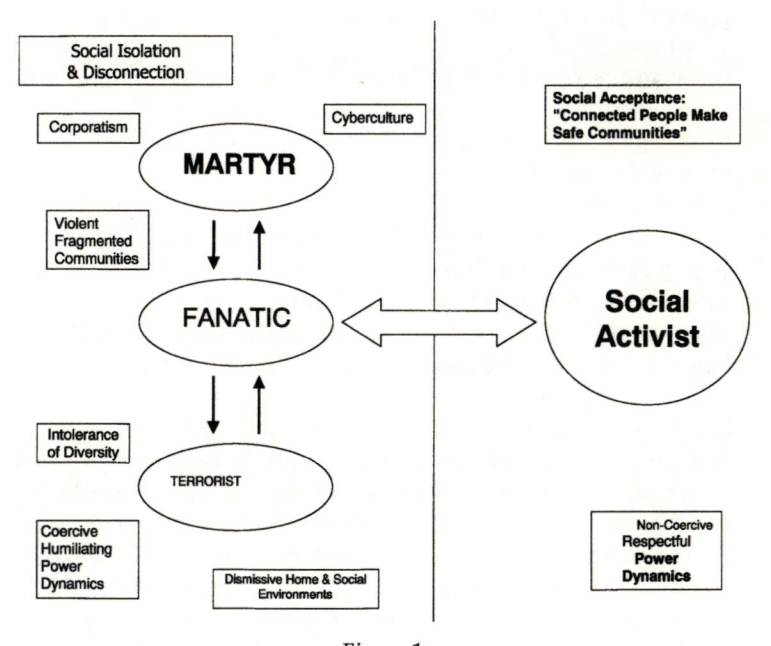

Figure 1.

flames of which are fanned by the bystanding audience, i.e. the culture and context in which the battle rages. A deeper understanding of the preconscious and unconscious roots of the desire for war other than as a biological given of predatory animals is to see it resulting from group pressures and social customs. Thus, the fanaticizer and the fanaticized are mirror images of each other, each seeing the other as a victimizer and each feeling the victim of that victimization. These co-created roles create behaviours that are grossly irrational, both in developed as well as developing countries, and leaders in both worlds can unwittingly get caught up in the process. Leaders with a deeper understanding and respect for the enemy and of the implications of conflict are more likely to fight a war that can be ended and that will be minimally destructive. If it is, as Barber (1995) suggests, Jihad vs. McWorld, then the Bystander is the abdicating social democracy, the necessary and basic antidote, urgently needed.

Notes

1. *Harpers Magazine*, January 2002, p. 19.
2. *USA Today*, 07–05–01.
3. A documentary was made of the march: *People Reaching Out* by Cathy Zeutlin.
4. Speech given Session Septidi, 7. Prairial, Year II of the One and Indivisible French Republic.
5. *Time Magazine*, April 8, 2002, p. 39.
6. *Newsweek*, February 15, 1993, p. 2, 28–29, *ibid.*, February 15, 1994, p. 28.
7. Jack Kelly, *USA Today*, 7/5/01.
8. *Harper's Magazine*, January 2002, pp. 25–27.
9. The word terrorist first appeared in English in 1795, in reference to the Jacobins of France, who ruled France from 1793 till 1794 in what was called the Reign of Terror. www.wordorigins.org
10. In July 1999, the FBI, and U.S. Attorney General Janet Reno convened a think tank with the authors and other experts on violence from around the world, together with staff from eighteen school districts where there had been killings or killings avoided and police, district attorneys, and FBI profilers. A publication summarized the findings; O'Toole (2000).
11. School and Juvenile Violence: A View of the Literature, 1999, US Dept. Justice, FBI National Centre for the Analysis of Violent Crime. School shooting, Oct. 1, 1997—Pearl, Mississippi, pp. 150–151.

12. Suicide Terrorism: An Overview: Boaz Ganor, ICT Executive Director—2-15-2000.
13. Personal communication, SSA Dr Mary Ellen O'Toole, Critical Incident Response Group, Federal Bureau of Investigation.
14. Martin Miller, "A dark reflection", *Los Angeles Times*, 2/27/02.
15. *Berkshire Eagle*, 2–13–02.
16. *Harper's Magazine*, January 2002, pp. 13–18.
17. Gerard Fromm, Ph.D, Erik Erikson Institute for Education and Research, Austen Riggs Centre, Stockbridge, MA, assisted in these conceptualizations.
18. *New Yorker*, October 15, 2001, p. 53.

HATRED, ENMITY AND REVENGE

Introduction

Jean Arundale

Within the psychoanalytic tradition many attempts have been made to understand the roots of aggression in the human mind, beginning with Freud's contention that hatred and the desire to annihilate are as basic to our instinctual make-up as their opposite, love. Although he recognized that there are environmental factors that aggravate and increase hatred, such as violence in the family or culture and competition for precious resources, Freud held that hate is an elemental, survival-related drive, inborn and incubated in the nursery when the infant feels love toward the nurturing mother and hatred toward her absence. The idea of innate aggression was taken even further by Freud, and given prominence by the influential Melanie Klein, in the notion of the so-called "death instinct". This force opposes the drive to live, is linked with envy, and is so threatening that it requires deflecting outward where it makes the individual anxious in relation to others and fearful of attack. This view is not accepted by all psychoanalysts and has been widely debated. More recently, theorists such as Hans Kohut have pointed out the origins of hatred in "narcissistic wounds" and Ronald Fairbairn held that frustrating relationships fostered hatred, both representing a viewpoint in the debate that sees the death instinct as too speculative and unnecessary, holding that frustrated love is sufficient to account for hatred and aggression. Nevertheless, a conclusion that hatred is part of our basic constitution as humans is difficult to deny in the face of its ubiquity and abiding presence.

The papers in this section address various aspects of the dynamic of hatred and its role in destructiveness. Kurt Eissler, in his classic paper, "On hatred: with comments on the revolutionary, the saint, and the terrorist", turns this question on its head and looks at the capacity to hate as an important measure of a healthy personality. The danger, according to Eissler, comes when a person or a group, "identify with the aggressor", so that "inadvertently one is dominated by what one is fighting to eliminate."

Integration between love and hate occurs normally in human development, however when bad experiences predominate, hatred can become a core feature of identity as well as a useful defense. Ping-Nie Pao writes of the role of hatred as a cover for unwanted feelings of fear, guilt, dependency, helplessness or forming the drive to dominate and control. Pao's exploration of hatred is based on disturbed, hospitalized patients, illustrating in individuals that which is magnified in the dynamics of groups or nations.

Ronald Britton's paper highlights splitting as a central activity of the mind, an activity that organizes good loving experiences and bad hating experiences by separating them into different mental spaces, beginning early in the life of the infant. Splitting in this way is an attempt by the developing human to deal with hatred, destructive phantasy and the death instinct by keeping them safely apart from good, cherished ideas and loved ones. When this defence inevitably fails, the self gets rid of the dangerous hatred by disowning it and attributing the badness to others, giving rise to the false view that all badness originates outside the self (or nation). Religions, Britton goes on to say, offer a symbolic binding of the splits, but beneath all civilizing structures there persist primitive fissures that re-open when there is trauma, re-creating polarizations and hatred of the "other". Britton outlines a particular kind of defensive split between the word and the image, yielding two different orientations toward experience: idealism and materialism. Understanding between adherents to these two mutually exclusive orientations becomes impossible as each view is felt to repel and annihilate the other, so that "otherness" becomes intolerable.

In the last paper in this section, Coline Covington writes further of the hatred of "otherness" and explores the hostility that develops even in relation to those who live nearby us in whom we perceive only minor differences. She argues that "when our impulse to form a loving relation with an other has been thwarted, our love turns to hatred of the other". This can lead to excessive self-love, over-valuation of one's identity, and malignant narcissism.

CHAPTER EIGHT

On hatred: with comments on the revolutionary, the saint, and the terrorist

K. R. Eissler

It is common to base an assessment of psychological health on an individual's ability to love. However, the ability to hate is no less important a manifestation of the healthy personality. The author investigates the psychology of hatred and the possible effects of psychoanalytic treatment on the development of the capacity to hate and, by extension, to engage in revolutionary political activity.

In ruminating about history, politics and psychoanalysis, a controversial topic comes to mind that is of psychoanalytic relevance. It would be interesting to know the political opinions, convictions, or tendencies of patients before and after analysis and the political opinions of their analysts. What proportion of patients change their political colours? If changes occur, what is their direction: from progressive to conservative, or the reverse? And what is the correlation with the analyst's political convictions? Do patients convert to their analyst's convictions without noticing it? If such a correlation exists, I would doubt that it is due to the direct influence of the analyst. But under what circumstances does the analyst intentionally try to change his patient's political opinions? Do political subjects come up in the course of treatment with some frequency? Are political opinions subjected to interpretations? Many other questions are attached to the group of problems I raise. They do not need to be spelled out. Is the equation here similar to that applicable to training candidates, most of whom as analysts pursue that brand of psychoanalysis in which their training analysts believe, as Glover (1955, pp. 262–64) maintained?

I am reasonably certain that only rarely in this country will a successfully analysed subject be discharged from treatment as a convinced revolutionary. As I have suggested, the tendency among analysts is to look at a patient's engaging in revolutionary activities or believing in revolutionary persuasion as a form of acting out. Thus, Winnicott (Khan, 1986, p. 11) wrote of a patient who had made a good recovery. "I would say that the only non-satisfactory feature from my point of view is that he is a communist." But evidently in contrast to what he really thought, he added, "but of course, it is not necessary that membership of this party should be a symptom of illness." An evaluation of actions stemming from revolutionary inclinations as acting out would be over-hasty, for only when an act is dissocial or self-destructive, or when the quality of an act suffers as a result of the bearing on it of the repressed, should one speak of acting out. To be sure, there is a reasonable chance that a revolutionary attitude toward authority is a derivative of an infantile aggressive impulse against the father, but this alone does not suffice to categorise it as acting out. If the infantile background *per se* would suffice to diagnose behaviour as acting out, then every wedding night would fall into that category, since it is hardly possible that it can be successfully consummated without gratifying unconscious infantile imagery.

The probability is that in the ranks of the analysed, only rarely is a person encountered who favours a militant revolutionary struggle. Revolutionary philosophies are looked at askance in Western democracies. More than that, indeed, they are in bad repute, but that is not sufficient reason to condemn them. Whatever the analyst's own political views are, he should have the inner freedom and certainty of letting the patient make his own choices, even if they are quite contrary to his own. In other words, he must treat that issue in an analytic way—that is, in the same way that he treats all other issues.

Among the many reasons that revolutionary outlooks are absent from psychoanalysis is a never-mentioned defect in psychoanalytic mental hygiene (*sit venia verbis*). Not only psychoanalysts but all workers in the field, I am sure, would concur that the capacity to love is a measure of health. Impairments of that function, as everyone seems to agree, belong to psychopathology, and if a patient approaches a state of unambivalent love, this is a welcome sign of progress that makes termination of treatment feasible. Freud, too, is sometimes quoted to the effect that a restored ability to love is a criterion of recovered health. There is much truth in that, but it remains a one-sided, narrow truth. Would it not be more accurate to say that a patient is cured when his ability to love *and* to hate is restored?

The favourable emphasis on love and the implied critical, if not contemptuous, neglect of hatred are due to the moralistic pre- and mis-conception that love is good, ethical, and preferable whereas hatred is a sign of a defect. I doubt this was Freud's opinion, for he had a list of seven or eight people he hated, as Jones reports (1953–57, vol. 3, p. 159). I surmise that Freud was a 'good' hater too, that he possessed the full capacity to hate with great intensity, which I believe belongs to health as much as the freedom to love passionately.

There are people who hate on little provocation and with great frequency but in whom the feeling evaporates as quickly as it has arisen. This sequence certainly betokens psychopathology. I am thinking, not of them, but of those who are capable of a deep, all-pervasive feeling of hatred. From Wittels' essay on 'great haters' (1929), one can learn how strong are the obstacles to the formation of a hatred that is, so to speak, uncontaminated by love—love, after all, would transform blind hatred into ambivalence. The historical examples he investigates, those of the Biblical Judith and of Brutus, hate in defence against another impulse. Usually it is unrequited love that leads to hatred. Love easily contaminates hatred and *vice versa*. Therefore, a true all-consuming passion and a true all-consuming hatred are rare. In general, presumably, analysts look on hatred as something immoral, probably essentially unsound and unhealthy, which it is not. But like love, it may be misdirected and lead to all kinds of symptoms and psychopathological irregularities. The most outstanding example is the hatred of some paranoiacs, which can be all-consuming and insatiable.

It may happen that the capacity to love has been restored by treatment at the expense of the capacity to hate. Hatred is the emotional equivalent of the wish to destroy. Aggression, the impulse to destroy, and the action of destroying may flare up on the spur of the moment, as happens so frequently in the *crime passionel*, without support of a rational system: a consistent yearning and scheming to destroy must be founded on hatred if it is to be effective.

The following may serve as a clinical example of pure hatred uncontaminated by any positive admixture:

> I have hated you in every hour that has gone by, I hate you so that I would happily give my life for your death, and happily go to my own doom if only I could witness yours, take you with me into the depths. When I let this hate free, I am almost overcome by it, but I cannot change this and do not really know how it could be otherwise. Let no-one deprecate this, nor fool himself about the power of such hatred. Hate drives to reality. Hate is the father of action. The way out of our defiled and desecrated house is through the command to hate Satan. Only so will we obtain the right to search in the darkness for the way of love.

And further:

> In their immense vanity, Satan's own have overreached themselves, and now they are in the net and they will never free themselves again. That is the fact, and this it is that rejoices my heart. I hate you. I hate you waking and sleeping. I hate you for undoing men's souls, and for spoiling their lives: I hate you, as the sworn enemy of the laughter of men ... Oh, it is God's deadly enemy which I see, and hate in you.

> In every one of your speeches you make a mockery of the Spirit, which you have silenced, and you forget that the private thought, the thought born in sorrow and loneliness, can be more deadly than all your implements of torture. You threaten all who oppose you with death, but you forget: our hatred is a deadly poison, it will creep into your blood, and we will die shouting with joy when our hate pulls you down with us into the depths.

> Let my life be fulfilled in this way, and let my death come when this task is completed. (my translation)

Here is a full and exclusive commitment to hatred and the destruction of an enemy whom the author equates with Satan. The words are those of Friedrich Percyval Reck-Malleczewen (1966, p. 85, 127f.), the 52-year-old scion of an East Prussian Juncker family; they appeared in his diary covering the period from May 1936 to October 1944. He was shot at Dachau on February 23, 1945.

I came across that example accidentally; perhaps better ones can be found. However, it is not only the manifestation and intensity of hatred that would serve as a paradigm. Iago's monologue of hatred in Arrigo Boito's libretto of Verdi's *Otello* is a magnificent pronouncement of hatred; Richard III outdoes Iago in the ferocity of his hatred, and Medusa's killing of her children may be upheld as the zenith of cruelty born out of hatred. But Iago acts out of jealousy—he loves Othello or Desdemona, and Richard III, out of resentment of his own repellent physical appearance and out of self-love. Medusa, of course, is impassioned by love of Jason and jealousy. The libidinal background of their hatred can be detected. The diarist I have quoted seems to have been a man ready and able to enjoy life and love, but he was under the curse of living in a malignant historical period that made irrequitable hatred a healthy reality response.

In what follows I shall try to adumbrate a few aspects of the psychopathology of hatred.

When discussing forms of love, it is asked whether the feeling is commensurate with the object. The clinical evaluation of drives and passions depends, in general, on the quality of the object. Thus, des Grieux's love for Manon is not appraised in positive terms because of Manon's psychopathology; to the contrary, Manon's unworthiness makes des Grieux's attachment to her suggestive of psychopathology. Similar considerations, oddly enough, enter into the problem of hate. Von Reck's passionate hatred was directed at the German dictatorship. Indeed, one wonders that there were not more of his stamp, inasmuch as most educated Westerners agree that the National Socialist regime was an absolute evil, certainly one of the worst civilisation has suffered. It is remarkable that a total dedication to hatred, as observed in Von Reck, occurs, if at all, only under extreme conditions, as when atrocities reach an intolerable peak. This challenges another aspect of a comparison between love and hate. Everyone is supposed to find someone worthy of his love. If a male were never able to find a woman who lives up to his needs and expectations, or went so far as to state that women in general have characteristics that make them unlovable, this would rightly be taken as a sign of a deficiency in that he is unable to find a proper outlet for libidinal strivings. Is the equivalent thought, *mutatis mutandis*, applicable to hatred?

To be sure, hatred aplenty is operative in the world in the form of bigotry, mendacity, ingratitude, racism, vindictiveness, and whatnot, but in these instances the hatred *per se* is often camouflaged, usually denied, even misrepresented as objectively justified, and if possible occasionally rationalised as an expression of love, as happens so frequently in parent–child and marital relations. Clinically, one speaks of free-floating anxiety which attaches itself unselectively to all occasions reality offers; correspondingly, one may speak of free-floating hatred that is unselectively aroused by all sorts of things. But again, it is then a case of hatred being frittered away on matters that are by and large indifferent and not worthy of a strong response. In almost all such instances it turns out that the hatred is petty, based on prejudice, dictated by plainly selfish concerns, and not in the service of a worthy goal.

Since hatred is in general in disrepute, most subjects try to keep its manifestations at a low level. However, the damage which covert hatred may cause in reality is more frequently than not considerable and out of proportion to the gravity of the factors that provoked it. Von Reck lost his life as a result of his hatred, but this sacrifice was in proportion to the enormity of the evil against which it was directed. There are parents, teachers, spouses who are unaware of their inimical motives and discharge them subliminally in a way often not noticeable to the victim and therefore all the more deleterious because the victim cannot bring defences into play. In the instance of Von Reck, however, hatred filled the entire inner world and directed all actions. It was not born out of a lack of *joie de vivre*. There seems to have been a minimum of narcissism involved. It is questionable that he would have experienced Hitler's downfall as a 'narcissistic' triumph, had he survived a few more months. His hatred seems to have been made 'impersonal' and implied in its entirety a grand effort against a structure that had to be destroyed under all circumstances. Had he been alive at the time of Hitler's defeat and experienced it as a triumph, this might have indicated that, after all, more of personal conflicts had been involved than would have been inferred from the diary.

I approach here the question of whether Von Reck's syndrome of hatred was 'healthy' because it was directed at an entity whose elimination was vital for him, his country, and the world at large, or whether one deals here with an unusual personality who was endowed with a particular, rarely encountered ability. Was it that unusual and tragic complexity—only rarely encountered in history, as many will say—that necessitated and justified Von Reck's complete surrender to hatred? Under ordinary circumstances one may maintain that there is no place for such responses. This I shall show to be a deception.

Only by virtue of extensive illusions or, better, scotomata can man pass by the perception of atrocities that occur around him. Nature is for many a consolation and a source of delight. Not only poets and artists but romantic lovers expand their souls and experience waves of bliss in response to a magnificent sunset or the agitations of a wild storm. But the person who is truly sensitive to injustice will not permit himself to be deceived by beautiful sense impressions and will refuse to find consolation in nature. It is not just a hypochondriacal oddity on Werther's part when he is thrown into despair by the thought that with each step he takes on a simple walk through the countryside he is extinguishing countless living organisms. Living *per se* means destruction of others.

And there is more to it than that. Even though it sticks compulsively to separation of classes, Nature is a gigantic bordello and a gigantic, classless slaughterhouse. There is no morality or restraint in nature. At its inception life was tolerable. The unicellular organisms, those early indestructible carriers of life, imperturbably propagated and survived without causing ostensible suffering or experiencing such. Yet the higher the forms life's evolution achieved, the greater became the victim's capacity to suffer (it is scarcely necessary to point out that the aggressors who cause pain themselves become the victims of more powerful aggressors). The final evolutionary product, man, holds the highest potential of suffering and of causing suffering.

The romantic spirit must deny the sufferings to which most living creatures are exposed: their mutual destructiveness, the horrendous torment when highly organised sentient beings are devoured alive by the stronger, who are forced to do it for survival's sake. Some animals achieve the extraordinary in the service of their progeny: even when driven by life-threatening deprivations they will grant precedence to their young. In view of the basic selfishness that pervades nature, it is moving to observe birds that, ignoring their own metabolic needs, fly over long distances seeking food which they reserve for their nest-bound young. Of course, good souls try to console by pointing to the numerous acts of co-operation, mutual help, and the like that are observed in the kingdom of animals. Those acts may make many a human being feel better, but they do not console the zebra that is devoured alive by a pride of lions.

The revolutionary realist will not be lured into illusion by soothing observations. He is aware that sacrifices by animals do not forestall later suffering of the brood and that they in their turn cause suffering in others. The knowledge of acts of love, the caring of some animals for their progeny, and like actions will not offset the knowledge of the unbearable anguish caused by the unmerciful cruelty that fills nature's every nook and cranny. The agony to which creatures are made to submit by the laws of nature is surpassed only by that which man inflicts on them. For the sake of lucre, over five thousand animals in this country alone are exposed daily to an excruciating death brought about by steel-jawed leg-hold traps.[1] These instruments of medieval cruelty create for their victims, terror-stricken and left to writhe for hours or even days in their clutch, an agony surpassing that of the Lord on the Cross and of dissidents on the stake.

Wherever one looks, there is failure. The heavenly bodies that arouse man's awe and adulation collapse, die, explode; formed out of dust, they decay again—no permanence and harmony are found. In the human world brutal force wins, and justice is a rarity. In human society as elsewhere in nature, those who need help the most remain unprotected. The old and the young are preferred targets of cruelty. Bizarreness accumulates on bizarreness. A saint-like Joan of Arc, condemned by a court composed of good Christians and even clerics, was burned to death, only to be declared innocent by another tribunal, in its turn composed of good Christians and even clerics. Was not Joan of Arc canonised? The deed affords the recognition that burning by Christians sometimes grants a saintly seat in Heaven.

Disorder, cruelty, injustice are to be found everywhere in the human world, but there are also acts of heroism and self-sacrifice. Jesus is upheld as God come to earth, who mercifully freed mankind of original sin. Unfortunately for the thousands burned and killed by his representatives on earth, he left a doctrine so ambiguously couched that the greatest scholars cannot agree on what he wanted us to do and believe. Alas, rather than leaving a proof of his divinity, he left a man more reasons to torment his brethren. Zola rising and alone fighting a whole nation is certainly a glorious chapter in the history of the West, but a unique exception; he knew well that God is not to be recommended as a guardian of justice on earth.

In earlier millennia personalities arose that made themselves the leaders of groups and promised their members redemption and a glorious future if they acknowledged and integrated certain systems of belief recommended by the leaders. But nothing seems to have an effect on mankind's basic misery. Since societies are not static but are in constant flux in most historical periods, the external facts of that misery change. When looked at from the outside, mankind's misery is unjustly distributed. A minority seems to escape almost unscathed while the vast majority is exposed to excessive deprivation. How long should mankind put up with scandalous calamities, wars, hunger, tyranny, intolerance, hypocrisy without shame? Each generation is told that conditions will get better—we should only be patient and have confidence in those who are in power. Each generation also finds its preachers and cajolers who persuade and exhort citizens to serve as good examples to others by their submissive conduct while those who are in power snuff out the weak as well as dissenters who are ready to execute tyrants.

In response there arise stiff-necked impatient ones who cry out, "Enough of waiting". Waiting means the death of the poor and the innocent, and preparations for new wars and suppression. The impatient ones are possessed by the urge to defeat evil. They appear at times as assassins who lie in ambush for a dignitary and take his destruction as a symbol of defeating universal wickedness. Sometimes great haters appear, like Robespierre, who gave history a new face. On the day when Lenin's adored older brother was executed at the age of 21, the fate of the Czar and his family was decided, for they in turn were executed 31 years later, years which Lenin had used for the preparation of revenge in the form of his great revolution. The desire for revenge certainly was not Lenin's only motive, but it may have made him the implacable enemy of Czarism and induced him to exterminate the Czar and his family. Great revolutionaries are great haters.

There are those who find injustice, whatever the form in which it makes its appearance, unbearable; many could call them overly sensitive to injustice. It took a long time until a full feeling for injustice evolved. Even today poverty is looked at by some as the poor man's fault or a proof of sin. It is strange to register Virgil's banishing to the most miserable place of the underworld those who had been executed despite their innocence.[2] Here is an accumulation of gravest injustices, an outrage to our feelings. We may take it as a symbol of what the majority of mankind has to suffer.

Even today the majority of the elite is not dedicated to the restoration of justice. In the eyes of most injustice is preferable to the convulsion of revolution. A person who desires to combat injustice must interfere with the course of events that appear serene and well ordered to the naked eye. If one tried to re-establish justice, those who had been unjustly executed would return to cause the downfall of governments, the loosening of the ties between citizens, the degradation of authority—that is, disorder, unrest. But disorder and unrest are exactly what the austere mind anathematises: the older it grows, the less it is inclined toward courageous, rejuvenating action, a sombre side effect of the present over-aging of most populations.

There are however, minds that are young and courageous and that impatiently and ardently long for action, like those of the *Sturm und Drang*. They are not terrorists, not even revolutionaries, but young idealists who would storm into the underworld to vindicate the unjustly executed. They champion the victim, whether it is nature or society that has discriminated against him.

Freud expressed his doubt in the adequacy of such moral tenets as "Love thy neighbour as thyself", but he never went so far as to acknowledge, as a legitimate way of handling reality, a life driven by hatred and absorbed in the one purpose of realising its goal. There is not much more than a short remark acknowledging the necessity of the existence of "men of action unshakeable in their convictions" (Freud, 1933a, p. 181). In concluding his treatise on civilisation, Freud declared that he could not offer mankind any consolation, which "at bottom ... is what they are all demanding—the wildest revolutionaries no less passionately than the most virtuous believers" (1930a, p. 145).

There are personalities at the fringes of society—terrorists, revolutionaries, and saints—about whom little is known but who are exceedingly interesting. Revolutionaries find consolation in the conviction that their schemes will be realised on an early occasion, but the true revolutionary seeks primarily not consolation but destruction—the destruction of all that stands in the way of the realisation of a higher societal state. This is not of small compass but includes a profound change in the very foundation of society. For that reason revolutions are looked at as a pathological societal excess and shunned by the majority.

But revolutions are part and parcel of mankind's history. They are not merely legitimate processes but even more—Great Moments, perhaps the greatest, that suddenly offer mankind an unmerited blessing. When a revolution occurs the gods hold their breath and watch man in order to see what he will do with the short interval of sudden freedom after an inherently unjust and frivolous society has lost its grip and he is given the opportunity of a new choice. When a society's revolutionary spirit is stamped out, it is usually a sign that the society's arteries have become sclerotic and it is taking a declining course. When that royal head fell in 1793, western absolutism fell with it. Tyrants appeared, and terrible excesses occurred thereafter, but the conviction of godliness that had surrounded royalty suffered an incurable injury. Revolutions go astray, tend toward excesses, kill too many, but in spite of all, the glorious French Revolution paved the way for the common man.[3]

The revolutionary evokes by contrast the image of the saint. One might expect that at a time of the deepest moral depravity since Christ's birth and the almost complete disappearance of Christian standards of behaviour, some saints might arise in order to redeem their times. Simone Weil (1909–43) was one of those rare exceptions. She exposed herself to the most severe deprivation of food, akin to what she knew some of her contemporaries to be suffering, and died a living death. In the search for saints one may think of Father Daniel Berrigan, S.J., and that tragic young man who lost both legs trying to stop an armament train by placing himself across the rails. There can be no question that St. Justin, the authoritative apologist of the second century, was utterly wrong in assuring the emperor that a kingdom of peace was coming. Did not he and the Church rely on Isaiah's prophecy that the Christians "shall beat their swords into plowshares, and their spears into pruninghooks" (Isaiah 2:4)? Did not the Christians do the opposite and beat plowshares into swords? By now everyone knows that Isaiah's prophecy that "nation shall not lift up sword against nation" was utterly wrong. No other religion encouraged as many and as cruel wars as the Christian. If Justin had known what his brethren in faith would do to one another, as well as to others, he would have hidden his face in shame and praised the ancient gods.

Thus, it becomes cogent to infer that it would be folly to expect redemption and salvation on earth from religious institutions that are in power. On the other hand, Father Berrigan and his followers, who by negative actions try to convert swords into plowshares, are true Christians, perhaps even saints. No doubt, in court they find their Pilate and are sent to prison as Christ predicted would happen to some of his disciples (Luke 21:12). There are very few who by sacrificing their lives to Divinity try to draw its blessings to earth. The saintly person's true experience reaches into the future without borders. He is certain that one day salvation will come upon mankind, no matter how long it is delayed by evildoers. God's mercy is bound to conquer Satan, and the saint, by sacrificing all claim to pleasures and gratifications of the world, is ready to accelerate the second coming of Christ.

The terrorist, too, is ready to sacrifice his life—but also that of others—for the attainment of a limited goal. His time experience is the opposite of that of the saint and the revolutionary (who, like the saint, bides his time, lying in wait for the moment the revolution will break out). The terrorist does not wait for salvation or revolution. His life is made insufferable by the presence of a certain condition, or several well-circumscribed conditions, and he insists upon repair now and here. He has a narrow horizon (unlike revolutionaries and saints, whose horizon bears no limitation) and will resort to any actions whatsoever to reduce the impact of the obstacle that stands in the way of his desire. He is ostracised and execrated by society and treated like a common criminal—unjustly, I surmise, in many, perhaps most, instances. What looks like unregenerate crime may cover an unquenchable thirst to realise a demand that has been placed upon him by his superego.[4]

The revolutionary and the saint both believe in the preacher's word: "Vanity of vanities ... all is vanity" (Ecclesiastes 1:2). And for both there is a point in the future when more or less suddenly the bleak turns into radiant light.

At any rate, revolutionaries and saints do not figure in Freud's work.

In religious and secular literature one encounters fantasies about man's end stage which embrace entire cultures. The most frequent in the Christian West has been the formidable image of the Last Judgement. For centuries it has haunted the faithful, and only recently has it lost the terror it struck in the hearts of the virtuous as well as of sinners. It is in its own way most characteristic of his time to note how Freud imagined his encounter with his maker: "I should add", he wrote to James J. Putnam on 8 July 1915,

> that I stand in no aware whatever of the Almighty. If we were ever to meet, I should have more reproaches to make to Him than He could to me. I would ask Him why He hadn't endowed me with a better intellectual equipment, and He couldn't complain that I have failed to make the best use of my so-called freedom ... I have always been dissatisfied with my intellectual endowment. [Freud, 1915e, pp. 307–308]

Times have radically changed since man invented monotheistic religion. Freud speaks with great respect of the birth of the idea that there is only one God, without due emphasis on the travesty that monotheistic religions apparently can avoid no more successfully than their predecessors did. Freud's imagery about his encounter with God is comforting. For centuries, if not millennia, when in a synagogue God is supposed to count with satisfaction the number of Jewish boys who are circumcised and learn the Torah by heart; but when in a Catholic church he is delighted by those who swallow wafers in the belief that they are his son's body; he also takes delight when those who believe it to be only a symbol of his body are burned to death. The Lord's Prayer, in its injunction "Do not lead us into temptation", contains—all theological gainsaying and wrangling notwithstanding—a blasphemy, at least in the sense any contemporary is forced to attribute to it. The imagery and rituals the monotheistic idea evoked in the various churches illustrate man's folly and disposition to be overcome by superstition.

Yet it seems that the days of such tomfoolery are numbered. At last man seems to be growing, however gradually, into a creature no longer afraid of facing the Lord, and nowadays it seems that the Lord must be a bit nervous when meeting his image.

There is a strong, rebellious, defiant recalcitrance in Freud's vision of his final confrontation with his God. Man is no longer willing to figure as a *figurante*; he has acquired a hitherto unthinkable freedom, at least of thought, which stands in the centre of his mission on earth as he sees it. He is no longer inhibited from pouring out his disgust and accusations in a gigantic outcry, even though society still shackles action, as ever in the past.

It is otherwise for the true revolutionary. His confrontation with God will be much wilder and will lead to a true tumult. The true revolutionary does not make compromises; he will not only execrate nature, he will raise his fist against Heaven, for he knows that, contrary to what all religions preach, nothing that God created has been good. Even the angels he formed deteriorated, and one of them became Satan. Why he made another try with man after he failed with the angels, who, after all, as we are told, are so much better as prospects than mortals, remains a mystery even a theologian cannot solve.

This constant failure of the Lord insofar as his best intentions come regularly to naught and cause the unending trail of suffering in his works will be in the centre of the revolutionary's tirade. Contrary to Freud, he is satisfied with the power of his intellect, but he will reproach his maker for having left a superhuman task for him insofar as his conscience demands that he undo all the Lord's failures. God gave him so little power to act effectively! Finally, he will scorn God for making so little use of his power to create the perfect, reserving perfection for men who, rare as they may be, achieve it in poetry and music whereas God's works always stumble into the impure and defective.

Returning from theology to psychology, on 27 May 1937 Freud wrote to Marie Bonaparte, "One could imagine a pretty schematic idea of all libido being at the beginning of life directed inward and all aggression outward, and that gradually changes in the course of life. But perhaps that is not correct" (Jones, 1953–1957, p. 464f.). It impresses me as a valid scheme: the infant's relationship to external reality, notwithstanding the rudiments of autoerotic libidinous gratification, is aggression as unmitigated as it is uninstigated. It wants to devour—that is, deprive of existence—what it encounters with its palate. This primitive state of all libido turned inward and all aggression outward, which Freud implied was the earliest model, sounds like a prototype of the Von Reck syndrome. This distribution of cathexis is the opposite of the ego's libidinal depletion, which has been described by Freud in conjunction with extreme love (1921, pp. 111–14). Then the self enters a state of bondage, and the beloved object, by absorbing the subject's entire libido, acquires irresistible power. In the Von Reck syndrome all libido is withdrawn and fills the self. Now all aggression is free to flow toward the outer world. A person with this constellation is the ideal hater and will ignore no opportunity to subdue his enemy.

The Von Reck syndrome must not be confused with the end-of-the-world hallucination in paranoid psychosis, as described by Freud in the Schreber paper (1911a). In a paranoid psychosis a serious regression occurs in the ego, whereas in the Von Reck syndrome cathexis are distributed in an extreme fashion without affecting or endangering the ego's developmental state. yet in the end-of-the-world hallucination, by the interruption of his relationship with the world the patient has lost adequate functioning of the reality principle. In the case of Von Reck this calamity did not occur. There is no reduction, not to speak of abolition, of the reality principle: the aggressive cathexis of the world is maintained, and all ego functions that serve, or could potentially serve, the purpose of destroying the opponent are alerted, activated, and even over-cathected. The loss of reality is avoided. The ideal hater is extremely efficient in managing reality, however one-sided that contact remains.[5]

If in the course of history more of this had lived, if more had been uncompromisingly dedicated to fighting the egregious injustices and cruelties done to the weak, would mankind's course have been more satisfactory? What one observes in reality is a general use of aggressivity for self-aggrandisement and the arrogation of personal power, but not for the betterment of the human plight. Unfortunately, the discharge of aggression gratifies narcissism at the same time, and narcissism seems unquenchable and asks for ever-increasing gratifications, which often leads to the overriding of basic moral principles. When I maintain that it is difficult to put aggression into the service of an ideal, it will be objected that those who act *ad majorem Dei gloriam* (in which *Dei* may be replaced by any other ideal) put their own welfare in second place and are ready to sacrifice even their lives for an ideal. An individual of this stamp is not so infrequent, but he acts under the tutelage and guidance of a person or a power which he has made a part of himself. He has not evaded serving his own selfish purposes.

The ideal revolutionary is alone or a member of a small coterie and does not expect rewards. He wants to see abusive power defeated, not for his own aggrandisement, but for the sake of others who suffer and will no longer suffer as soon as he has been victorious. But he is far less, if at all, concerned with the sufferers themselves. They form, contrary to what one would expect, an abstract entity on whose behalf he is ready to bear sacrifice. The activation of compassion would only diminish the impetus of his attack against superior power. This self-negating idealist directing all aggression toward the realisation of an ideal is rare. When this stage has been achieved, there is no room for neurotic symptomatology: all feelings of guilt have been eliminated despite maximal activation of aggression. Understandably the revolutionary will not need analysis.

In discussing the psychology of hatred, I must draw attention to a psychological factor that spells danger to the person who hates. Since Ferenczi (1933) discovered identification with the aggressor, this mechanism has become well known (cf. A. Freud, 1936). The hated person is always conceived of as an aggressor, and there is the danger that inadvertently one is dominated exactly by what one is fighting to eliminate. I do not want to delve into the engaging problem of why this often happens but rather point to an exception: namely, that if an absolute evil is hated, identification becomes improbable, even impossible. The one who identifies with the aggressor is indeed a very poor hater.

Furthermore, there is the danger of overvaluing the aggressor. Freud discovered that the love object is as a rule overvalued. The same occurs with the enemy. But whereas the overvaluation of the love object has its utilitarian advantage, since it makes the tie to the love object firmer, the overvaluation of the enemy leads to a detrimental squandering of energy. In Von Reck's situation identification with the aggressor and his overvaluation could not take place. His disgust with fascism was so great, and his recognition of the enormous destruction that would have been brought about had fascism been victorious so keen, that overvaluation was impossible.

I must mention another caveat in relation to hatred. The spirit of puritan democracy proposes recourse to the imagery of absolute evil and in general tempers strong emotions. We are supposed neither to fall into passionate love nor to hate to an excessive degree. And according to the Catholic Church, hatred *per se* is a sin.

Thus, hatred becomes a risky affair: it easily may rebound and lower the quality of the hater's actions, and it may falsify the image of the detested adversary, thus leading to squandering of energy. Most people evade insight into the abyss into which man has been born. It is much easier to hate trivialities than the very society in which one lives. Fear of isolation and retribution makes people petty and shallow haters who bypass those insufferable problems whose acknowledgement would make existence unbearable because they do not permit compromise.

Evidently there are many reasons for the absence of the revolutionary spirit in those who are connected with psychoanalysis. If that absence were due to an aversion against revolution, a moral and ethical reproof and disapprobation, this would amount to a defect in the psychoanalytic outlook, which should encompass the broadest possible unbiased evaluation of, and attitude toward, the great variety of channels through which man takes action in coming to terms with his reality. However, it may be claimed that the psychoanalytic style *per se* of approaching reality may counteract the formation of ideal revolutionaries: psychoanalysis, with its great stress on insight and the investigation of unconscious motives, may engender a prudent attitude toward action that possibly stands in the way of maximal insight. Thinking, after all, requires the decathexis of the motor systems; in ideal instances the concentration of all available energy on thought processes is required. However, the revolutionary is foremost an action person. He will refrain from action only when this is required for the sake of subsequent action, and he never loses sight of occasions that can be used for preparing and carrying out action. Archimedes concentrating on a mathematical problem and not noticing the sack of Syracuse is the extreme opposite. A man so strongly involved in thinking may produce thoughts of revolutionary calibre, but planning and carrying out revolutionary actions will be beyond him.

Ferdinand Lassale (1925–64), a man of action, provided Freud with the motto[6] of his most important work, the dreambook, but would not serve as a model of the way to live. Freud's identification with Moses never tempted him to strike the rock in impatience, as Moses did: I sometimes wonder whether Freud would have taken a professional revolutionary into analysis. In any event, there is no doubt that analysts themselves are closer to Archimedes in their lifestyles; they ponder and think and deliberate. The centre of their professional existence is to find correct interpretations in the service of an improved understanding of the mind's working.

This preponderance of thinking versus action in the analyst's way of living may give one cause to suspect that the analyst's example automatically creates a similar tendency in the analysed person and that therefore the chances that psychoanalytic treatment will engender a revolutionary spirit are almost reduced to zero, but this would be a wrong inference. Psychoanalysis, despite the analyst's relative passivity, does not in general diminish the analysed individual's tendency toward action. The effect of unduly prolonged deliberation prior to action certainly should not be anticipated as a result to be expected from treatment *per se*. To be sure, during the treatment period, when the subject's attention is maximally geared to observation and understanding of inner processes that sometimes go far back into the past, restraint upon actions may become advisable in order to avoid acting out. Once the process is ended and motivations are brought into proper order, actions more forceful and more effective than previously (though not rash) would be among the expectable results.

Thus, nothing is observed in the psychoanalytic procedure as such that would permit the expectation that a person's revolutionary potential will be reduced. One may, however, assume with some certainty that in this country the probability of a patient leaving a successful analysis as a revolutionary is minimal. The revolutionary spirit is so alien to the present political atmosphere that hardly a patient will enter treatment with the ambition or desire to become one. However, one would feel entitled to expect that in the course of treatment some patients will spontaneously embark on a revolutionary career. One has to admit that here the analyst's own retrenchment of horizon will unintentionally steer the patient into quieter waters.

Notes

1. Editors' note: According to the Friends of Animals, a non-profit animal protection group, in 1988 approximately 17 million animals had been trapped in the United States alone; in 1995 this number had declined to 2 million.
2. *Falso damnati crimine mortis* [on false acusal slain], *Aeneid*, VI, 430.
3. Cf. Shelley's comments on the French Revolution in his preface to *The Revolt of Islam* (1817): "Can he who the day before was a trampled slave suddenly become liberal-minded, forbearing and independent?" [Editor's footnote]
4. It turns out that the captive terrorist is an even greater danger than the one who is free because the former's captivity inspires his colleagues again and again to commit new acts of terror to achieve his freedom.
5. It would be important to know whether Von Reck ever resorted to revolutionary action.
6. *Flecteresi nequeo Superos, Acheronta movebo* (Virgil, *Aeneid*, VII, 312). See Freud's letter of 30 January 1927 to Werner Achelis: "I had borrowed the quotation from Lassalle" (Freud, 1927a, p. 375).

CHAPTER NINE

The role of hatred in the ego

Ping-Nie Pao

In the treatment of hospitalised and severely disturbed patients, I have had the opportunity to observe the rise and fall of intense feelings of hatred. Sometimes I was the target of these feelings; at other times I was accused of hating the patient. This exposure to the feeling of hatred led me to consider that it is so complex a human phenomenon that it cannot be encompassed by such common expressions as anger, rage, aggression, hostility, or destructiveness though these expressions often are used interchangeably with hatred.

Hatred and rage

Spitz (1953, 1963) noted that rage in the form of screaming can be observed in infants of two to three months. It is an ego-organised expression of frustration of instinctual needs. And as the mother repeatedly responds to the infant's rage by modifying his frustration, he learns that his rage has an intimidating effect on her. In this sense rage is an ego response to the conflict between the ego and the object.

With the acquisition of new ego functions, rage gradually undergoes a metamorphosis (Fenichel, 1954; Jacobson, 1953), and eventually transforms into hatred which involves the participation of all three psychic structures: id, ego, and super-ego. In hatred the ego is not only in conflict with objects in the external world, as in the case of rage, but with internalised objects as well.

Although hatred and rage are both organised affective responses of the ego to frustration, they can be distinguished (Jacobson, 1953; Novey, 1959). Unlike hatred, the earlier and less complicated human experience of rage in a form of communication. Both hatred and rage reflect a conflict between the ego and outside objects, but hatred also reflects a conflict between the ego and internalised objects. In rage there is concern only with the power and status of the external object without going beyond realistic bounds; in hatred, influenced by the internalised object, there is a tendency to ascribe enormous status and power to the external object, often accompanied by a feeling that one's own existence depends on the object. In rage the instinctual drives seek immediate muscular action, such as shouting, kicking, or hitting; in hatred the interposition of the ideational process results in suppression of muscular release. Rage tends to come and go with the exciting cause; hatred can linger on and grow in intensity. In rage one attempts to modify the object's frustrating behaviour in order to insure immediate gratification, using past knowledge only to help modify the object's frustrating action; in hatred one dwells on the past, thinks of revenge in the future, and is not concerned with the present. Rage serves no ego-syntonic defensive purpose; hatred, in linking past and future, establishes a sense of continuity and may be used as an ego-syntonic defence, as a basis of relationship, and as the core of a person's identity.

Hatred as an experience of entrapment

Freud (1926) said, "The affective states have been incorporated in the mind as precipitates of primeval traumatic experiences, and when a similar situation occurs they are revived in the form of memory symbols." Hatred as an affective state results from old traumatic experiences and can be revived in similar situations in

THE ROLE OF HATRED IN THE EGO   153

later life. In this section we are concerned only with the phenomenology of the ego state of hatred as it is revived.

When hatred becomes a conscious experience, the one who hates is beset with fears and feels pulled in different directions. The hater tends to ascribe unrealistic power and importance to the object of his hate and believes it would be disastrous to offend the omnipotent and omniscient object. But he feels wronged by the object and 'wants to get even with it'. Thus he finds himself in a state of bondage. If he remains close to the object, he may betray his hatred and provoke the wrath of the object, who could crush him. On the other hand, if he attempts to avoid the hated object, he is denying himself needed libidinal supplies. Caught in a dilemma, the hater feels trapped and schizophrenic regression, manic flight, suicide or homicide, promiscuity, perversion, or crime may ensue.

Two cases show how hatred is experienced as entrapment.

> For about four months following the birth of her second child, a patient was physically weakened by recurrent bleeding. Although she was very fond of the baby, she developed fears about not being able to care for her. Then she began to feel that her husband neglected her, that he was too engrossed in his work. She entangled him in quarrels but when he still failed to heed her, she hated him. She threatened to leave him, made two tentative attempts to see a lawyer about divorce, and after several months decided to act promptly. Instead she drove around aimlessly for several hours and then returned home. That evening she was found sitting alone in the car in the garage. She was catatonic and was taken to a hospital. In the course of therapy she explained that she hated her husband and wanted to leave him. On the day she had driven around aimlessly, she had intended to check into a hotel but as she approached the hotel she became more and more alarmed and reluctantly returned home. She could not remember what happened after that.

> A manic depressive woman accompanied her husband to a business meeting in a distant city. Left alone for four days while he was engaged in 'talks with the boys', she complained. Her husband, in turn, criticised her for lack of understanding. They then went on a vacation trip and she felt that her husband continued to neglect her by playing golf and drinking with strangers. She hated her husband for not loving her, and hated herself for living with him. She thought

of divorce but dreaded being alone and did not want to see her husband happily remarried. Feeling trapped, she attributed all her unhappiness to him. Before the vacation was over she became excessively energetic, loud, flirtatious, irritable, and argumentative. This behaviour was followed by such a degree of disorganisation and incoherence that she had to be hospitalised.

These two patients illustrate how the ego state of hatred locked each in a type of bondage with the most significant person in their lives. Neither could move close to, nor away from, this significant person. Bak (1954) has postulated that "the aggressive drive is instrumental in bringing about the [schizophrenic] regression". In the two cases cited it seems that the aggressive drive was instrumental in bringing about the ego state of hatred, which may be an intermediate step to further regression and psychosis.

Ego syntonic uses of hatred

That hatred can be used for ego syntonic purposes has been described in the literature. Ernest Jones (1929) showed how hatred can serve to cover fear or guilt. Hill (1938) observed that it can serve to avoid "feelings of dependency, of a need to be loved, of passivity and helplessness, or a desire to dominate and control (as a reaction-formation against passivity), and even feelings of affection". Searles (1956, 1962) indicated that vengefulness or scorn can serve as a defence against repressed grief and separation anxiety.

To hate is to feel something, which is far better than feeling purposeless, empty, amorphous, or swamped by anxieties. Hatred may become an essential element from which one derives a sense of self-sameness and upon which one formulates one's identity. Thus a young paranoid man said to me, "I don't like to hate but I have to. If I am not a hater, I am nobody. And I don't want to be nobody." When his hatred receded he became more disorganised and paranoid. Similarly another young schizophrenic man said, "I hate my mother. Even though at times I think she is not too bad, I still hate her. For hatred is a pleasant emotion." In his case hatred served to relieve him of all sorts of unmanageable emotions and uncertainties.

That hatred has great power to sustain one's life is seen in the following case.

> A borderline patient entered the hospital voluntarily because of an uncontrollable urge to injure her body. One year later she decided to leave the hospital and her analyst. After six months she sought outpatient treatment with the same analyst and stayed with him for six years. She explained: "When I left the hospital, I hated it. I did not hate you. I had no idea if I could hold out on my own, but I knew I had no choice. I simply had to do what I did... But I managed all right. I found an apartment and a job which occupied me in the daytime. At night I was often seized with the urge to kill myself. But I couldn't do it because I hated the hospital and didn't want to live up to the hospital's prophecy that I could not manage outside."

An important aspect of this case was the displacement of the patient's hatred from her analyst to the hospital which allowed her to form a bond with the analyst to whom she could return and eventually work through her problems. Displacement of hatred to an object of lesser significance is a common experience. In setting up national, racial, or personal enemies one can then live more peacefully with one's loved ones.

Hatred as a basis of human relationship

Hatred tends to incite hatred in others. And he who hates detests most those who feel indifferent toward his hatred, and will make every effort to goad the other person into hatred too. A young schizophrenic woman expressed her hatred for her husband through incessant tirades. Following one such tirade, the husband told her with sincerity that he loved her. Her hatred mounted and she pushed her fist through a pane of glass. She said, "He was so superior. I hate him even more."

When hatred becomes the basis of a human relationship it can perpetuate the relationship as durably as love. One can grow accustomed to such a relationship and feel lost without it. The manic depressive patient mentioned earlier and her husband were in a hateful state of bondage for most of the twenty years of their marriage. Until the wife became psychotic, they were considered by others to be happily married and both were outgoing and successful. However, they scarcely communicated and each did his best to expose the other's weaknesses. When they did speak to each other, a bitter quarrel would soon break out. Each secretly thought of leaving the other. For a time the husband shared a more peaceful life with another woman, but finding this life unexciting, returned to his wife and they resumed the hateful struggle. It is to be noted that a relationship perpetuated by hatred is not like a sadomasochistic relationship where there is fusion of libidinal and aggressive drives. In hatred there is little libidinal component.

> For several years two elderly women occupied adjacent rooms on a ward. Every day they complained to the nursing staff of the other's behaviour in the shared bathroom. They made no attempt to resolve their differences, refused to talk to each other, and would not accept suggestions from the nursing staff when they tried to arbitrate. They hated each other. When one was transferred to another hospital, the patient who remained said, "I am sad because Mrs. A is my only friend".

As stated above, when one is accustomed to a hateful bond with another, one feels lost without it. It is not always wise for the analyst to disturb the bond. Sullivan (1956) observed that in some instances manic depressive patients who had been previously analysed committed suicide after resuming treatment; he did not offer any explanation of this observation. Others have suggested that the new analyst may fall short of the patient's expectations and thus extinguish the patient's last hope. I should like to suggest that re-entering treatment may weaken the bond of hatred which the patient has already firmly established with his particular significant object and thus create a disequilibrium that leads the patient to drastic action.

Hatred in the course of treatment

In the course of treatment that is inherently frustrating, many patients will turn their hatred toward their analyst. When the analyst, in turn, does not hate them, these patients feel an even greater sense of frustration. For instance when I began working with a patient who had begun to emerge from a severe catatonic reaction, she stood in the doorway during each session and cursed me. When I maintained my detachment, she attacked me physically. After eight months of this behaviour, she one day scornfully cried out: "You are full of hatred. You hate me. You have a heart full of black blood". By this time I did hate her and I realised that often in the past months when restraining her, I had had an urge to strangle her. I said: "You may be happy to find someone who hates as much as you do, but you are the only one of us who is ashamed of feelings of hatred." It is uncertain whether my statement influenced her so that she was no longer ashamed of her hatred, or whether she was gratified by her success in making me hate her. In any event that particular hour was a turning point in the treatment and thereafter her behaviour markedly improved: she stopped being assaultive, ceased soiling her clothes, and began taking care of her person.

As the analyst helps his patient to rid himself of his hatred, he must discern what the hatred means to the patient. The untimely removal of such a useful ego syntonic defence may leave the patient completely deprived and invite undesirable complications. Unpleasant as it is for the analyst when he becomes the target of the patient's hatred, it is necessary for him to recognise that when the patient allows himself to reveal this affective state, the patient is more committed to attempting a constructive personality change. To quote Novey: "It is of considerable importance to envision [affective states] as being not only disruptive psychopathological experiences but also as attempts at the re-establishing of a more stable and more constructive integration of the personality."

CHAPTER TEN

Fundamentalism and idolatry

Ronald Britton

I n this paper I am using religious terms for psychoanalytic purposes because I think we try to deal in psychological terms with, what had been before the "Enlightenment" the subject matter of theology; just as the writers of the Romantic movement did in philosophical or poetic terms.

As M. H. Abrams wrote in Natural Supernaturalism

> much of what distinguishes writers I call Romantic derives from the fact that they undertook whatever their religious creed or lack of creed to save traditional concepts, schemes and values which had been based on the relation of the Creator to his creature and creation, but to reformulate them within the prevailing two-term system of subject and object, ego and non-ego, the human mind ... and its transactions with nature.

Freud had a good deal to say about religion. Mythology was a favourite study of his and produced traffic in both directions. The implication was that study of one should provide material for the other. He wrote:

> I believe that a great part of the mythological view of the world, which reaches far into most modern religions is nothing other than

psychological processes projected into the outer world. The obscure apprehending of the psychical factors and relationships of the unconscious is mirrored ... in the construction of a supersensible reality, which science has to re-translate into the psychology of the unconscious. One could venture in this manner to resolve the myths of Paradise, the Fall of Man, of God, of Good and Evil, of Immortality, and so on thus transforming Meta-physics into Metapsychology. [Freud, 1904]

In his paper on Leonardo da Vinci he stated, "Psychoanalysis... has taught us that the personal God is psychologically nothing other than a magnified father" (1910). He regarded monotheism as a great achievement of the Jews because it took them nearer to what he thought was religion's origin—the Father nucleus. "Now that God was a single person man's relations to him could recover the intimacy and intensity of the child's relation to the father" (*ibid*.).

The infantile supremacy of the father complex was later questioned and with it the reasons for God the father being placed in solitary state on the heavenly throne. Barag (1947) suggested that Jewish monotheism was impelled by a defensive repudiation of an otherwise dangerous mother fixation. In Kleinian terms this would be the desire to remove from mother the qualities of omnipotence, omnipresence, and omniscience felt by the infant to be hers and to transfer them first to father and then to God the father. Thus these super-natural qualities are separated from their infantile source in mother whose body is destined to be the proto-type of the Natural world—mother earth—and become the possessions of the father in heaven.

There is a hint in Freud's paper on "A seventeenth century demonological neurosis" (Freud, 1923b) that God might be unambiguously father but the devil is more doubtful. Freud took the view that God and the Devil were originally one figure that became divided into absolute goodness and absolute evil personified. This is his version of the kind of primal splitting which Melanie Klein elaborated into the theory of the origin of goodness and badness from the infantile experience of a good nurturing breast and bad persecuting breast. In this paper Freud gave an account of the painter Christoph Haizmann who painted his hallucinatory meetings with the Devil. Freud postulated that the Devil was a substitute for the painter's lost father for whom he longed, but towards whom he was ambivalent, and he suggested that Haizmann suffered a severe melancholia as a neurotic form of mourning and in this state formally concluded a pact with the Devil as a father substitute. This explanation is in line with Freud's father complex which during this period he was strongly urging. However, he drew attention to something that struck him as strange and requiring explanation. The Devil has breasts! In one picture he has in addition, "A large penis ending in a snake". Freud's explanation for this was two-fold: one that the breasts are a projection of the man's own femininity on to the father substitute; and two that, "The child's tender feelings towards his mother have been displaced on to his father", as there had previously been a strong fixation on the mother. Indeed Haizmann had declared that only the Holy Mother of God of Mariazell could release him from his pact with the devil, on her day of Nativity (Freud, 1923b).

I think that only the physical appearance of mother in her own form as the Holy Mother distinct and separate from father could save him because the Devil was a phantasy of what Klein called a combined object. Klein wrote, "the infant's capacity to enjoy ... its relation to both parents ...depends on his feeling that they are separate individuals" this she thought was a "precondition for the infant's hope that he can bring them together and unite them in a happy way" (Klein, 1952, p. 79).

In some cases there is difficulty in the individual infant establishing a distinction between unequivocally good and bad experience and therefore instituting the normal primal split between a good and a bad object. If that is so I think then all other distinctions between the parental objects are then compromised and prone to fusion and confusion. If this has been the case then regression in later life can lead to the re-emergence of primitive phantasies of combined objects or their disintegration. This is in turn leads to an arbitrarily imposed defensive splitting to keep apart these archaic objects and the values they represent.

Perhaps the dream of a patient of mine who faced just such problems will make my point. In his dream my patient was holding in one hand a candelabra and in the other a vase. His associations revealed that the candelabra was from his father's piano and the vase was one his mother had always locked away because it was an heirloom from her own mother. In his dream he slowly brought his hands together and as they touched both objects disintegrated into tiny fragments. It was apt commentary on what had been the trouble in his thinking and the problem of his analysis, that is that bringing any two different basic ideas together led to a fragmentation of thought.

The fear of such catastrophic moral or cognitive disintegration can lead to some ruthlessly self-imposed division of the mind to keep things apart, often along some over determined or natural line of cleavage. The boundaries formed by different modes of self-object experience, like fault lines in the formation of the earth's crust, provide such lines of cleavage in development for later ruptures in the continuity of self and object relations. Such a line of cleavage I am suggesting is that between a parental object experienced as the source of solace and comfort and the parental object perceived as the source of knowledge. Goodness is then felt either to reside in material objects or in pure spirituality, often seen as conflicting powers.

I think this holds true for the symbolic representations of these attributes of a collective kind as they are found in religion, philosophy or political ideology. In religions there is a common tendency for conflict to arise between sacramental theology (with emphasis on material objects, ritual practices, and sacred places) and a contrary tendency to anti-material, idealistic, textual, spiritual, Puritanism. In the Student's Catholic Doctrine we see that an attempt is made to bind word and thing within a sacrament.

> The word Sacrament means something sacred or holy ... the outward signs of the Sacraments not only signify grace ... they actually impart the grace they signify ... when, in Baptism we see the Priest pouring the water, and hear the words that he pronounces at the same time, we know that the soul of the child is at that very moment really cleansed from original sin. [Hart, 1916, pp. 254–255]

Such an attribution of sacred significance to a physical substance is regarded as idolatrous by those bible based Protestants who regard text alone as holy and spiritual activity as exemplified only in prayer, preaching and reading.

I see this as reflecting a psychic conflict between the earliest attachment to a maternal object later represented by sacred, material objects and activities on the one hand, and on the other a father object represented as the source of words, power and law.

I am inclined to think that such latent conflict becomes manifest and supercharged when confusion threatens and moral certainty is lost; that is, when the confident sense of the primal split between good and bad is lost and resort is taken to splitting along some other plane. I am further suggesting that this particular split into different modes of object relating, though institutionalized by the psychic manipulation of the Oedipus situation into worship of earthly mother or spiritual father, has its origins in the relationship to the primary maternal object. In this relationship where there is failure to establish an unequivocally good experience of the infant–mother interaction to contrast with the bad experience of being deprived of it, some arbitrary split is made to enshrine the notion of good and to segregate it from the bad.

One such split is the one I am describing. In a context where there is a passionate desire for the mother's presence and an overwhelming need for her functions as a mother but an actual experience of a dysfunctional relationship, the concept of a good maternal object might be salvaged by treating her as two figures; one a presence and the other a function; one regarded as goodness the other as badness. I have encountered this split clinically both ways around. We could schematize it as a division which instead of resulting in a good breast and a bad breast as moral prototypes we have either a good breast with bad milk, or good milk from a bad breast. I have found the clinical permutations of this in the individual psychopathology of addictions, perversions, and eating disorders fascinating, but I want to use it to explore what I am calling fundamentalism and fetishism or idolatry in the transference.

The term fundamentalism is derived from a series of tracts "The Fundamentals" published in the USA in 1909 which base their authority on the infallibility of the Bible because every word in it is the Word of God. The movement had two particular objects of enmity, Modernism and Roman Catholicism. The latter was regarded as idolatrous particularly in regard to the central doctrine of the Roman Catholic Church of the "Real Presence" in the sacramental bread and wine signifying the body and blood of Christ. The term fundamentalism is applied widely now to a variety of religions including Judaism and the Muslim religion usually denoting literalism and worship of religious texts.

It is almost invariably accompanied by condemnation of

modernism (linked with materialism) and idolatry. Christendom and Islam have both had historical wars between Puritan members of their religion and co-religionists they regarded as Idolaters.

An idol has been variously defined as an image of a deity; any material object adored; and any thing or person that is the object of excessive or supreme devotion (*OED*).

In this paper I will describe "Fundamentalism" as "Word Worship" and Idolatry as "Thing Worship". I suggest that they are bound together in mutual hostility and always co-exist. This I hold to be the case not only in their religious and social forms but also where they are manifested in the personal psychology or more precisely psychopathology of individuals. They are rival absolutes each asserting that ultimate reality and goodness exists in the form it alone professes. They assert it is a monistic universe with one good object and one good modality. A similar mutually hostile tendency in philosophy between "idealism" and "realism" was commented on by J. S. Mill (1950), between those who look to innate ideas as the source of knowledge and those who assert that "sensation and experience are the sole materials of our knowledge". As he puts it:

> Neither side is sparing in the imputation of intellectual and moral obliquity ... and of the pernicious consequences of the "creed" of its antagonists. Sensualism is the common term of abuse for the one philosophy, mysticism for the other. The one doctrine is accused of making men beasts, the other lunatics. [p. 111]

Plato represents it as the:

> Battle of gods and giants—one side drags everything down from heaven and the unseen to earth, rudely grasping rocks and trees in their hands. For they get their grip on all such things, and they maintain that alone exists which can be handled and touched ... terrible men ... those who battle against them defend themselves very carefully from somewhere above in the unseen, contending that true existence consists in certain incorporeal forms which are the objects of the mind. [1979, p. 36]

Blake in the "Marriage of Heaven and Hell" proclaims the necessity of this conflict making a virtue of it and condemning formal religions for attempting to unite them:

These two classes of men are always upon the earth and they should be enemies: whatever tries to reconcile them seeks to destroy existence. [Blake, 1825, pp. 16–17]

You will see that I have equated the constantly recurrent conflict in philosophy between idealism and materialism with that in theology between scriptural and sacramental authority. I would like to relate them both to a psychological conflict we meet in practice between "word worship" and "thing worship" which I will attempt to illustrate from psychoanalytic experience. Further I will suggest that this arises from failure in the infantile experience of containment leading to a particular form of splitting which, in turn, leads to difficulties of integration in the depressive position with a consequent failure of symbolization.

The true symbol (as understood in the German and English Romantic movement and now in psycho-analysis) is the meeting place of meaning and matter, or of spirit and substance. It is the place where something is simultaneously what it is in its substance and is also what it signifies. The symbol is more than signifier and more than metaphor, as Coleridge put it, "It partakes of reality of the original", without being identified with it.

This sounds abstract so let me flesh it out. As an analyst my experience of how I am regarded and treated by the hour varies. One of the parameters of this variation is how much my actual physical and mental self is included by the patient in what we call the "transference". Another way of putting this might be to say how much of my manifest existence is included in the patient's conception of me and how much am I entirely a product of the patient's mind. Here we have materialism and idealism in practice. When all goes well I feel perceived as recognizably myself doing what I think I am doing and yet know that in a way peculiar to this particular patient at this particular time I am shaped into a transference figure. There is always a tension in it; I think the symbol is always a point of tension where ideas and things meet. But in a favourable analytic situation the coexistence of my patient's ideas about me and my sense of my self are tolerably close. It is not always so in any analysis and with some patients it is not so for a long time.

I want to discuss situations where such compatibility is lost;

where such extreme discrepancies, between the patient's idea of the analyst and the analyst's idea of himself, are found that there seems to be no hope of their being reconciled, without destruction of one of them.

It is in such discrepant situations, when the normal process of interaction between phantasy and reality has broken down, that "Fundamentalism" and "Idolatry" appear. They appear, I believe, where Ideality and Reality or if you prefer it, Internal and External Objects are felt to be not only incompatible but that one will be the death of the other. At such times the countertransference phantasy of the analyst is that if he adopts the psychic reality of his patient his own psychic reality will be annihilated; the patient believes that if there is an effort made by the analyst to assert his version of their shared situation this will crush the patient's sense of self. The only way out of such an impasse is by the analyst's recognition of the nature of his own countertransference anxiety and his need to struggle to accommodate both his own and the patient's psychic reality. It is that difficult work which needs to be done, otherwise inevitably the analyst tries to compel the patient accept his reality and since it is the patient's fear of this that has created the problem in the first place, this is fruitless. It is a great deal easier to describe this than to do it and it was a failure of mine to contain such a situation which first really acquainted me with the dimensions of this problem.

Subsequent similar failures of mine to contain such situations has fortified my belief in the generality of this point and experiences of supervising other analyst's encounters with similar clinical situations has convinced me of it.

My reason for describing it now is that with some patients it led to a re-enactment within analysis of the psychic catastrophe that had caused their ontological and epistemological problems in the first place. These problems could be characterized as finding it impossible to think for themselves and to be themselves at the same time, as if the two were incompatible. Sequential, logical, thought came from a different place internally than sensation, assumption, desire, and fear. Thinking, in fact was couched in terms of what should be thought; belief was a matter of adherence to principles and not arising from inner convictions; action was not prompted by desire but by obedience. There were other beliefs but they were only existent as silent assumptions embedded in the imagery of day dreams or in unarticulated physical gratification and instinctual action.

In terms of Freud's structural theory the ego had divided itself together with its object relationships into an Id-complex and a Super-ego complex. From the point of view of this discussion the aspect of this I wish to emphasize is that the mode of the "Id-self" was feeling or action and that its objects were things evoking desire, fear, or worship; whereas the mode of the "super-ego" self was obedience, disobedience or reverence and its objects were words. One could say that for the latter, to paraphrase Wittgenstein, there were no things only facts, but that it was complemented by a self for which there were no facts only things.

I will now return to the scene of the "catastrophe" within the analysis which re-enacted a primitive psychic catastrophe. It followed an interpretation of mine which my patient took to be a pronouncement.

> I had said that my patient wished to have a physically contiguous and continuous relationship with me and was trying by various efforts to give himself the sense that this was so. I added that this would not serve him well because it required my eternal presence and that what he needed was to take in some understanding from me so that he had it available inside. One could think this portentous, or one might think it right but unwelcome or that it was wrong or simply naive.

> I entertained all those views, at different moments afterwards, but it was what my patient thought that mattered. This was that I had attacked his mode of relating to me and that I sought to impose on him, in its place, my religion. As he saw it I was forbidding the one kind of link he really believed in and that I was demanding that instead he accept my words as gospel, sustenance, and the only source of good. His reaction was a violent severance of any verbal contact with me and he extended this at times by removing himself physically from the consulting room. This evoked in the transference/countertransference relationship a sense of desolation. It left him without any link to an outside figure for his quintessential self and attempts on my part to establish verbal connections were likely to lead to further ruptures. His own solution to this eventuality was to form a relationship to me which excluded those elements he could

not tolerate and to enhance those he could. I am calling this transference relationship idolatry. I was, as an idol, the source of goodness but as the origin of the word, I was anathema. My physical presence and the contents and walls of my room were the principal elements of this object relationship but he managed to include in it my speech, by treating it as conveying voice qualities but not meaning. It communicated tactile qualities such as soft or hard.

He split his object world by keeping his perceptions of the one object in different sensory modalities apart, treating them as if they were from different objects. He further institutionalized this segregation by attaching these different object relationships to the different members of the basic Oedipus situation. In this way words had become father's things in a realm of ideas without substance or texture. Mother's things on the other hand had substance: shape, texture and qualities such as colour, softness, warmth, firmness and pliability, which provided comfort and security but not meaning.

In the light of this clinical material I would like to discuss further this polarization of representation into fundamentalism and idolatry. I have described them as word-worship and thing worship. In the former the words of the text are treated as powerful, sacred and inviolable beyond their function of conveying, inexactly, like all words, a meaning. In idolatry the thing itself though a material object is treated as possessing psychic or spiritual power.

In his 1915 paper on "The unconscious" (1915a) Freud, in attempting to describe the form of representation in the conscious and unconscious mind, distinguishes between word-presentation and thing presentation. He believed that in the normal state of affairs that the two are brought together in the preconscious and that this conjunction gives them the potential for consciousness. When they are separate word-presentation is preconscious but thing-presentation is unconscious. However he suggested in schizophrenia it was different: repression in this condition, he wrote "had nothing in common" with "the repression which takes place in the transference neuroses". In schizophrenia, he thought, the ego had taken flight more drastically from the object thus abolishing potential connection with the representation of the "thing" itself; instead word-representation was given the investment and significance that usually belonged to thing-representation.

Thus word abstractions were treated as things. He added, "we may, on the other hand, attempt a characterization of the schizophrenic's mode of thought by saying that he treats concrete things as though they were abstract". So in this mental world Freud describes, words are the real things, language is a form of action and to name it is to do it: in contrast to this thing-representations are only the furniture of thought. Freud added "When we think in abstractions there is a danger that we may neglect the relations of words to unconscious thing presentations, and it must be confessed that the expression and content of our philosophising then begins to acquire an unwelcome resemblance to the mode or operation of schizophrenics".

His final comment on this was even more perspicacious when he suggested that this endowment of words with "thing" status was an attempt at cure, an endeavour, he wrote, "directed towards regaining the lost object" (1915a). He followed this in his paper a "Metapsychological supplement to the theory of dreams" written immediately after "The unconscious" with the suggestion that hallucination in schizophrenia may also be an attempt at restitution: this time of the lost ideas of objects (1915b). Thus he proposed that in schizophrenia words may be endowed with material status, to restore the object they represent and hallucination may be an attempt to reinstate the lost ideas of the object.

These two papers were written in conjunction with his great paper on the vicissitudes of loss, "Mourning and melancholia" (1915c). In all three of these papers he makes a connection between the loss of the primal object and a process which gives thing status to words or perceptual status to thoughts. This is so whether the primal object is lost from the individual's external world, as a person, or whether it is lost from the individual's internal world as what as an Melanie Klein called an internal object (Klein, 1929).

I have found that if the concept of non-verbal unconscious phantasy is used for what Freud called "thing-representation" it becomes easier to discuss mental content. Unconscious phantasy has become a term to describe the mental representation of drives (wishes and needs), early somatic and perceptual experience, anxieties and all other affects, such as hope or despair, and of the various defensive manoeuvres such as projection, denial etc. which might be called on to protect the individual from his own mental content. Most of all unconscious phantasy creates what we call internal objects some of which become incorporated into our core sense of self; sometimes as what we have inside us; sometimes as what envelopes us. Unconscious phantasy also creates the sense we have of the external world both of other people and of inanimate things. We begin as believers in animism so that the distinction between living and non-living things is an accomplishment. The notion of their being thinking things other than ourselves is a considerable achievement. (Fonagy & Morgan, 1991) The real acceptance of the fact that other people's minds are truly independent of ours and just as real is something that I think we vary in our ability to truly accept.

It is this conception of another person that is meant by the phrase "whole object". We begin, however, with part object relationships in which other people and things are simply personifications of ideas or qualities. Thus you might say we have an Angry god, a Loving god, a Jealous god, an Evil god, a Good god, and so on.

In the most primitive part object world where time does not exist, where part is whole, there is only self and object; i.e. there is just a sense of the object as the entirety of the universe. I think that in relation to this primary object in its most primitive form there is only one parameter of relating; either I am inside it or it is inside me. The first form of projection is of the total self into the object and the most primitive introjection is the incorporation of the entire object into the self. Desire is expressed as a phantasy of total introjection or self-projection. The negative of this is total repulsion; I repel the object and the object repels me. Whilst absoluteness reigns when I repel the object it is annihilated, when the object repels me I am annihilated. This state of affairs begins to be changed by two developments in infantile mentation which are linked.

1. Both object and self acquire continuity so that the object is believed to go on existing even when not perceived.
2. The self and the object can put parts of themselves into one another whilst continuing to exist outside each other: function and being, in a primitive way, begin to be separable. The verb "to be" acquires the two distinctive meanings we ascribe to it: that is as identity and as descriptive of possession. I am begins to be separable from, I am-full, empty, good, bad happy, sad etc.

Whether this step is going to be negotiable depends on what

Bion (1962a) described in his theory of containment. Given that in phantasy our infant can now put part of himself into his mother and receive part of her into him without either of them ceasing to exist outside each other then this first primitive interaction of container/ contained can take place. In this the infant's raw experience is directed towards the mother who not only receives this but also makes meaning out of it which by her response she communicates to the infant. If she fails to do this the infant feels as if its attempt to find meaning has been attacked and destroyed by some other meaning of the mother. In analysis such a situation is relived when the patient has attempted to communicate to the analyst by projective identification and feels that the analyst has ignored this and annihilated the patient's attempt at meaning and enforced an alien understanding through words.

In other words if the infant feels his projections have been repelled he feels his sense of himself has been annihilated. If he repels the mother's projections he feels he has abolished the meaning of her psychic world and his place in it.

To sum up, I am suggesting one particular arbitrary division of mental life which shapes some of the psychic organizations we find in analysis and which structure our philosophies and religions: there are obviously other splits with other sequels.

1. There is a primal object felt to be the source of life and on whose existence the existence of the self depends. This would correspond to what Winnicott described as a state of "Absolute Dependence" (1960).
2. As development takes place this object is perceived to exist with functions. One of these is to provide meaning. If this function of the object is unbearable and this provokes a wish to annihilate this function there is felt to be a risk of losing the primal object—the source of life itself.
3. To avoid this the one object is seen as two: one the source of life the other the source of meaning. One whose nature is simply to exist, i.e. to have substance but not meaning, and the other object whose nature is only to personify meaning, i.e. to have significance but not substance.
4. The emergence of awareness of the Oedipal situation with its cast of three whilst further challenging our tolerance of reality

also presents an opportunity for this defensive split to be institutionalized. We could call it the "sexing of God". In theological rather than psychological terms we then have God as the source of light and ideas, and mother Nature as the source of everything else. If Puritanism develops then the true religion will be all in the mind. If materialism develops in all its religious and secular forms then some form of "sacramental" catering will be provided.

5. I have suggested that such junctures in our mental lives as that where our relationship with the physical world meets our relationship with the psychic world are like natural fault lines in the earth's crust, places where tension accumulates and where eruptions or dehiscence can occur.

6. It is where Freud placed the "ego"—"as a frontier-creature, the ego tries to mediate between the world and the id" (Freud, 1923a). As he wrote in the "Ego and the Id",

> Whereas the ego is essentially the representative of the external world, of reality, the Super-ego stands in contrast to it as the representative of the internal world, of the id. Conflicts between the ego and the ideal will ... ultimately reflect the contrast between what is real and what is psychical, between the external world and the internal world. [*ibid.*]

In the same passage he argues that the ego-ideal, "as a substitute for a longing for a father ... contains the germ from which all religions have evolved". What I have argued in this paper is that behind this conflict between "what is real and what is psychical" and prior to the "father-complex" (*ibid.*) lies the conflict between attachment to mother as a physical object and mother as a psychic object between mother as a source of physical comfort and mother as a source of meaning.

7. In personalities where for innate or environmental reasons mother's psychic functions and her physical presence cannot be integrated as mutually good, splitting produces a good maternal presence coupled with a bad maternal function or vice-versa, this is replicated in the transference. There it takes the form of analytic idolatry or analytic fundamentalism. In the former the analyst is personally idolised with a craving for his physical presence or its tokens[1] (this may be covertly combined with

aversion to his ideas or words). In the latter there is an idealization of the analysts words and presumed thoughts (this may be coupled with a covert aversion to the analyst's physicality). I think that this antipathetic tendency to word-worship or thing-worship has significance not only for individual cases but also for psycho-analytic theory which so readily seems to divide along such lines.

Note

1. I am conscious that these explorations are taking place close to the ground on which Winnicott built his theory of "Transitional Objects and Transitional Phenomena" (1953) but an adequate discussion of the latter is beyond the scope of this paper.

CHAPTER ELEVEN

The benign and malignant other

Coline Covington

An essential, ever present dynamic within any conflict is the juxtaposition of "us" and "them". When this happens, the "other" turns from being a relatively benign or even familiar object into a malignant or "other" object. Similarly, the familiar and benign "other" that enables us to form an identity and to differentiate ourselves from others, individually and collectively (and most fundamentally, sexually) can be transformed, or perverted, into a malignant "other" that also serves to establish and consolidate identity. The difference between what I call benign and malignant "others" is perhaps best described in terms of the different motivations that underlie the two. In the case of the benign other, there is a desire to relate to the object and to grow from that relationship. In the case of the malignant other, the desire is primarily to defend against the object (seen as hostile) and it is not in the service of growth or development.

In thinking about the ways in which we relate to the "other", I would like to focus on one aspect of "otherness" in particular and this is its companion, narcissism, for I do not think it is possible to consider one idea without the other. It also means thinking of "otherness" from a developmental point of view—as a state of awareness that comes about through separation, that can lead either to differentiation and individuation or, conversely, to the erection of rigid defence structures that deny reality and difference. And this brings us to Freud's "narcissism of minor differences". I would like to explore this idea and specifically the relationship between narcissism and tolerance of difference and how the perception of otherness evolves and develops in the mind.

Freud first used the phrase, "narcissism of minor differences", in the course of an essay titled, "The taboo of virginity", that he wrote in 1917. This was toward the end of the First World War and mankind's aggression towards one another was powerfully evident and foremost in peoples' minds. Freud observed that:

> it is precisely the minor differences in people who are otherwise alike that form the basis of feelings of strangeness and hostility between them ... it would be tempting to pursue this idea and to derive from this "narcissism of minor differences" the hostility which in every human relation we see fighting against feelings of fellowship and overpowering the commandment that all men should love one another. [Freud, 1917, p. 48 I.]

Freud elaborated on this idea in terms of his clinical experience and his observation of the anxiety caused by the perception of difference between the sexes. In his patients' material, Freud found that the sheer difference or otherness presented by the opposite sex was threatening and produced hostility.

Extending his views to groups, Freud wrote five years later in his essay, "Group psychology and the analysis of the ego", with the observation that the closer the relation between the individual or the group, the greater is the potential hostility. He stated:

> Of two neighbouring towns each is the other's most jealous rival; every little canton looks down upon the others with contempt. Closely related races keep one another at arm's length; the South German cannot endure the North German, the Englishman casts every kind of aspersion upon the Scot, the Spaniard despises the Portuguese. We are no longer astonished that greater differences should lead to an almost insuperable repugnance, such as the Gaelic people feel for the German, the Aryan for the Semite and the white races for the coloured. [Freud, 1922, p. 49 I.]

By 1922, when Freud wrote this passage, he had lived through his own painful experience of witnessing how differences had turned into hostilities and split his own group—a pattern that we continue to repeat within our psychoanalytic profession today. It is also striking that Freud wrote this in the dawning of Hitler's Germany and the widespread transformation of minor racial difference to major difference—from the benign, familiar other to the hostile, malignant other. In this same essay on group psychology, Freud links this phenomenon directly to narcissism. He writes:

> In the undisguised antipathies and aversion which people feel towards strangers with whom they have to do we may recognize the expression of self-love—of narcissism. This self-love works for the preservation of the individual, and behaves as though the occurrence of any divergence from his own particular lines of development involved a criticism of them and a demand for their alteration. [*Ibid.*, p. 50 I.]

This statement is later echoed in Freud's essay "Civilisation and its discontents", in which he makes the connection between narcissism and intolerance explicit. He writes: "It is always possible to bind together a considerable number of people in love, so long as there are other people left over to receive the manifestations of their aggressiveness" (1930a). When Freud was writing these essays he had already changed his views on the nature and function of instinctual drives and the importance of external reality. He gave much greater prominence to the role of fantasy in the internal world and had espoused the idea of the death instinct and innate destructiveness. While the "other" could be seen as a threat to survival, and hence a cause of anxiety, it's role as an object for growth and development was secondary. Freud explains aversion towards strangers as a defensive function of narcissism in the service of self-preservation—but the self-preservation is concerned with fending off or diverting innate aggression into the "other", whether it is an individual or a group. Klein was later to develop Freud's ideas in her conceptualization of early infancy and the paranoid–schizoid position. It is, however, also possible to understand such aversion or hostility to strangers as a return or regression to primary narcissism (in Freud's original meaning of this term as referring to the stage between primitive auto-erotism and object-love) in which there can only be a two person relation, in which separation and differentiation cannot be tolerated and as a specific reaction to external reality. In the case of groups, as in the case of individuals, this can be triggered when there is the threat of frustration and deprivation, when there is literally not enough to go around, or when there is a particular history of deprivation. But this understanding places much greater emphasis on the importance of environmental conditions and the extent to which these foster or inhibit narcissistic development and, ultimately, the way in which the "other" is related to.

The way in which we understand our relation to the "other" and "otherness" does in fact differ according to our model of the psyche and, within that, our view of narcissistic development and object relations. It was Fairbairn who in 1930 countered the dualistic, Platonic view of man in which energy and structure are perceived as separate, opposing forces with an integrated or holistic conception of man, more in accord with Aristotelian psychology. In this view, man is an integrated being in whom "matter is potentiality, form actuality" (Aristotle, De Anima II, 421a, 10 in Fairbairn, 1994, Vol. 1, xvi). The meaning of actuality encompasses "the relationship of the individual psyche to personal experience of external relationships" (xvi). Adaptation, for Fairbairn, was a response to reality. The roots of aggression were therefore traced directly back to their source as a reaction to frustration—frustration caused by the object that fails to respond adequately to the subject and its needs. The importance of the object and the impulse to relate to the object is paramount in Fairbairn's model of the psyche and ego development. This is in contrast to Freud, Klein, and Jung's view of the psyche in which environmental conditions undoubtedly influence development but are not considered necessary constituents for development. Both Freud and Klein considered instinctual drive as the main motivating factor in development, while Jung viewed the teleological or purposive aspect of the archetype of the self as the prime impetus towards development in both its instinctual and spiritual manifestations.

Fairbairn's view of impulses as directed towards an object also challenged Freud's idea of primary narcissism as an objectless state. (Balint elaborates this argument in his paper, "Early developmental states of the ego. Primary object-love', 1937). Within this framework, the infant is conceived as experiencing separateness from the start and as having some rudimentary awareness not only of an external environment but also, by implication, of the existence of an "other". There is increasing evidence from infant research to indicate that the infant is more self aware than has been previously hypothesized in psychoanalytic theory. Referring to this early state, the Peruvian psychoanalyst, Gustavo Delgado-Aparicio has proposed the idea that the depressive position, along with the accompanying awareness of dependency on an "other", comes before the paranoid–schizoid position (personal communication). The paranoid–schizoid position then develops as an adaptation to the frustrations and impingements of reality. As reality can be increasingly tolerated and managed, the infant will fluctuate between the depressive position and the paranoid–schizoid position—a process that continues throughout an individual's life. However, the degree to which reality can be tolerated and managed at this early stage is highly dependent on the extent to which the infant is able to internalize a secure object relation that can then serve to support the ego so that separation becomes increasingly bearable.

Here I am reminded of a paper on the archetype of separation written by the Jungian analyst, Ruth Strauss, delivered to the second international Congress in Zurich in 1962. In this paper, Strauss explores the paradoxical nature of separation as containing within it both aspects of union and of separateness, of oneness and of otherness. She begins by distinguishing between two states of union, "referred to as the self by Jung:" the first is the "original self" (later to be developed by Fordham in his work with children) and the second is "the conjunctio, the union of the opposites in individuation." While recognizing the integral part that separation plays in the process of ego development, she writes that the "growth of ego boundaries cannot come into being without the experience of primary union or oneness which Jung (1954) has also referred to as 'abaissement du niveau mental.'" Strauss goes on to write: "I have gradually come to regard the experience of oneness ..., which may be looked upon as regression, as the prerequisite for any process leading to transformation" (pp. 104–105).

Winnicott's observations of infants with their mothers also led him to postulate on the importance for the baby to experience an illusion of omnipotence, or oneness, in order to begin to establish object constancy and a sense of "I-ness", or of going-on-being, that is also necessary for healthy narcissistic development. Without such an experience of primary identification, no real differentiation can take place in which it is safe to become disillusioned. Instead a malignant narcissism forms in which grandiosity serves a defensive purpose (as opposed to a developmental one)—to protect the ego from its reality. In this way, the defensive or malignant narcissism becomes part of the ego's defence system.

I'd like to return once again to Freud's "narcissism of minor differences" and the connection Freud makes between narcissism and intolerance. The historian, Michael Ignatieff, writing about ethnic war in his book *The Warrior's Honour* (1998), devotes a chapter to the "narcissism of minor difference". He concludes that "the root of intolerance lies in our tendency to overvalue our own identities." He explains: "by overvalue, I mean we insist that we have nothing in common, nothing to share. At the heart of this insistence lurks the fantasy of purity, of boundaries that can never be crossed" (p. 62). It is clear that Ignatieff is referring to the pathological form of narcissism I have described above in which grandiosity—the overvaluing of our own identities—serves a defensive purpose. Within an individual, such narcissism is the symptom of a fragile ego that is indeed threatened by difference and needs to keep out that which is other. In this case, boundaries must also be clearly—and rigidly—delineated and imposed because of the lack of a secure internal identity with its own experience of boundaries that can be relied upon. The narcissistic psyche will also more often than not be governed by a severe superego that has had to develop in a Gestapo-like way in order to control the impulses (the id) that the ego cannot manage. Safety is then achieved through a kind of political correctness that transforms minor differences into major ones. Examples of this abound in political contexts around the world from ethnic warfare in the Balkans to the self-ghettoisation of homosexuality in San Francisco. Crude distinctions are made, based on minor difference, as an attempt, ironically, to eradicate real differentiation. In psychoanalytic terms, the paranoid–schizoid position is maintained when the experience of separateness is too costly.

In commenting on the "us–them" dichotomy that is set up under the "narcissism of minor difference", Ignatieff writes:

Individuality only complicates the picture, indeed makes prejudice more difficult to sustain, since it is at the individual level that empathy often subverts the primal group opposition. Intolerance, from this perspective, is a willed refusal to focus on individual difference, and a perverse insistence that individual identity be subsumed in the group. If intolerant groups are unable to perceive those they despise as individuals, it may be because intolerant groups are unable or unwilling to perceive themselves as such, either. The narcissism of minor difference is thus a leap into collective fantasy that enables threatened or anxious individuals to avoid the burden of thinking for themselves or even of thinking of themselves as individuals. Toleration depends, critically, on being able to individualise oneself and others, to be able to "see" oneself and others—or to put it another way, to be able to focus on "major" difference, which is individual, and to relativise "minor" difference, which is collective. [p. 63]

Ignatieff illustrates how major and minor difference become distorted and perverted, transforming the benign "other" into a malignant "other". In this case, group differences, as Ignatieff points out, are highlighted at the expense of individual difference in order to create a political boundary. As Ignatieff stresses, the effect of this form of difference or otherness is to stop the individual from thinking. In the contexts I have referred to of ethnic cleansing in the Balkans or the establishment of the concept of homosexual nationality in San Francisco, the reality of hatred and what has been missing in these people's lives is so painful that it is not difficult to understand why thinking and consciousness would need to be denied and suppressed.

We can see in our consulting rooms and in our own experience that people tend to treat others in the way that they have themselves been treated—whether it is in a loving way or an abusive one. When our impulse to form a loving relation with an other has been thwarted, our love turns to hatred of the other and when we come to expect this response, this is what we provoke in others. Perhaps our main task as analysts is to enable our patients to see the ways in which they have been treated, how this has affected their own way of relating to others (and their own internal identifications), and to experience a different way of relating within the analytic context so that they can separate from their past and have a mind of their own.

This also means being able to differentiate between self and other, between internal and external reality, and between past and present. As I argued earlier, differentiation can only be achieved within a safe environment in which the individual can experience his own individuality, or otherness, as fully accepted—without the pressure to be different or other than who he is. Thanks to Freud and Jung, their colleagues and their followers, we have the tools to provide this—we can offer our patients the possibility of benign regression in which a healthy narcissism can develop that allows for difference and otherness to be accepted, tolerated and valued. How we achieve this in a wider political context remains to be seen.

WHY WAR?

Introduction

Paul Williams

The question "Why War?" more often than not yields to questions like "why this war"? or "what to do about such and such a war", due to the complexity of problems of definition. It is a hubris for a single discipline to claim privilege in explaining the origins of war, given their multiple socio-political, biological, and psychological determinants. However, psychoanalysis is unique in providing insights into the role of the unconscious in war-making. These insights have helped us to grasp the persistent, magnetic appeal of war and how we rationalize the destructive acts committed in the name of war. If internal destructiveness cannot be managed within the psyche, it is likely to result in forms of externalization and cycles of psychological and physical violence.

The capacity to transform primitive impulses into food for contained reflection is a compelling goal for a militarily over-armed, post-modern world. Our psychoanalytic knowledge of such issues has been accumulated slowly but surely, and renders the question "Why War?" naive as well as elemental. We might just as well ask "Why not War?", in the light of the seemingly ineradicable aggression that characterizes humankind: there is no inquiry more important than identifying the conditions under which people abandon themselves to the embrace of hatred and conflict. This is the subject of the discussion between Freud and Einstein. Freud's chink of optimism is derived from the notion of a gradual internalization of aggression under the evolutionary impact of civilizing processes and the growth of identifications amongst those who value thought and reason. Archaic loyalties to violence as a response to conflict may gradually be displaced by the increased capacity for reflection, Freud thought, although he was clearly referring to a time-frame extending over many generations. Freud's view is bolstered today by growing evidence from psychoanalytic work that structural change within the personality is certainly possible and that this can help individuals to integrate aspects of their deepest negativity in the service of life. How far this carries itself into the social sphere is not known, although analysts and patients have long testified to the "ripple effect" of psychoanalytic therapy on families and the wider milieu.

The papers in this section of the book take up Freud's theme of "Why War?" in several ways. Carl Jung offers perspectives on war written after World War II. Donald Kaplan pursues interdisciplinary questions arising from an inquiry into how the social context relates to how the mind can function in times of war. Diana Birkett reviews a number of classical and later psychoanalytic understandings of the precipitants of war in the light of the how we deal with basic internal mental states. Isobel Hunter-Brown offers her response to Birkett's paper. Bob Hinshelwood draws on the work of Elliot Jacques and Melanie Klein to link unconscious states of mind in the individual to collective attitudes and defences. Lastly, Hanna Segal's paper is a denunciation of the policy of deterrence in a nuclear world. Her argument is grounded in psychoanalytic theory and clinical experience and is employed in a sophisticated manner to underline contradictions and paradoxes in military policy. The extrapolation from individual object relations to group dynamics is prevalent in the papers in this section and implies that an interdisciplinary link between psychoanalysis and anthropology and sociology is of relevance in this area.

CHAPTER TWELVE

Freud/Einstein correspondence

Caputh, near Potsdam, 30 July, 1932

Dear Professor Freud,

The proposal of the League of Nations and its International Institute of Intellectual Co-operation at Paris that I should invite a person, to be chosen by myself, to a frank exchange of views on any problem that I might select affords me a very welcome opportunity of conferring with you upon a question which, as things now are, seems the most insistent of all the problems civilisation has to face. This is the problem: Is there any way of delivering mankind from the menace of war? Is it common knowledge that, with the advance of modern science, this issue has come to mean a matter of life and death for civilisation as we know it, nevertheless, for all the zeal displayed, every attempt at its solution has ended in a lamentable breakdown.

I believe, moreover, that those whose duty it is to tackle the problem professionally and practically are growing only too aware of their impotence to deal with it, and have now a very lively desire to learn the views of men who, absorbed in the pursuit of science, can see world-problems in the perspective distance lends. As for me, the normal objective of my thought affords no insight into the dark places of human will and feeling. Thus, in the enquiry now proposed, I can do little more than seek to clarify the question at issue and, clearing the ground of the more obvious solutions, enable you to bring the light of your far-reaching knowledge of man's instinctive life to bear upon the problem. There are certain psychological obstacles whose existence a layman in the mental sciences may dimly surmise, but whose interrelations and vagaries he is incompetent to fathom; you, I am convinced, will be able to suggest educative methods, lying more or less outside the scope of politics, which will eliminate these obstacles.

As one immune from nationalist bias, I personally see a simple way of dealing with the superficial (i.e. administrative) aspect of the problem: the setting up, by international consent, of a legislative and judicial body to settle every conflict arising between nations. Each nation would undertake to abide by the orders issued by this legislative body, to invoke its decision in every dispute, to accept its judgements unreservedly and to carry out every measure the tribunal deems necessary for the execution of its decrees. But here, at the outset, I come up against a difficulty; a tribunal is a human institution which, in proportion as the power at its disposal is inadequate to enforce its verdicts, is all the more prone to suffer these to be deflected by extrajudicial pressure. This is a fact with which we have to reckon; law and might inevitably go hand in hand, and juridical decisions approach more nearly the ideal justice demanded by the community (in whose name and interests these verdicts are pronounced) insofar as the community has effective power to compel respect of its juridical ideal. But at present we are far from possessing any supranational organisation competent to render verdicts of incontestable authority and enforce absolute submission to the execution of its verdicts. Thus I am led to my first axiom: the quest of international security involves the unconditional surrender by every nation, in a certain measure, of its liberty of action, its sovereignty that is to say, and it is clear beyond all doubt that no other road can lead to such security.

The ill-success, despite their obvious sincerity, of all the efforts made during the last decade to reach this goal leaves us no room to doubt that strong psychological factors are at work, which paralyse these efforts. Some of these factors are not far to seek. The craving for power which characterises the governing class in every nation is hostile to any limitation of the national sovereignty. This political power-hunger is wont to batten on the activities of another group, whose aspirations are on purely mercenary, economic lines. I have specially in mind that small but determined group, active in every nation, composed of individuals who, indifferent to social considerations and restraints, regard warfare, the manufacture and sale of arms, simply as an occasion to advance their personal interests and enlarge their personal authority.

But recognition of this obvious fact is merely the first step towards an appreciation of the actual state of affairs. Another question follows hard upon it: How is it possible for this small clique to bend the will of the majority, who stand to lose and suffer by a state of war, to the service of their ambitions? (In speaking of the majority, I do not exclude soldiers of every rank who have chosen war as their profession, in the belief that they are serving to defend the highest interests of their race, and that attack is often the best method of defence.) An obvious answer to this question would seem to be that the minority, the ruling class at present, has the schools and press, usually the Church as well, under its thumb. This enables it to organise and sway the emotions of the masses, and make its tool of them.

Yet even this answer does not provide a complete solution. Another question arises from it: How is it these devices succeed so well in rousing men to such wild enthusiasm, even to sacrifice their lives? Only one answer is possible. Because man has within him a lust for hatred and destruction. In normal times this passion exists in a latent state, it emerges only in unusual circumstances; but it is a comparatively easy task to call it into play and raise it to the power of a collective psychosis. Here lies, perhaps, the crux of all the complex of factors we are considering, an enigma that only the expert in the lore of human instincts can resolve.

And so we come to our last question. Is it possible to control man's mental evolution so as to make him proof against the psychoses of hate and destructiveness? Here I am thinking by no means only of the so-called uncultured masses. Experience proves that it is rather the so-called 'Intelligentsia' that is most apt to yield to these disastrous collective suggestions, since the intellectual has no direct contact with life in the raw, but encounters it in its easiest synthetic form—upon the printed page.

To conclude: I have so far been speaking only of wars between nations; what are known as international conflicts. But I am well aware that the aggressive instinct operates under other forms and in other circumstances. (I am thinking of civil wars, for instance, due in earlier days to religious zeal, but nowadays to social factors; or, again, the persecution of racial minorities.) But my insistence on what is the most typical, most cruel and extravagant form of conflict between man and man was deliberate, for here we have the best occasion of discovering ways and means to render all armed conflicts impossible.

I know that in your writings we may find answers, explicit or implied, to all the issues of this urgent and absorbing problem. But it would be of the greatest service to us all were you to present the problem of world peace in the light of your most recent discoveries, for such a presentation well might blaze the trail for new and fruitful modes of action.

Yours very sincerely,

A. EINSTEIN

Vienna, September, 1932

Dear Professor Einstein,

When I heard that you intended to invite me to an exchange of views on some subject that interested you and that seemed to deserve the interest of others besides yourself, I readily agreed. I expected you to choose a problem on the frontiers of what is knowable today, a problem to which each of us, a physicist and a psychologist, might have our own particular angle of approach and where we might come together from different directions upon the same ground. You have taken me by surprise, however, by posing the question of what can be done to protect mankind from the curse of war.[1] I was scared at first by the thought of my—I had almost written 'our'—incapacity for dealing with what seemed to be a practical problem, a concern for statesmen. But I then realised that you had raised the question not as a natural scientist and physicist but as a philanthropist: you were following the promptings of the League of Nations just as Fridtjof Nansen, the polar explorer, took on the work of bringing help to the starving and homeless victims of the World War. I reflected, moreover, that I was not being asked to make practical proposals but only to set out the problem of avoiding war as it appears to a psychological observer. Here again you yourself have said almost all there is to say on the subject. But though you have taken the wind out of my sails I shall be glad to follow in your wake and content myself with confirming all you have said by amplifying it to the best of my knowledge—or conjecture.

You begin with the relation between Right and Might.[2] There can be no doubt that that is the correct starting-point for our investigation. But may I replace the word 'might' by the bolder and harsher word 'violence'? Today right and violence appear to us as antitheses. It can easily be shown, however, that the one has developed out of the other; and, if we go back to the earliest beginnings and see how that first came about, the problem is easily solved. You must forgive me if in what follows I go over familiar and commonly accepted ground as though it were new, but the thread of my argument requires it.

It is a general principle, then, that conflicts of interest between men are settled by the use of violence. This is true of the whole animal kingdom, from which men have no business to exclude themselves. In the case of men, no doubt, conflicts of *opinion* occur as well which may reach the highest pitch of abstraction and which seem to demand some other technique for their settlement. That, however, is a later complication. To begin with, in a small human horde, it was superior muscular strength which decided who owned things or whose will should prevail. Muscular strength was soon supplemented and replaced by the use of tools: the winner was the one who had the better weapons or who used them the more skilfully. From the moment at which weapons were introduced, intellectual superiority already began to replace brute muscular strength; but the final purpose of the fight remained the same—one side or the other was to be compelled to abandon his claim or his objection by the damage inflicted on him and by the crippling of his strength. That purpose was most completely achieved if the victor's violence eliminated his opponent permanently—that is to say, killed him. This had two advantages: he could not renew his opposition and his fate deterred others from following his example. In addition to this, killing an enemy satisfied an instinctual inclination which I shall have to mention later. The intention to kill might be countered by a reflection that the enemy could be employed in performing useful services if he were left alive in an intimidated condition. In that case the victor's violence was content with subjugating him instead of killing him. This was a first beginning of the idea of sparing an enemy's life, but thereafter the victor had to reckon with his defeated opponent's lurking thirst for revenge and sacrificed some of his own security.

Such, then, was the original state of things: domination by whoever had the greater might—domination by brute violence or by violence supported by intellect. As we know, this regime was altered in the course of evolution. There was a path that led from violence to right or law. What was that path? It is my belief that there was only one: the path which led by the way of the fact that the superior strength of a single individual could be rivalled by the union of several weak ones. '*L'union fait la force.*' Violence could be broken by union, and the power of those who were united now represented law in contrast to the violence of the single individual. Thus we see that right is the might of a community. It is still violence, ready to be directed against any individual who resists it; it works by the same methods and follows the same purposes. The only real difference lies in the fact that what prevails is no longer the violence of an individual but that of a community. But in order that the transition from violence to this new right or justice may be effected, on psychological condition must be fulfilled. The union of the majority must be a stable and lasting one. If it were only brought about for the purpose of combating a single dominant individual and were dissolved after his defeat, nothing would have been accomplished. The next person who thought himself superior in strength would once more seek to set up a dominion by violence and the game would be repeated *ad infinitum*. The community must be maintained permanently, must be organised, must draw up regulations to anticipate the risk of rebellion and must institute authorities to see that those regulations—the laws—are respected and to superintend the execution of legal acts of violence. The recognition of a community of interests such as these leads to the growth of emotional ties between the members of a united group of people—communal feelings which are the true source of its strength.

Here, I believe, we already have all the essentials: violence overcome by the transference of power to a larger unity, which is held together by emotional ties between its members. What remains to be said is no more than an expansion and a repetition of this.

The situation is simple so long as the community consists only of a number of equally strong individuals. The laws of such an association will determine the extent to which, if the security of communal life is to be guaranteed, each individual must surrender his personal liberty to turn his strength to violent uses. But a state of rest of that kind is only theoretically conceivable. In actuality the position is complicated by the fact that from its very beginning the community comprises elements of unequal strength—men and women, parents and children—and soon, as a result of war and conquest, it also comes to include victors and vanquished, who turn into masters and slaves. The justice of the community then becomes an expression of the unequal degrees of power obtaining within it; the laws are made by and for the ruling members and find little room for the rights of those in subjection. From that time forward there are two factors at work in the community which are sources of unrest over matters of law but tend at the same time to a further grow of law. First, attempts are made by certain of the rulers to set themselves above the prohibitions which apply to everyone—they seek, that is, to go back from a dominion of law to a dominion of violence. Secondly, the oppressed members of the group make constant efforts to obtain more power and to have any changes that are brought about in that direction recognised in the laws—the press forward, that is, from unequal justice to equal justice for all. This second tendency becomes especially important if a real shift of power occurs within a community, as may happen as a result of a number of historical factors. In that case right may gradually adapt itself to the new distribution of power; or, as is more frequent, the ruling class is unwilling to recognise the change, and rebellion and civil war follow, with a temporary suspension of law and new attempts at a solution by violence, ending in the establishment of a fresh rule of law. There is yet another source from which modifications of law may arise, and one of which the expression is invariably peaceful: it lies in the cultural transformation of the members of the community. This, however, belongs properly in another connection and must be considered later.

Thus we see that the violent solution of conflicts of interest is not avoided even inside a community. But the everyday necessities and common concerns that are inevitable where people live together in one place tend to bring such struggles to a swift conclusion and under such conditions there is an increasing probability that a peaceful solution will be found. Yet a glance at the history of the human race reveals an endless series of conflicts between one community and another or several others, between larger and smaller units—between cities, provinces, races, nations, empires—which have almost always been settled by force of arms. Wars of this kind end either in the spoliation or in the complete overthrow and conquest of one of the parties. It is impossible to make any sweeping judgement upon wars of conquest. Some, such as those waged by the Mongols and Turks, have brought nothing but evil. Others, on the contrary, have contributed to the transformation of violence into law by establishing larger units within which the use of violence was made impossible and in which a fresh system of law led to the solution of conflicts. In this way the conquests of the Romans gave the countries round the Mediterranean the priceless *pax Romana*, and the greed of the French kings to extend their dominions created a peacefully united and flourishing France. Paradoxical as it may sound, it must be admitted that war might be a far from inappropriate means of establishing the eagerly desired reign of 'everlasting' peace, since it is in a position to create the large units within which a powerful central government makes further wars impossible. Nevertheless it fails in this purpose, for the results of conquest are as a rule short-lived: the newly created units fall apart once again, usually owing to a lack of cohesion between the portions that have been united by violence. Hitherto, moreover, the unifications created by conquest, though of considerable extent, have only been *partial*, and the conflicts between these have called out more than ever for violent solution. Thus the result of all these warlike efforts has only been that the human race has exchanged numerous, and indeed unending, minor wars for wars on a grand scale that are rare but all the more destructive.

If we turn to our own times, we arrive at the same conclusion which you have reached by a shorter path. Wars will only be prevented with certainty if mankind unites in setting up a central authority to which the right of giving judgement upon all conflicts of interest shall be handed over. There are clearly two separate requirements involved in this: the creation of a supreme agency and its endowment with the necessary power. One without the other would be useless. The League of Nations is designed as an agency of this kind, but the second condition has not been fulfilled: the League of Nations has no power of its own and can only acquire it if the members of the new union, the separate States, are ready to resign it. And at the moment there seems very little prospect of this. The institution of the League of Nations would, however, be wholly unintelligible if one ignored the fact that here was a bold attempt such as has seldom (perhaps, indeed, never on such a scale) been made before. It is an attempt to base upon an appeal to certain idealistic attitudes of mind the authority (that is, the coercive influence) which otherwise rests on the possession of power. We have seen that a community is held together by two things: the compelling force of violence and the emotional ties (identifications is the technical name) between its members. If one of the factors is absent, the community may possibly be held together by the other. The ideas that are appealed to can, of course, only have significance if they give expression to important affinities between the members, and the question arises of how mush strength such ideas can exert. History teaches us that they have been to some extent effective. For instance, the Panhellenic idea, the sense of being superior to the surrounding barbarians—an idea which was so powerfully expressed in the Amphictyonic Council, the Oracles and the Games—was sufficiently strong to mitigate the customs of war among Greeks, although evidently not sufficiently strong to prevent warlike disputes between the different sections of the Greek nation or even to restrain a city or confederation of cities from allying itself with the Persian foe in order to gain an advantage over a rival. The community of feeling among Christians, powerful though it was, was equally unable at the time of the Renaissance to deter Christian States, whether large or small, from seeking the Sultan's aid in their wars with one another. Nor does any idea exist today which could be expected to exert a unifying authority of the sort. Indeed it is all too clear that the national ideals by which nations are at present swayed operate in a contrary direction. Some people are inclined to prophesy that it will not be possible to make an end of war until Communist ways of thinking have found universal acceptance. But that aim is in any case a very remote one today, and perhaps it could only be reached after the most fearful civil wars. Thus the attempt to replace actual force by the force of ideas seems at present to be doomed to failure. We shall be making a false calculation if we disregard the fact that law was originally brute violence and that even today it cannot do without the support of violence.

I can now proceed to add a gloss to another of your remarks. You express astonishment at the fact that it is so easy to make men enthusiastic about a war and add your suspicions that there is something at work in them—an instinct for hatred and destruction—which goes halfway to meet the efforts of the warmongers. Once again, I can only express my entire agreement. We believe in the existence of an instinct of that kind and have in fact been occupied during the last few years in studying its manifestations. Will you allow me to take this opportunity of putting before you a portion of the theory of the instincts which, after much tentative groping and many fluctuations of opinion, has been reached by workers in the field of psycho-analysis?

According to our hypothesis human instincts are of only two kinds: those which seek to preserve and unite—which we call 'erotic', exactly in the sense in which Plato uses the word 'Eros' in his *Symposium*, or 'sexual', with a deliberate extension of the popular conception of 'sexuality'—and those which seek to destroy and kill and which we group together as the aggressive or destructive instinct. As you see, this is in fact no more than a theoretical clarification of the universally familiar opposition between Love and Hate which may perhaps have some fundamental relation tot he polarity of attraction and repulsion that plays a part in your own field of knowledge. But we must not be too hasty in introducing ethical judgements of good and evil. Neither of these instincts is any less essential than the other; the phenomena of life arise from the concurrent or mutually opposing action of both. Now it seems as though an instinct of the one sort can scarcely ever operate in isolation: it is always accompanied—or, as we say, alloyed—with a certain quota from the other side, which modifies its aim or it, in some cases, what enables it to achieve that aim. Thus, for instance, the instinct of self-preservation is certainly of an erotic kind, but it must nevertheless have aggressiveness at its disposal if it is to fulfil its purpose. So, too, the instinct of love, when it is directed towards an object, stands in need of some contribution from the instinct for mastery if it is in any way to obtain possession of that object. The difficulty of isolating the two classes of instinct in their actual manifestations is indeed what has so long prevented us from recognising them.

If you will follow me a little further, you will see that human actions are subject to another complication of a different kind. It is very rarely that an action is the work of a *single* instinctual impulse (which must in itself be compounded of Eros and destructiveness). In order to make an action possible there must be as a rule a combination of such compounded motives. This was perceived long ago by a specialist in your own subject, a Profession G. C. Lichtenberg who taught physics at Göttingen during our classical age—though perhaps he was even more remarkable as a psychologist than as a physicist. He invented a Compass of Motives, for he wrote: "The motives that lead us to do anything might be arranged like the thirty-two winds and might be given names in a similar way: for instance, 'bread-bread-fame' or 'fame-fame-bread". So that when human beings are incited to war they may have a whole number of motives for assenting—some noble and some base, some which are openly declared and others which are never mentioned. There is no need to enumerate them all. A lust for aggression and destruction is certainly among them: the countless cruelties in history and in our everyday lives vouch for its existence and its strength. The satisfaction of these destructive impulses is of course facilitated by their admixture with others of an erotic and idealistic kind. When we read of the atrocities of the past, it sometimes seems as though the idealistic motives served only as an excuse for the destructive appetites; and sometimes—in the case, for instance, of the cruelties of the Inquisition—it seems as though the idealistic motives had pushed themselves forward in consciousness, while the destructive ones lent them an unconscious reinforcement. Both may be true.

I fear I may be abusing your interest, which is after all concerned with the prevention of war and not with our theories. Nevertheless I should like to linger for a moment over our destructive instinct, whose popularity is by no means equal to its importance. As a result of a little speculation, we have come to suppose that this instinct is at work in every living creature and is striving to bring it to ruin and to reduce life to its original condition of inanimate matter. Thus it quite seriously deserves to be called a death instinct, while the erotic instincts represent the effort to live. The death instinct turns into the destructive instinct when, with the help of special organs, it is directed outwards, on to its objects. The organism preserves its own life, so to say, by destroying an extraneous one. Some portion of the death instinct, however, remains operative *within* the organism, and we have sought to trace quite a number of normal and pathological phenomena to this internalisation of the destructive instinct. We have even been guilty of the heresy of attributing the origin of conscience to this diversion inwards of aggressiveness. You will notice that it is by no means a trivial matter if this process is carried too far: it is positively unhealthy. On the other hand if these forces are turned to destruction in the external world, the organism will be relieved and the effect must be beneficial. This would serve as a biological justification for all the ugly and dangerous impulses against which we are struggling. It must be admitted that they stand nearer to Nature than does our resistance to them for which an explanation also needs to be found. It may perhaps seem to you as though our theories are a kind of mythology and, in the present case, not even an agreeable one. But does not every science come in the end to a kind of mythology like this? Cannot the same be said today of your own Physics?

For our immediate purpose then, this much follows from what has been said: there is no use in trying to get rid of men's aggressive inclinations. We are told that in certain happy regions of the earth, where nature provides in abundance everything that man requires, there are races whose life is passed in tranquillity and who know neither coercion nor aggression. I can scarcely believe it and I should be glad to hear more of these fortunate beings. The Russian Communists, too, hope to be able to cause human aggressiveness to disappear by guaranteeing the satisfaction of all material needs and by establishing equality in other respects among all the members of the community. That, in my opinion, is an illusion. They themselves are armed today with the most scrupulous care and not the least important of the methods by which they keep their supporters together is hatred of everyone beyond their frontiers. In any case, as you yourself have remarked, there is no question of getting rid entirely of human aggressive impulses; it is enough to try to divert them to such an extent that they need not find expression in war.

Our mythological theory of instincts makes it easy for us to find a formula for *indirect* methods of combating war. If willingness to engage in war is an effect of the destructive instinct, the most obvious plan will be to bring Eros, its antagonist, into play against it. Anything that encourages the growth of emotional ties between men must operate against war. These ties may be of two kinds. In the first place they may be relations resembling those towards a loved object, though without having a sexual aim. There is no need for psycho-analysis to be ashamed to speak of love in this connection, for religion itself uses the same words: "Thou shalt love thy neighbour as thyself". This, however, is more easily said than done.[3] The second kind of emotional tie is by means of identification. Whatever leads men to share important interests produces this community of feeling, these identifications. And the structure of human society is to a large extent based on them.

A complaint which you make about the abuse of authority brings me to another suggestion for the indirect combating of the propensity to war. One instance of the innate and ineradicable inequality of men is their tendency to fall into the two classes of leaders and followers. The latter constitute the vast majority; they stand in need of an authority which will make decisions for them and to which they for the most part offer an unqualified submission. This suggests that more care should be taken than hitherto to educate an upper stratum of men with independent minds, not open to intimidation and eager in the pursuit of truth, whose business it would be to give direction to the dependent masses. It goes without saying that the encroachments made by the executive power of the State and the prohibition laid by the Church upon freedom of thought are far from propitious for the production of a class of this kind. The ideal condition of things would of course be a community of men who had subordinated their instinctual life to the dictatorship of reason. Nothing else could unite men so completely and so tenaciously, even if there were no emotional ties between them. But in all probability that is a Utopian expectation. No doubt the other indirect methods of preventing war are more practicable, though they promise no rapid success. An unpleasant picture comes to one's mind of mills that grind so slowly that people may starve before they get their flour.

The result, as you see, is not very fruitful when an unworldly theoretician is called in to advise on an urgent practical problem. It is a better plan to devote oneself in every particular case to meeting the danger with whatever means lie to hand. I should like, however, to discuss one more question, which you do not mention in your letter but which specially interests me. Why do you and I and so many other people rebel so violently against war? Why do we not accept it as another of the many painful calamities of life? After all, it seems to be quite a natural thing, to have a good biological basis and in practice to be scarcely avoidable. There is no need to be shocked at my raising this question. For the purpose of an investigation such as this, one may perhaps be allowed to wear a mask of assumed detachment. The answer to my question will be that we react to war in this way because everyone has a right to his own life, because war puts an end to human lives that are full of hope, because it brings individual men into humiliating situations, because it compels them against their will to murder other men, and because it destroys precious material objects which have been produced by the labours of humanity. Other reasons besides might be given, such as that in its present-day form war is no longer an opportunity for achieving the old ideas of heroism and that owing to the perfection of instruments of destruction a future war might involve the extermination of one or perhaps both of the antagonists. All this is true, and so incontestably true that one can only feel astonished that the waging of war has not yet been unanimously repudiated. No doubt debate is possible upon one or two of these points. It may be questioned whether a community ought not to have a right to dispose of individual lives; every war is not open to condemnation to an equal degree; so long as there exist countries and nations that are prepared for the ruthless destruction of others, those others must be armed for war. But I will not linger over any of these issues; they are not what you want to discuss with me, and I have something different in mind. It is my opinion that the main reason why we rebel against war is that we cannot help doing so. We are pacifists because we are obliged to be for organic reasons. And we then find no difficulty in producing arguments to justify our attitude.

No doubt this requires some explanation. My belief is this. For incalculable ages mankind has been passing through a process of evolution of culture. (Some people, I know, prefer to use the term 'civilisation'.) We owe to that process the best of what we have become, as well as a good part of what we suffer from. Though its causes and beginnings are obscure and its outcome uncertain, some of its characteristics are easy to perceive. It may perhaps be leading to the extinction of the human race, for in more than one way it impairs the sexual function; uncultivated races and backward strata of the population are already multiplying more rapidly than highly cultivated ones. The process is perhaps comparable to the domestication of certain species of animals and it is undoubtedly accompanied by physical alterations; but we are still unfamiliar with the notion that the evolution of civilisation is an organic process of this kind. The *psychical* modifications that go along with the process of civilisation are striking and unambiguous. They consist in a progressive displacement of instinctual aims and a restriction of instinctual impulses. Sensations which were pleasurable to our ancestors have become indifferent or even intolerable to ourselves; there are organic grounds for the changes in our ethical and aesthetic ideals. Of the psychological characteristics of civilisation two appear to be the most important: a strengthening of the intellect, which is beginning go govern instinctual life, and an internalisation of the aggressive impulses, with all its consequent advantages and perils. Now war is in the crassest opposition to the psychical attitude imposed on us by the process of civilisation, and for that reason we are bound to rebel against it; we simply cannot any longer put up with it. This is not merely an intellectual and emotional repudiation; we pacifists have a *constitutional* intolerance of war, an idiosyncrasy magnified, as it were, to the highest degree. It seems, indeed, as though the lowering of aesthetic standards in war plays a scarcely smaller part in our rebellion than do its cruelties.

And how long shall we have to wait before the rest of mankind become pacifists too? There is no telling. But it may not be Utopian to hope that these two factors, the cultural attitude and the justified dread of the consequences of a future war, may result within a measurable time in putting an end to the waging of war. By what paths or by what side-tracks this will come about we cannot guess. But one thing we *can* say: whatever fosters the growth of civilisation works at the same time against war.

I trust you will forgive me if what I have said has disappointed you, and I remain, with kindest regards,

Sincerely yours,

SIGM. FREUD

Notes

1. ["Das Verhängnis des Krieges." Freud quotes Einstein's actual words, which are, however, translated differently in Einstein's letter above.]
2. [In the original the words 'Recht' and 'Macht' are used throughout Freud's letter and in Einstein's. It has unfortunately been necessary to sacrifice this stylistic unity in the translation. 'Recht' has been rendered indifferently by 'right', 'law' and 'justice'; and 'Macht' by 'might', 'force' and 'power'.]
3. [Cf. the discussion of this in Chapter V of 'Civilisation and its Discontents' (1930a), 109ff.]

CHAPTER THIRTEEN

Jung correspondence: Letter to Dorothy Thompson

[Original in English]
23 September 1949

To Dorothy Thompson

Dear Mrs Thompson,

It is a pleasure to receive the letter of a normally intelligent person in contrast to the evil flood of idiotic and malevolent insinuations I seemed to have released in the USA.[1]

Well, you know I am just as deeply concerned with the extraordinary as well as uncanny situation of the world as you are yourself. (By the way, I have read quite a number of your political comments and admired their practical intelligence and common sense!)

I could say quite a lot about the actual dilemma of the world from my psychological point of view. But I am afraid it would lead too far afield into realms of psychological intricacies which would demand a great amount of explanation.

I will try to be simple. A political situation is the manifestation of a parallel psychological problem in millions of individuals. This problem is largely *unconscious* (which makes it a particularly dangerous one!). It consists of a conflict between a conscious (ethical, religious, philosophical, social, political, and psychological) standpoint and an unconscious one which is characterised by the same aspects but represented in a 'lower', i.e., more archaic form. Instead of 'high' Christian ethics, the laws of the herd, suppression of individual responsibility and submission to the tribal chief (totalitarian ethics). Instead of religion, superstitious belief in an *ad hoc* doctrine or truth; instead of philosophy, a low-grade doctrinary system which 'rationalises' the appetites of the herd; instead of a differentiated social organisation, a meaningless chaotic agglomeration of uprooted individuals kept under by sheer force and terror and blindfolded by appropriate lies; instead of a constructive use of political power with the aim of attaining an equilibrium of freely developing forces, a destructive tendency to extend suppression over the whole world through attaining mere superiority of power; instead of psychology, use of psychological means to extinguish the individual spark and to inhibit the development of consciousness and intelligence.

You find this conflict in nearly every citizen of any Western nation. But one is mostly unconscious of it. In Russia, which has always been a barbarous country, the unconscious half of the conflict has reached the surface and has replaced civilised consciousness. That is what we fear might happen to ourselves too. We are afraid of this schizophrenia all the more since Germany has clearly demonstrated that even a civilised community can be seized by such a mental catastrophe as it were overnight (which proves my point).

Thus we have got to realise:

1. We are not immune.
2. The destructive powers are right there in ourselves.
3. The more unconscious they are, the more dangerous.
4. We are threatened from within as well as from without.
5. We cannot destroy the enemy by force; we should not even try to overcome Russia, because we would destroy ourselves, since Russia is—as it were—identical with our unconscious, which contains our instincts and all the germs of our future development.

6. The unconscious must be slowly integrated without violence and with due respect for our ethical values. This needs many alterations in our religious and philosophical views.

The West is forced to rearmament. We have to be ready for the worst. Europe must be organised by the USA *à tort et à travers* if needs be. And it will be of vital importance to the USA. *But no attack! Under no condition!* Russia can only defeat herself. We cannot defeat our instincts, but they can inhibit each other and they do if you allow them to run freely within certain limits, i.e., only so far that they don't just kill you. You shoot when you are threatened in your very existence, not when you are merely hurt in your feelings or in your traditional convictions.

The accumulation of weapons, though indispensable, is a great temptation to use them. Therefore watch the military advisers! They will itch to pull the trigger. Russia is certainly on the warpath and it is only fear of those who are in the know that holds her back. Your country is already at war with Russia, like the *drôle de guerre* 1939/40. *There is no reason and no diplomacy that will effectively deal with Russia*, because there is an *elementary drive* in her (as was the case with Hitler!).

I see the main trouble not in Russia but in Europe, which has become a vital extension of the USA. The great question is whether the historically differentiated nations of Europe can be sufficiently welded together to form a unified bloc. Apart from military defensive measures the organisation of Europe forms the foremost and most difficult task of American policy.

I should like to call your attention to my little book: *Essays on Contemporary Events* (Kegan Paul, London, 1947), where you will find some further contributions to the great problem of our time. It seems to me that at the bottom of all these problems lies the development of science and technology, which has destroyed man's metaphysical foundation. *Social welfare has replaced the kingdom of God*.

Earthly happiness can only be attained through somebody else's misfortune, as wealth grows at the expense of poverty. 'Social welfare' has become the lure, the bait and the slogan for the uprooted masses, which can only think in terms of personal needs and resentments, but they don't see that there is no escape from the law of compensation. Their Marxist philosophy is based upon the conviction that the river once in the future can be persuaded to flow upwards. They don't see that they themselves have to pay for this stunt by unending suffering. Much better to know, therefore, that life on this earth is balanced between an equal amount of pleasure and misery, even when it is at its best, and that *real progress* is only the psychological adaptation to the various forms of individual misery. Misery is relative. When many people possess two cars, the man with only one car is a proletarian deprived of the goods of this world and therefore entitled to overthrow the social order. Germany was not in possession of world-supremacy, therefore she was a 'have-not'.

We all think in terms of social welfare. That is the big mistake, because the more you economise on the vulgar forms of misery, the more you are ensnared by new, unexpected, complicated, intricate, incomprehensible variants of unhappiness such as you have never dreamt of before. Think of the almost uncanny increase of divorces and neuroses! I must say I prefer a modest poverty or any tangible discomfort (f.i. no bathroom, no electricity, no car, etc.) to those pests. The bit of social progress attained by Nazi Germany and Russia is compensated for by police terror, a new and very considerable item on the list of miseries, but an inevitable consequence of 'social welfare'. Why not 'spiritual welfare'? There is no government on earth bothering much about it. yet spiritual adjustment is *the* problem.

If we understand what Russia is in ourselves, we know how to deal with her politically.

Ancient Rome, not knowing how to deal with its own social problem, *viz*. slavery, succumbed to the onslaught of barbarous tribes. The Christian Middle Ages withstood the first Asiatic wave and the second (the Turks). Now the world is confronted with the third. The great danger is that we are not up to our own spiritual problem like old Rome. Technology and 'social welfare' provide nothing to overcome our spiritual stagnation, and they give us no answer to our spiritual dissatisfaction and restlessness, on account of which we are threatened from within as from without. We have not understood yet that the discovery of the unconscious means an enormous spiritual task, which *must* be accomplished if we wish to preserve our civilisation.

I hope you will forgive the unsystematic way in which I represent my ideas you wanted to hear of. My attempt is, I know, very incomplete, but I cannot write a whole book. Nevertheless I hope that you can perceive at least something.

Yours sincerely,

C. G. JUNG

Note

1. An acrimonious controversy had arisen in the USA over the award, by the Fellows in American Letters of the Library of Congress, of the Bollingen Prize in Poetry to the poet Ezra Pound in 1949. Articles published in *The Saturday Review of Literature* (11 and 18 June) arbitrarily dragged Jung into the conflict, presenting him as a Nazi and anti-Semite by the method of misquotation, quotation out of context, and insinuation. The only connection with Jung lay in the name of the award, in which the name 'Bollingen' appears simply because it was the Bollingen Foundation (named after the village where Jung had his country retreat) that had put the money ($1000) at the disposal of the Library. The articles were followed by a long correspondence in which, again quite arbitrarily and without relevance to the original issues, opponents of Jung came up with unfounded accusations based on the same methods of falsification. Concerning the award to Pound cf. 'The Case against the Saturday Review of Literature', *Poetry* (Chicago), 1949. Dorothy Thompson mentioned the controversy in her letter (10 Sept.) to Jung, referring to the "mendacity and malice" of his opponents.

CHAPTER FOURTEEN

Thoughts for the times on war and death: a psychoanalytic address on an interdisciplinary problem

Donald M. Kaplan

I want to begin by congratulating the members of the Programme Committee of The New York Freudian Society not only for conceiving of this particular programme but also for surviving the understandable apprehensions of their colleagues in the Society over a proposal to convene a meeting before so large a community on a subject with which the Society has had no experience. Psychoanalysts are also, of course, ordinary citizens and therefore no less beleaguered witnesses to the agitations of international affairs and the awesome spectre of nuclear diplomacy that has long since complicated the very difficult idea that even ordinarily we all live on borrowed time.

Each of us owes Nature one death, Freud was given to say, and this being so, one's only heroism in this matter can be to pay the debt as fully on one's own terms as possible. In conveying a sense of a total communalisation of sudden death, the present nuclear situation threatens the very possibility of this fundamental heroism Freud perceived in the death of every human being. However, such a line of thought is rather faint and brief. For it is merely an existential consideration in a vast turbulence of political, historical and technological problems, among which it is not readily apparent how psychoanalysis itself might figure, if at all, in a view the analyst takes of the plight he shares with every other citizen at this most fraught moment in the history of civilisation. To suppose that the urgency alone of an issue, regardless of its source or nature, is sufficient to arouse a relevant psychoanalytic commentary is to expect that psychoanalytic discourse can endure any dislocation from the contexts in which its technical meaning is furnished. There is a difference between speaking psychoanalytically and psychoanalysis in a manner of speaking. While the difference is always worth bearing in mind, not all subjects compel us to retain the difference to the same extent. However, to address the problems that have brought us together on this occasion in simply a manner of speaking would amount to irreverence.

To be sure, analogies from the clinical to the social and cultural realms are common in Freud's work. Freud likened religion to a collective obsessional neurosis; he allowed that Hamlet suffered unduly from an Oedipus complex; he diagnosed Lady Macbeth a fate neurotic. Indeed such exercises of analogy are what we mean by applied psychoanalysis. On the other hand, there were certain crucial points in his concerns with social, political and cultural processes where Freud was careful to disanalogise individual and social psychology, insisting that the explanatory principles appropriate to each were different. Toward the end of 'Civilisation and its Discontents', for example, where Freud (1930a) was drawing similarities and differences between the development of the individual and of society, he had this to say:

> May we not be justified in reaching the diagnosis that, under the influence of cultural urges, some civilisations, or some epochs of civilisation—possibly the whole of mankind—have become 'neurotic'? ... I would not say that an attempt of this kind to carry psychoanalysis over to the cultural community was absurd or doomed to be fruitless. But we should have to be very cautious and not forget that, after all, we are only dealing with analogies and that it is dangerous, not only with men but also with concepts, to tear them from the sphere in which they have originated and been evolved ... And as regards the therapeutic application of our knowledge, what would be the use of the most correct analysis of social neuroses, since no one possesses authority to impose ... a therapy upon the group? [p. 144]

Thus from a technically psychoanalytic point of view it is fatuous to speak of society as neurotic or self-destructive or sadistic in the sense in which we speak of such outcomes in the development of individual patients studied in the clinical situation. To describe a particular political state of affairs as a state of insanity is a manner of speaking but it is not an analysis. Nor is the dissemination of information for the well-being or improvement of a community, through whatever tactics this takes place, a particularly edifying analogy to the analyst's attempts by means of interpretation to alter a patient's defensive self-deceptions.

What I mean to suggest in these opening remarks are the cautions I believe one should keep in mind in preparing to advance some lines of Freud's thoughts for the times on war and death. Whoever speaks for psychoanalysis on issues of social and political moment must be prepared to allow psychoanalysis to expire with dignity at the limits of its pertinence and to leave to other callings the huge remainders that exceed psychoanalytic reflection.

Since my discussion, like Freud's own manner of dealing with the issues before us, will not be systematic but rather fugitive, a statement about these limits and remainders should be helpful at the outset. Much that I shall be pursuing in a wide-ranging reading of Freud can be contained in the following thesis: as a psychology, psychoanalysis is concerned with an account of how mind transforms the biological into the social. Psychoanalytic principles and concepts are pertinent essentially to mind and only incidentally, if at all, to biology and society. Though the concepts id and superego, for example, conjure something biological and social respectively, their technical meanings are limited to psychological circuits of desire and morality. Since psychoanalysis is also a clinical psychology—a psychology of conflict and its outcomes in symptoms and character—the issues of conflict include the biological and social, for these are issues with which mind reckons. But, again, with respect to this, the pertinent principles and concepts answer only to mind as the theatre of conflict. As for society as one of the terms in mental conflict psychoanalysis simply takes what it needs. For the most part, it treats social structure as a received fact and the varieties of social structure as contingencies in a general problem of mental development and adaptation. What psychoanalysis assumes about the social is only what it requires in order to maintain an account of mind in society or society in mind. Thus mind in society is a vicissitude of object relations, while society in mind is a process of internalisation. However, such assumptions of psychoanalysis, which are independent of any compelling social accounts of its own, are hardly extensive compared to the interests of sociology, anthropology, political science, history. This is not to say that psychoanalysis has contributed nothing to an account of social structure itself. Freud's ideas about group psychology embody great explanatory power with respect, for example, to the liberation of individually proscribed behaviour by the communalising processes of social institutions. Nor are Freud's ideas about art and other aspects of culture negligible. However, it is no detraction from such achievements to observe that vast realms of social, political, economic, historical, cultural and technological processes are opaque to psychoanalytic inquiry.

One of the problems this statement assigns to a reading of Freud on social and cultural matters is the nature of his many excursions into these matters. When was he on business? When was he on pleasure? That is, which commentaries were imperative to the structure of his thought[1] and which were simply the musings of a brilliant spirit worth attending to on virtually any subject? Such questions, I expect, will answer themselves in the course of things. But at the outset I must insist that a significant amount of intellectual traffic Freud conducted at the interface of psychoanalysis and society was imperative. One reason for this was that from a psychoanalytic point of view the civilising processes of a developing mental life leading to its engagements of social structure inevitably entail conflict. Hence such processes and their outcomes in socialisation become considerations in a general psychoanalytic theory of pathogenesis.

In a comprehensive statement on the non-clinical value of psychoanalysis—'The claims of psychoanalysis to scientific interest' —Freud (1913b) notes: "It is true that psycho-analysis has taken the individual mind as its subject, but in investigating the individual it could not avoid dealing with the emotional basis of the relationship of the individual to society" (p. 188). If it is the emotional basis of the relationship of mind to society that concerns psychoanalysis, then psychoanalysis entertains a psychopathology of conformity precisely as it does a psychopathology of object relations. That is, precisely as we speak of the development from one psychosexual stage to another as an enlargement of the libidinal object in the mental life, so we may speak of the social structure, with which mind interacts developmentally and in connection with narcissistic and anaclitic supplies, as an aspect of the enlarging, libidinal object of mind. In 'Mourning and melancholia' Freud (1915c) made the point explicitly: "Mourning is regularly the reaction to the loss of a loved person, or to the loss of some abstraction which has taken the place of one, such as one's country, liberty, an ideal, and so on. In some people the same influences produce melancholia instead of mourning and we consequently suspect them of a pathological disposition" (p. 243). A psychopathology of conformity would then consist of the emotional costs and conflicts—the intra-psychic means—with which one maintained the fact of belonging to one or another social order. Indeed Freud spoke of neurosis as a psychopathology of socialisation no different from a psychopathology of object relations. He went on in the 1913b passage I have been quoting: "Psycho-analysis has recognised that in general the neuroses are asocial in their nature and that they always aim at driving the individual out of society and at replacing the safe monastic seclusion of earlier days by the isolation of illness" (p. 188). It is worth stressing here that Freud is not describing neurosis as a social protest in the political sense, an equation that informs that brand of Soviet psychiatry in which political dissent has become diagnostic of mental illness. Freud simply means that neurosis can be regarded as a psychopathology of the process of socialisation.

This is not to say that Freud deemed every social order, each in its own way, hospitable to mind. Since psychoanalysis embodies no predictive power in these matters on the experimental order 'if a, then b', Freud's ideas of what is and is not socially salutary are a species of common sense. From the point of view of mental health he held that the simpler the social order the individual deals with the better. When one of his colleagues—Theodor Reik—complained in a letter that Freud had made it seem in his study of Dostoevsky that any dull and unimaginative Philistine was morally superior to Dostoevsky, Freud (1928) replied, "I should not wish to deny the excellent Philistine a certificate of good ethical conduct, even though it has cost him little self-discipline" (p. 196). As for Dostoevsky in life, as against art, Freud was unimpressed by the great writer's complicated arrival at some resolution of his problem with authority, "a position which lesser minds have reached with smaller effort" (p. 177). To the end of his life, Freud regarded social complication sceptically. In his posthumous 'Outline' (1940) he continued to insist: "We must not forget to include the influence of civilisation among the determinants of neurosis. It is easy, as we can see, for a barbarian to be healthy; for a civilised man the task is hard" (p. 185). Clearly, social structure is a crucial consideration in the psychoanalytic theory of development and adaptation no less than any of the other factors of fate and chance that figured in Freud's account of the aetiology of neurosis. Moreover, he believed that a favourable set of social structures could transform a neurosis that various childhood experiences would otherwise lead to, much as certain favourable conditions at any stage of development could transform what was pathogenic at some other stage (Freud, 1913b, p. 188). I stress this because there still lingers over Freud's thought a reputation for a peculiar biologism that pre-empted all other determinants in his considerations of the mental life.

However, that society embodies reciprocities, opportunities and regulations continuous with various conditions for mental development and adaptation, places mind and society in a relationship so intimate that they are apt to be thought of as mirror images of each other inviting conceptualisations by a single set of principles. Yet we know that the principles that govern the environment are not synonymous with the subject's version of those principles. The primal scene of the oedipal child is only a selection of its parents' version of sex. Similarly, society has a way of its own, independent of mind in the psychoanalytic sense, and Freud was careful to keep these accounts straight. I quote at length from 'Thoughts for the times on war and death' because Freud's point here will be important for much that follows:

> The development of mind shows a peculiarity which is present in no other developmental process. When a village grows into a town or a child into a man, the village and the child become lost in the town and the man ... the old materials or forms have been got rid of and replaced by new ones. It is otherwise with the development of the mind. Here one can describe the state of affairs, which has nothing to compare with it, only by saying that in this case every earlier stage of development persists alongside the later stage which

has arisen from it; here succession also involves co-existence, although it is to the same materials that the whole series of transformations has applied ... This extraordinary plasticity of mental developments is not unrestricted as regards direction; it may be described as a special capacity for involution—for regression— since it may well happen that a later and higher stage of development, once abandoned, cannot be reached again. But the primitive stages can always be re-established; the primitive mind is, in the fullest meaning of the word, imperishable. [1915, pp. 285–286]

In this passage, the difference between mind, on the one hand, and cultural and maturational structures, on the other, is a function of the process of regression, which Freud assigns exclusively to mind. I shall not pause over the technicalities of the concept of regression except to note that regression is an access to one's past whose conservation in mind determines what it is in the present that affords a continuity of personal development in thought, action and experience. Such a conservation of the past does not take the form of replications of original immaturities but rather of restorations in present fantasies of longstanding desires that have become attenuated in successive considerations of reality. It is in a comparison of fantasy with other modes of thought directly implicated in the operational rules of reality that psychoanalysis differentiates primary and secondary process and speaks of the primitive as a function of primary process and as an imperishable characteristic of the mental life. Thus primitiveness is not immaturity. Dreams, for example, do not consist of immature but rather of primitive modes of thought. Nor do dreams represent mind in ruins. The past that survives in the mental life by virtue of regression is merely that which psychologically contradicts certain actualities—perceptions—that constitute the present, in particular actualities that seem, for various reasons, inconsistent with one's version of personal existence. Yet regression also fosters memories of those pleasures of one's past in the broadest sense that match opportunities in the present for their repetitions, which guarantee an experience of personal continuity. If the contradiction of regression with which Freud was concerned in the passage I have just quoted was dire—a contradiction of vast parts of reality in a permanent psychosis—it was because Freud was addressing the most dire political event in his life to that moment—World War I.

However, the extreme crises of the mental and the political in this essay were largely associative. Ordinarily regression is an expectable process of mind enabling the plasticity required for problem solving, creativity, recovery from the improbable and other adjuncts to the maintenance of one's bearings in the odyssey of development. Much that is primitive in mental life is not necessarily pre-emptive or catastrophic.

With society and its institutions things are different. When a village develops into a town, which was Freud's metaphor here for a social process, an earthquake, or, for that matter, an economic depression, does not reinstate anything remotely resembling the village it once was. An accident in the social structure does not set in motion processes representing a reversion to a past useful to a reparation in the present. The burnt-out tenements of the South Bronx do not exist for the sake of those rural expanses that preceded them in the history of that urban region. Nor does an unemployed population exist for the sake of the opportunities it once had as carefree school children. There is nothing comparable in society to the provisional fantasies of mind, which do exist for the sake of something individually historical; a persecutory delusion, for example, may exist for the sake of some dreadful excitement of once having been the absolute centre of parental attention, but we distinguish a persecutory delusion even in a social order of total persecution—a paranoic is no less so because of the fact of an actual plot against him, while the plot, on the other hand, exists only for purposes of the present. And though the plot was assuredly hatched in the past, this past is social history, not the past of primary process; hence it is the purview of the historian, not of the psychoanalyst.

Nor are our collateral ideas about social catastrophe to the effect that it only happens in the social realms of others a contradiction of primary process, since protection by social permanence is what society is constructed to assure. In 'Civilisation and its Discontents' Freud (1930a) singled out three sources of existential danger to the individual: the indifference of nature and its elements to the individual's survival; the limitation to the individual's psychic power; and the disadvantage of that limited power in relation to the power of a collectivity—"the family, the state and society" (p. 86). Because the social order is not a wish-fulfilment but a fact, we give credence to such assurance. Though Freud referred to such credence as illusion, he gave it no diagnostic import; for nothing so reduces our sense of exposure to the dangers Freud enumerated than our participation in our various social orders. Reality-testing requires only that we differentiate wishes and perceptions to the extent that we achieve a sense of reality. It does not require any far-reaching truth value for our perceptions. Even with respect to extreme circumstance, such as the political action of the Nazi regime against its Jewish population, we can understand why the great majority of Jews, whose final fate was as yet unknown to them, behaved in the belief that trust in the social order, as demonstrated by increasing compliance, would guarantee their survival, even as this belief was tried to its limits by the knowledge that Jews qua Jews were already beginning to perish. That many Jews had the apparent perspicacity to flee the Nazis cannot serve as a critique of the sense of reality of those who stayed behind. What such flight may represent is a fortunate capacity to exchange one social order for another. However, that the majority of European Jews stood fast by their various social orders only demonstrates that tragedy is one of the outcomes of necessity. For a social order does not exist in relation to any other alternative except that fortuitous alternative of another social order. With respect to mind, a social order is always a present stage of reality whether it is in a state of ruin, stability or development.

In one of his Norton Lectures, Czeslaw Milosz, the 1980 Nobel Laureate for Literature, recalled the social and cultural disintegration in Poland following the pact concluded by Hitler and Stalin in August 1939. Milosz (1983) observed how very far things had to go in Poland and how many years they had to be that way before the general population responded to a change in perception. "People always live within a certain order", he wrote, "and are unable to visualise a time when that order might cease to exist. The sudden crumbling of all current notions and criteria is a rare occurrence and is characteristic only of the most stormy periods of history" (p. 20). It is amazing how the business of 'notions and criteria'—customs and standards of behaviour—goes on as usual, while the social order itself has already undergone radical change from top to bottom or is imminently about to. In the midst of the Cuban Missile Crisis, how many Americans fled to the Andes, the Alps or other localities reputed to be proof against massive radioactive fallout? Indeed, how many Americans interrupted the routine comings and goings of their everyday lives in consideration of the fact that for a week in 1962 their very existences hung by a thread?

Nor does subsequent outcome decide anything about the relative merits of the judgements of those who stay put as against those who do not in social, political, military or economic crises—assuming that judgement is being exercised. Here I call upon a piece of academic psychology. One of the more modest conclusions that Kahneman et al. (1982) make in Judgement Under Uncertainty: Heuristics and Biases is that while acts of human judgement about situations embodying uncertainty are not without systematic features, the quality of such judgement is absolutely no good. Moreover, our suspicions of this limitation in ourselves is why we do not exert ourselves to exercise judgement precisely when uncertainty arises in our prevailing circumstances. The alternative to an exercise of judgement that will be poor anyway is to persist in behaviour that is more tried and true, which is our ordinary behaviour even in extraordinary situations. This is hardly denial. It is rather a considered risk that a situation that has passed into uncertainty will revert to our favour in good time. Thereafter we relate to the situation as though it were an object in its own right, and we enlist the measures of object relations—submission, compliance, idealisation, identification and so forth—in the service of regulating anxiety. And through these measures combined with personal character and social status we become variously victims, victimisers, isolates, free-loaders, refugees.

With this we have returned to Freud's idea that the relationship of mind to society is always an emotional one. What psychoanalysis includes in this idea is that the relationship always entails measures of ambivalence. To this extent mind in society is also a plight, and we suffer this by universal necessity. Freud's views on this particular problem involved ideas about the origins of civilisation, which I shall return to shortly.

But in our relationship to society we suffer also by universal accident, and this was by far the more alarming to Freud in the long course of his reflections on social problems. The accidental were those problems that followed unpredictably from the very solutions of any immediate social moment. Though Freud might just as well have made reference to urbanisation or economic events, for each creates its own forms of accident, he dwelled on the introduction of advanced industrialisation into human society and the massive disruptions this application of knowledge inflicted on all members of society. Freud's doubts about the unbridled complications to our lives by industrialisation is caught in a passage in 'Civilisation and its Discontents' where he (Freud, 1930a) was praising the telephone and the telegraph for enabling him to speak to his child hundreds of miles away and to be assured of the safe arrival of his friend who had embarked on a long and difficult journey. But he adds: "If there had been no railway to conquer distances, my child would never have left his native town and I should need no telephone to hear his voice; If travelling across the ocean by ship had not been introduced, my friend would not have embarked on his sea-voyage and I should not need to cable to relieve any anxiety about him" (p. 88). Though Man has become in Freud's phrase in this passage a 'prosthetic God', it is questionable that the attainment has contributed commensurably to his happiness, let alone to his actual survival. And among these issues Freud gave thought to war whose increasing violence was also an accidental factor of the ordinary pursuit of knowledge. Industrialisation imbues the inventions of society with violent potential, while their multiplication and their devastating effects on the natural environment follow principles independent of the designs of any mind or institution in society. The aeroplane was invented for purposes quite irrelevant to military ones, but Freud observed that since its invention the military relevance of the fact that England was an island suddenly came to an end.

If these were partly the musings of Freud in the guise of an ageing citizen who lived through the accelerations of social change characteristic of our present century, there was also an analytic principle at work here having to do with the reality-principle as the great detour through the contingencies of the "real object of satisfaction" (Freud, 1911b). According to Freud's thought, all satisfaction acquires contingencies in the course of development but the difference between the contingent and the accidental is not necessarily clear, so that we are never sure whether our efforts are advancements of our cause, whatever it may be, or departures from it in our assumptions of the digressive assignments of accident. Nor does society furnish any guidelines in the matter. And as for society itself do we not have a sense that the rate at which it works creates problems of an order geometrically greater than the capacities of our existing institutions to solve them? "An unpleasant picture comes to mind", Freud (1933b) remarked, "of mills that grind so slowly that people may starve before they get their flour" (p. 213).

On the issues of the origins of civilisation, where Freud located the necessity of the plight of mind in society, he spoke with more credentials, though only partially with those of a psychoanalyst. As I have said earlier, the issues concerned him because the problem of socialisation was synonymous with the problem of individual development in which society itself becomes a final stage in the construction of the libidinal object. Though Freud's approaches to a history of the process of civilisation—and it was only a history of process that concerned him—begin with elements of fancy, they initiate an account that becomes increasingly authoritative inasmuch as it becomes increasingly psychoanalytic. In giving a précis of this aspect of psychoanalytic thought, I shall bring matters to bear on the functions of force and violence, which figure crucially in Freud's theory of the development of society. We shall see that alternatives to these functions as accompaniments to civilisation are feeble indeed in Freud's thought and are better sought elsewhere than in psychoanalysis. Though Freud characterised himself a pacifist in his paper 'Why War?' (1933b), psychoanalysis does have a problem with the change from war to law, which it shares with Hobbes, Spinoza and Hegel.

In 'Totem and Taboo' (1913a), Freud's most extensive departure into social anthropology, he argued that early civilisation evolved in connection with the replacement of certain behaviour characterising a stage of human pre-history by certain laws interdicting such behaviour. A history of civilisation begins when ordinary slaughter and cohabitation among stipulated members of a human group achieve a conceptual status of murder and incest. Thereafter the social order itself takes on the devices of power and the right to exercise them upon its individual members in order to restrain the commission of acts that have acquired a moral quality. In the relations among the father, mother and sons of Darwin's primal horde, Freud deciphered the birth of society not as an extinction but as a deployment of force and violence at the service of a moral order. Force and violence became the properties of society and were kept in abeyance only to the extent that remorse and obedience regulated social organisation. An adjunct to force and violence is the institution of law, which gives external support to less than optimal internal developments of remorse and obedience among members of the community. In Freud's view law rests on society's power to enforce it. In brief, might makes right.

Indeed, it is through force that the individual first encounters ethics in development. Chapter VII of 'Civilisation and its Discontents' (Freud, 1930a) is an exegesis of this psychoanalytic principle of development. However, succinct statements of the principle can be found earlier in Freud's writing. In 'The Economic Problem of Masochism' (1924), for example, we come across the following passage:

> One might expect that if a man knows that he is in the habit of avoiding the commission of acts of aggression that are undesirable from a cultural standpoint he will for that reason have a good conscience and will watch over his ego less suspiciously. The situation is usually presented as though ethical requirements were the primary thing and the renunciation of instinct followed from them. This leaves the origin of the ethical sense unexplained. Actually, it seems to be the other way about. The first instinctual renunciation is enforced by external powers, and it is only this which creates the ethical sense, which expresses itself in conscience and demands a further renunciation of instinct. [p. 170]

In other words, to a child the advantage of a set of ideals that will fit him or her for a future social existence is not at once apparent. What is apparent is the superior power of the parents and the succession of other authorities who transmit the ideals that become motives for the restraint on impulse. It is only later in development that mind discovers the value of ideals as a wherewithal to achieve good standing in a community. However, a relationship between force and ethicality is a permanent vicissitude in mind. Indeed, the ironies and paradoxes of the moral life is a principal subject of Freud's thought from its very outset, becoming increasingly explicit from the years of the First World War in his elaborations of the superego concept.

Thus force and violence are the very instrumentalities of morality. However, it is also consistent with this principle that the prevalence of a moral order will subdue the necessity of force and violence. This is why Freud (1933b) is able to say in his reply to Einstein on the problem of war, "Whatever fosters the growth of civilisation works at the same time against war" (p. 215). And since it was possible for Freud to observe in the long course of history certain developments in the general mentality, specifically a strengthening of intellect corresponding to a greater internalisation of aggression, Freud is also able to say that pacifism is becoming 'a constitutional intolerance of war' (p. 215). Freud's evidence for this claim of social development, which he likens to the domestication of certain species of animals, is the fact that "sensations which were pleasurable to our ancestors have become indifferent or even intolerable to ourselves" (p. 214). In line with this he had already noted in 'The Future of an Illusion' (1927b) that of three former strivings that have acquired moral qualities in civilisation—cannibalism, incest and murder—only murder can still find a socially moral context for its justification (pp. 10–11). He does not mean, of course, that the other two are unheard of but only that they have lost all moral justifications in most human communities. Nor does Freud regard such evolution in communalisation without hazard, particularly to the sexual life of mankind in the way of sexual inhibition with consequences to genetic distributions in the population—the least civilised in the population in these respects will become the more represented. Such was Freud's habit not to lose sight of the probability that every silver lining has a cloud. Even so, he means to be sanguine.

It is this line of Freud's thought, as it points specifically to the problem of international violence, that I referred to earlier as feeble. Not that Freud's speculations on social evolution do not hold water. There is, for example, a burgeoning literature relating the incidence of stress diseases to the intellectual and moral complexities created by modern societies which a slower rate of biological evolution has not quite fitted us for. Nor is it far-fetched to regard stress disease as one of the clinical expressions of the discontent in civilisation Freud analysed in his monograph on the subject. However, that mind in modern society reveals a capacity to surpass direct physical conquest as a crucial endeavour of everyday life is an observation that offers too little too late. For the problem of war and the quality of death war incurs is not the problem of mind. It is the problem of society. Actually, in a larger view, this was always Freud's position, which is why psychoanalysis is an iconoclastic and revolutionary critique of society. The difficult inconsistencies of Victorian morality, which have not disappeared by any means, or the martial law that a totalitarian politics imposes on mind were appalling to Freud, and he laid much of our individual woes—our plight of necessity—at such doorsteps.

Still, was Freud not saying in his letter to Einstein that if mind has become more pacifist in its strivings, then civilisation must have become less violent in its ideals? For in psychoanalytic theory social ideals are as much motives of mind as superego contents, and social ideals as regards every form of oppression and cruelty have changed quite rapidly since the Enlightenment. Presently most governments are shamed by prevailing values into keeping secret the sanctions they impose on political dissent and the atrocities they carry out on prisoners deemed enemies of the state. I might interject in this connection that psychoanalysis itself has made an extraordinary contribution to the momentum of changing social values that took a new turn since the eighteenth century. In one historical perspective we read Freud as a continuity with Darwin, in another with Nietzsche and also Kant. But in still another, Freud's writings extend from John Locke's (1693) 'Some Thoughts Concerning Education', a fuse that exploded a whole liberal ideology that characterises our present century, including even the political tracts and manifestos of totalitarian states. In his poem memorialising Freud, W. H. Auden (1939) describes psychoanalysis in the public domain as a 'whole climate of opinion', a general threat to political perversity, "the concupiscence of the oppressor", as Auden put it:

> No wonder the ancient cultures of conceit
> in his technique of unsettlement foresaw
> the fall of princes, the collapse of
> their lucrative patterns of frustration:
> If he succeeded, why, the Generalised Life
> would become impossible, the monolith
> of State be broken and prevented
> the co-operation of avengers. [p. 216]

However, in the light of Freud's own psychological principles, what he observes of social

evolution as it bears on the problem of war does business both ways. Whatever fosters the growth of civilisation also makes for a superb military community. The army was one of the social orders Freud used to exemplify the psychoanalytic principles of communalisation in his study of group psychology (1921)—the church was another. An internalisation of aggression with its concomitant intellectualisation of impulses—the constitution of the pacifist Freud later spoke of—is also what fosters a passionate allegiance to group ideals. If the group in question is a military one, these psychological dispositions will make a good soldier. In fact, insofar as neurosis is, as we saw earlier, a psychopathology of socialisation, the more mentally healthy a recruit is, the better soldier he will become, all things being equal, including an absence of conflict with the moral order of the state served by the military.

But this line of thought may well be obsolete. Whether or not history or sociology can demonstrate that something like national character was a variable in different qualities of soldiering during the Second World War, for example, the problem currently is that modern military technology does not require significant differences in soldiering to bring havoc to the entire planet. Military communities of both more and less civilised dispositions are fast becoming able to wage wars of what for all intents and purposes are equally destructive to their enemies. Technology has eliminated the value of communal passion in the waging of the total war we presently dread.

Against such a note one might want to remember that the military is not, of course, synonymous with the state. It is merely a standing instrumentality of the state and does not represent the moral order of the state. No modern nation stock piles weapons with the claim that militarism is its national purpose. Its national purpose is always of a higher moral order, and military security is only a means of preserving national morality. Viewed this way, the hatred of all things military can signify that one does not believe that one has something moral to defend, that any one moral order is interchangeable with any other. But such a position on the arbitrary interchangeability of moral orders is contrary to the whole process of civilisation, which involves the attainment of values and ideals and their codifications in law. There is no human society in which such things are deemed arbitrary, because such things are the very particulars of socialisation itself. It is true that national purposes can be defended by alternatives to war, but such alternatives are the equivalents of force. Even the threat of martyrdom, which was Gandhi's strategy in his radicalisation of the national law of India, is ineffective in advancing a moral order unless it entails potential violence among the followers of a resistive leader.

Having arrived at such a conception of the problematic relationship between force and morality, Freud could imagine no other alternative than the deployment of force to a structure of law superordinate to separate national entities, a deployment to yet a higher moral order. He writes: "Here, I believe, we already have all the essentials: violence overcome by the transference of power to a larger unity, which is held together by emotional ties between its members. What remains to be said is no more than an expansion and a repetition of this" (1933b, p. 205). And he goes on to say:

> Wars will only be prevented with a certainty if mankind unites in setting up a central authority to which the right of giving judgement upon all conflicts of interest shall be handed over. There are clearly two separate requirements involved in this: the creation of a supreme agency and its endowment with the necessary power. One without the other would be useless. The League of Nations is designed as an agency of this kind, but the second condition has not been fulfilled. [p. 207]

To which he adds something quite crucial that rests on a principle somewhat as follows: once a communalising moral order is established, the largest share of the power behind its maintenance reverts to the family where the moral order of the community is passed on in child-rearing. But in the family, power need not be violence as a fact, only as a provisional fantasy in the mind of the child, which fantasy yields to a more benevolent experience with ideals in the course of development. This is the principle I surmise in Freud's suggestion that the value of ideals can gain a sufficient appreciation among nations to create affinities that become regulating in themselves. That is, the appreciation and adoption of an already existing moral order does not entail violence; on the contrary, it leads to restraint. There is something to be said for this final statement of Freud. Despite the mutual suspicions among nations poised for combat at this very moment, history has never seen a greater sharing among nations of a vocabulary of ideals. To be sure, there are vast hidden realms of hell on earth and terrible events of terrorism and belligerence. But this is not to deny an increasingly common discourse among nations about what constitutes a more salutary and fulfilling social and political order. Nor should we shrug as if such discourse is merely words. Words count heavily in human affairs, and there are more words passed among us now than ever before. As for this, I return to Freud once more. In 1893, in one of his earliest psychoanalytic papers, Freud quoted an unidentified English writer to this effect: "The man who first flung a word of abuse at his enemy instead of a spear was the founder of civilisation" (p. 36).

It is here that my subject of some of Freud's views on the relationship among mind, civilisation and war leaves off and branches out to a number of questions for political science, history and psychological theories other than psychoanalysis. However, I should like to repeat a point I was at pains to make near the outset. I had been mindful of yet another allegation against psychoanalysis for a doctrine of reductionism to the aggressive instinct as the deus ex machina in the affairs of social life. In separating mind and society, as was Freud's strategy, we can say that while an aggressive instinct is in mind, the instrumentalities of aggression come to reside in society where they exist as facts, not as mental representations, which is how instincts are seen in mind. By this I mean to suggest a line of thought that would unburden psychoanalysis of its alleged position that individuals by their very nature, by some obdurate determinism, are murderous and warlike. Were this so, there would be no repository of the unconscious whose very existence is what enables the common decency, heroism, reformatory commitment and other virtues that psychoanalysis remarks in the great round of human existence.

But I was about to end with a few questions raised by this reading of Freud but which cannot be answered by any further pursuit of psychoanalysis. For example, global communication has increased significantly over the past several decades. What are the ongoing effects of this on a standardisation of values and ideals across national boundaries? This bears on Freud's thought about the regulation of aggression in shared values.

Also, what is the actual extent of international regulatory agencies such as the international monetary system, international trade agreements, the international postal system, information exchange programmes and the myriad treaties pertaining to military and extra-military affairs? This also bears on the problem of increasing affinities among nations inasmuch as such matters are aspects of a superordinate legal system.

Furthermore, why are treaties between hostile nations so often obeyed? The international agreement, for example, to ban atmospheric testing of atomic weapons has not been violated since its inception nearly thirty years ago. This would bear on the problem of the variety of forces short of actual aggression that underlies the compliance with law by independent sovereignties.

Finally, what does a history of warfare reveal of the comparative incidence of war over the past decades? Has a large outline of a unifying moral order been sufficiently established to reduce its further promulgations by war? Was Vietnam a proving ground for the power of an existing moral order to compensate for an inferior military force? In other words, has there been a cultural evolution toward significantly less conflicting moral orders that reduces the justifications for extreme measures of conflict such as war?

I should not be surprised to hear that such questions are not the right ones. Perhaps they lack urgency and put us in mind of Freud's image of 'mills that grind so slowly that people may starve before they get their flour'. But, then, this would be as it should, because with such questions the psychoanalyst reverts to an ordinary citizen who now listens rather than speaks.

Note

1. This might be a place for some definition of the terms society, civilization and culture, though more often than not Freud used these terms interchangeably, since what psychoanalysis has to say about them does not require any hard and fast distinctions. By society I shall mean the system of relationships among persons regulated by institutionalizations of facts, manners, rules and practices. Needless to say, such institutionalizations, particularly in so-called modern societies,

are inconsistent and contradictory. Culture might then be thought of as the symbolic accounts in ideas and art that represent the experience of persons in social relationships. Civilization is the utilitarian process, involving the education of behaviour and skills, through which society and culture achieve a relationship. For a psychoanalytically more stringent explication of these differences cf. Ricoeur (1970, p. 248ff.).

CHAPTER FIFTEEN

Psychoanalysis and war

Diana Birkett

The earliest and some of the most creative developments in psychoanalysis took place in Europe at a time when the continent was devastated by two of the most destructive wars in history. Further, many of the most gifted practitioners and theorists in this field were, by virtue of their race or nationality, more than averagely affected by the splitting of families and the deaths of members resulting from fighting, persecution, invasion and separation.

One would think that any science which sought to explain human behaviour would be drawn to these issues. Yet they are addressed, in the psychoanalytic literature, almost exclusively in terms of the inner life of the individual. Psychoanalysis has curiously little to say about world events; in another context, that of political persecution in Argentina, Janine Puget (1980) comments: "the theoretical instrument does not allow for the formulation of theories about external reality", though she does qualify this in relation to group analysis. Indeed, it was in the field of groups that Freud took a leap in applying the insights of psychoanalysis to an understanding of society. This represented a one-way process, however, and there was little attempt to study the effects of society on the psyche.

Perhaps this should come as no surprise. Psychoanalysis in its early days never claimed to be a political or social theory, and has always concentrated on the inner world of the individual as determined by infantile conflicts. From its inception it has striven to fend off the claims of real-life events (as in Freud's abandonment of the seduction theory). In a passage from 'A Child is being Beaten' (1919), Freud seems to be paying lip-service to the impact of events in later life:

> at the present time theoretical knowledge is still far more important than therapeutic success, and anyone who neglects childhood analysis is bound to fall into the most disastrous errors. The emphasis which is laid here on the importance of the earliest experience does not imply any underestimation of the importance of later ones. But the later impressions of life speak loudly enough through the mouth of the patient, while it is the physician who has to raise his voice on behalf of the claims of childhood.

From this passionately theoretical standpoint, the effects of later trauma, such as sexual abuse or suffering in time of war, seemed to require no elucidation by psychoanalysis. But we know that, in spite of Freud's disclaimer, these experiences often do not "speak loudly enough through the mouth of the patient" and are subject to repression as of the 'inexpressible'. In more recent times several developments have served to modify this standpoint: the recognition of how serious was the psychic damage wrought by the experience of concentration camps on its victims, and often on their children; an increasing awareness of the very high incidence of sexual abuse of children; and the effects of political oppression on a flourishing psychoanalytic community in Argentina. All these have contributed to bringing actual trauma back into the psychoanalytic focus. Earlier, theories of maternal and environmental deprivation had also served to validate external influences at the expense of instinctual theory, though these too tended to stress the very early years.

Attitudes to war, too, have changed: consider Fairbairn's summary of the 'war neuroses' which he considers to be solely the result of separation-anxiety: 'All neurotic or psychotic symptoms are a persistence of, or a defence against, infantile dependence' (1943). He cites as his patients' two most common complaints: "I can't bear army food" (a longing for the mother's breast) and "I can't bear being shouted at" (a fear of the father's anger). For Fairbairn as war-psychiatrist (elsewhere he takes a more critical stance) war is a norm, and those who cannot tolerate what war imposes are judged to have been already neurotic, for reasons unconnected with war and the military life. The effects of war itself are seen as precipitants rather than causes of disturbance.

Later theorists, however, have seen the war neuroses as a failure in the individual to activate the paranoid defences that would enable him to be free from guilt and fear. But to return to Fairbairn: he relates the story of a seaman who had been traumatised in the following way: shipwrecked and badly burned, he was struggling to stay afloat in a sea full of bodies and wreckage, when a drowning Chinaman began to cling to him and almost pulled him under; he pushed the Chinaman's head under water until he drowned and subsequently haunted by guilt and recurring nightmares. Fairbairn's conclusion is that the neurosis was caused by the reactivation of the patient's unresolved hostility towards his father, identified with the man he killed. But war offers countless such opportunities for destructive phantasies to be acted out, or to be seen enacted on the world stage, and should therefore be seen as more than a mere precipitant of pre-existing neurosis. Eike Hinze (1986), in an article entitled 'The Influence of Historical Events on Psychoanalysis' remarks on this imbalance:

> In psychoanalytical practice it can be dangerous to regard the events of external reality simply as cues for the analysis of the inner psychic world. Thus on the one hand Scylla lies in waiting, overemphasising the spiritual world of the patient, and on the other hand Charybdis threatens to overshadow the unconscious life of the soul with a treatment which is leaning too heavily towards historical and social aspects.

Perhaps an approach more fruitful than sailing warily between Scylla and Charybdis would be to embrace the present reality as a respectable entity, one which is an important determinant of neurotic and psychotic behaviour in a *majority* of people when subjected to appalling circumstances. Psychoanalysis, in the name of 'the unconscious life of the soul', has tended to see as schismatic any emphasis on personal or social trauma rather than address the following central question: what happens when the individual's worst personal fantasies are confirmed by reality? What is the analytic response when images of destruction, or of personal dissolution, which had previously been contained within the sphere of private fantasy, and limited by the opposition of reality, seem to burst upon the world stage? Though it seems likely that much current practice, as evidenced by those working with the victims of torture and the concentration camps, diverges from the classical relegation of the trauma theory, there remains a strong theoretical opposition to a more interactive approach.

Causes of war

Where psychoanalysis has had a clearer contribution to make is in shedding light on the causes of war, as opposed to its effects. In the 1930's and 1940's, in particular, the relationship of psychoanalysis with the social sphere expanded in the direction not only of attempting to understand the origins of war, but of suggesting solutions to the problem of war prevention.

The attempt to understand why men go to war takes as its starting-point the reversal of values adhered to in times of peace. Here is Freud's radical description of the role of the state in time of war (1915d):

> The individual citizen can with horror convince himself in this war of what would occasionally cross his mind in time of peace—that the state has forbidden to the individual the practice of wrong-doing, not because it desires to abolish it, but because it desires to monopolise it, like salt and tobacco.

He attempts to console his readers for their disillusionment at the easy lapse of civilised men into barbarism in time of war: "In reality our fellow citizens have not sunk so low as we feared, because they had never risen to high as we believed". What had been relegated to the sphere of fantasy in order to make social living possible now re-emerges. The fragility of the social code in peacetime he explains in terms of aggression towards the father, repressed as a consequence of the Oedipus complex, in the beginnings of socialisation. War he sees as a re-acquisition of this aggression: "the power which the individual has lost through group relations is regained by the destructive capacities of the group". Freud sees the nation's interest, given as a cause for war, as mere rationalisation, serving the passions of its citizens rather than their preservation. But he remains perplexed as to "why the collective individuals should in fact despise, hate and detest one another—I cannot tell why that is so". This is a point on which Kleinian theory was later to elaborate.

Glover, in *War, Sadism and Pacifism* (1946), continues in the tradition of the Oedipal theory of war but takes further some of Freud's ideas. He shares with him a belief in the hypocrisy of objective causes: in this he starts from the individual's readiness to go to war, springing from repressed sadism and masochism. He is insistent that the end of war is destructive, not self-preservative, but makes the interesting distinction that, though morally speaking the defending nation may be justified, the mechanisms employed to mobilise psychologically for war are no less psychotic for fighting a 'just' war. Briefly, his main contribution is as follows: our rulers are father and mother substitutes; the war-crisis (i.e. the situation immediately preceding the outbreak of war) precipitates a loss of confidence in authority, a sense of not being sufficiently loved and loving. The outbreak of war allows for a split into the loving and protective father (political leader or commanding officer) and the aggressive and hated one (the enemy, in particular its leaders). Further, any attack on a small and defenceless nation re-evokes fantasies in which the good mother and child are attacked by the bad father. (Jaques, (1955) elaborates on this theory by suggesting that resentment against a ship's first officer enables the crew to co-operate with an idealised captain.)

The destructive element in war is an expression of unconscious sadism, while the capacity to tolerate situations of great suffering is seen as the masochism that serves as a primitive method of overcoming unconscious guilt. Thus the war neuroses indicate a breakdown in the ability to employ such psychic mechanisms for the avoidance of guilt and fear. When the state or the leader fail to replace the peace-time superego with an adequate parental imago that would justify killing and being killed, the individual has to re-appropriate all the violence and guilt expressed by the collective war phenomenon (a situation that seems to have contributed to the extraordinarily high level of suicide among veterans of the Vietnam war). The phenomenon of 'fragging' (killing one's own commanding officer) certainly did not make its first appearance in Vietnam, and had already been explained by Freud (1921) and later Fairbairn (1943) as a breakdown in the splitting of the father-figure, in which the good, protective father is suddenly perceived to be bad, wishing the death of his own sons.

This theory of war as 'mass insanity', in which insanity is seen as "a curative process initiated in the hope of preventing disruption, but ending in hopeless disintegration", nevertheless suggests that the cure lies in the individual as much as in society; and that psychoanalysis might have something to contribute to war prevention, by resolving the conflicts that find expression in the readiness to participate in war. Indeed, just after Munich, Glover sent a questionnaire to his colleagues in the British Psychoanalytical Society asking for information about their patients' response to the crisis. There was some agreement in the replies, in that most patients' reactions were seen in terms of infantile conflicts, and that political leaders were perceived as parental imagos. But Glover notes that changes occurring as a response to war are almost identical in pathological and normal groups. It remained for Ernest Jones to make the most damning observation that analysed people, including psychoanalysts, differed surprisingly little from unanalysed people in the use made of their intelligence in such matters as political controversy. Freud put it more succinctly when he spoke of the 'logical bedazzlement' of the best minds in time of war (1915d). So one contribution to war prevention, put forward at different times by Jones (1938), Money-Kyrle (1934) as well as Glover, that all political leaders be subjected to psychoanalytic vetting, would seem unlikely to yield positive results.

At a societal level, Glover suggests that another contribution would be in moves towards a greater inhibition of aggression—including the more humane upbringing of children. This, of course, is open to Freud's criticism that the more society inhibits aggression, the more likely it is to erupt in time of crisis. Alix Strachey (1957), in seeing the family as a prototype of the state, advocates a focus on creating happier families (*not* more powerful ones, which would increase the tendency to authoritarianism). And Bowlby (who incidentally was one of the analysts most influential in shifting the psychoanalytic focus from the inner to the outer world) echoed these proposals (Bowlby & Durbin, 1939).

The Kleinian contribution to the theory of war, as represented by Money-Kyrle (1937), lays less stress on the instinctual content (primitive aggression unleashed by the war-crisis), than on the psychic structures to which men regress in time of war. He sees the phenomenon not so much as an expression of innate aggression, relating mainly to the father, as in the Freudian view, but more as a return to the child's relation to its earliest environment, the mother, at a stage in which the splitting of the object holds sway. Thus the enemy becomes the repository of all bad impulses and will then be seen as persecutory and attacking. Conversely, identification with a bad object can confer a kind of manic strength and justify cruelty towards the enemy. Money-Kyrle gives an illustration of this mechanism: a child develops a phobic fear of a tree-stump which he imagines to be haunted by a lion, into which he projects all his own destructive wishes. But in time he begins to think that he too can be a lion, and fight the other one, thus re-introjecting at a manic level the power and violence he had projected.

This analysis goes some way towards answering Freud's perplexity as to "why the collective individuals should in fact despise, hate and detest one another". The bad impulses have to be projected outwards, and it is always easier to operate at a pre-ambivalent level towards a collective unknown without the reparative wishes to which knowledge gives rise. Equally, the appeal of the paranoiac leader to a demoralised nation becomes more understandable in the light of this theory: the evil and the guilt lie not in ourselves, but in a hated outsider, who takes on the projected feelings against which the nation can then with a clear conscience defend itself. The most obvious example of this mechanism is of course Hitler's use of the Jews, but it is a model that holds good for many historical conflicts: Europe during the Crusades, the French Revolution and its aftermath, and more recently the Cold War and the Gulf Crisis. It also serves to explain why the blood-bath often continues after a successful revolution; the guilt caused by the initial parricide or revolt against authority is so great that it must continue to be projected outwards onto erstwhile comrades, if the purity of the inner circle is to be maintained. Jaques (1955) expands the theory of projected aggression to include the relationship between the armed forces and the civilian population:

> ... the members of the Army are temporarily freed from depressive anxiety, because their own sadistic impulses can be denied by attributing their aggressiveness to doing their duty, that is expressing the aggressive impulses collected and introjected from all the community.

Money-Kyrle does not, any more than Glover, deny the existence of 'just' or truly defensive wars: but he too stresses that a psychotic distortion is necessary to enable men to go to war, and to consider it a justifiable resolution of real conflicts. He traces pacifism back to reparative mechanisms arising from depressive anxiety, based on the fantasy of having done real damage to one's good object. But pacifism, though representing a more advanced developmental position, is also open to paranoid regression, in that the political leaders who advocate war often serve as the recipients of aggressive projections, and are thus seen as the enemy of the good. Alternatively, pacifism can serve as a denial of the other's real hostility since if accepted this would mirror the pacifist's own, which has to be denied. Pacifism also serves another purpose, as Hinshelwood (1986) points out, which is to contain, in a harmless and denigrated way, the caring faculties of the community:

> The peace groups then represent the whole population's revulsion against war and are the receptacle for their guilt; and they are often persecuted as a token punishment (e.g. conscientious objectors in the First World War). For the social defence system, it is essential that the peace groups are a minority and weak—weak in the sense of sentimental and therefore slushy and unrealistic. The majority is seen as right. The denigrated 'caring' peace groups do not therefore threaten the mobilised aggressiveness which can then be guiltlessly idealised.

Turning to primitive communities, Money-Kyrle sees in them a clear example, because less obfuscated by modern economic relationships, of how war serves as a structure for projecting evil things into enemies who must be killed, and good things into the group's own leader, who thus becomes much more powerful. Fornari (1975) adds that many primitive communities are better equipped than modern states to re-own their destructive impulses by mourning the death of their enemies and attributing good qualities to them. Among head-hunting tribes, it is the custom to cherish and honour the heads of slain enemies, thus turning them into friends in an acknowledgement of their power, and of the guilt of having slain them. Similarly, in 'Totem and Taboo' (1913a), Freud describes the taboos imposed upon the warrior on his return from killing the enemy, in which he is treated as 'unclean' until the rites of purification have been carried out. Fornari suggests that projecting, then re-owning destructive impulses, is an effective way of maintaining the psychic health of both tribe and individual; and that one of the chief contributory factors to the decline of primitive communities coming into contact with the West is the suppression of tribal warfare through defeat and colonisation.

Perhaps this model of carefully sustained ambivalence is a more useful one for understanding the present situation, in which nuclear war threatens to destroy not only our enemies but ourselves, than the model of paranoid splitting that underpins conventional modern warfare. A leader whose main weapon for protecting us could also be the agent of our annihilation cannot be idealised in the same way, nor can a mainly civilian enemy passively experiencing total destruction be as easily transformed into aggressors fully deserving of their fate. On the other hand, as Segal (1987) points out, nuclear war feeds into a "typically schizoid mechanisation and dehumanisation ... Pushing a button to annihilate parts of the world we have never seen is a mechanised split-off activity", and therefore less accessible to ordinary morality, based on guilt and the need for reparation. It could be said that we have moved backwards from the depressive morality of primitive peoples, through the splitting mechanisms of conventional warfare, to even earlier mental structures organised around the omnipotent desire to annihilate the persecutor.

Another question arises in relation to this: if conventional war and its ideological accompaniments have offered the world such clear opportunities for dealing with internal guilt and anxiety by externalising them, what are we to do with these feelings in the absence of such a structure? Are the aggressive young men on the football terraces merely pining for war, and is racial hatred similarly motivated? As Fornari chillingly puts it: "If it were not for war, society would be apt to leave men defenceless before the emergence of the Terrifier as a purely internal foe". But he adds the more hopeful converse: "We can no longer cure our madness through war". If it is true that men tend to regress in time of crisis to earlier psychic structures (as in the Kleinian theory), or to liberate repressed psychic contents (as in the Oedipal theory), this tendency would have to be replaced by a more sophisticated response. Ironically, it could well be the very indiscriminate nature of the destruction wrought by nuclear war that will protect us from the 'innate madness' of seeing war as a solution to real conflicts.

Psychoanalysis and war— response to Diana Birkett

Isobel Hunter-Brown

Ms Birkett is to be congratulated on bringing to our attention important issues regarding Psychoanalysis and war [*British Journal of Psychotherapy*, 8(3)]. My own feeling like hers is that it would be good to see more psychoanalytic contributions on the effects of militarism (and of the lessening of humanitarianism in our present day society too). There are, however, a number of aspects of her article which require response.

She begins with two criticisms of psychoanalysis: (1) that, generally, it should have had more to say on the effects of social changes on the individual psyche; and (2) that it has an addiction to infantile fantasy and ignores the impact of current realities. In particular she mentions the realities of persecution, war, migration, and the concentration camp and holocaust.

She conveys the impression that psychoanalysts have only recently begun to realize the damage wrought by these disasters but, though there may be a relative paucity of literature, psychoanalysts have been writing about them for many years. Contributions are too numerous to mention but in 1968 a series of papers for a conference on the effects of social disaster was included in the *International Journal of Psychoanalysis*. On the nuclear threat, a six-page bibliography was published in the *International Review of Psychoanalysis* (1987) which included psychoanalytic papers dating back to 1946.

It is perhaps true as Ms Birkett says that Bettelheim is the only psychoanalyst to have written from his personal concentration camp experience, though in many ways others suffered greatly. It was a by-word after the barbarities of the First World war that ex-servicemen typically maintained a life-long silence on their sufferings. The effect of enduring horrors not shared by others seems to cause this reaction. Anna Freud dealt with her experience of becoming a "displaced person" by offering help to certain of the most vulnerable and impressionable of her host country's displaced persons—babies—for whom she set up several residential nurseries in London. Her writings show how she gave weight to the impact on the infants of war-time external realities, including the reality of their mothers' attitudes, as affecting their developing psychological functioning. All psychoanalysts, however, do stress that "the eye brings with it what it sees", Kleinians particularly emphasizing the phantasy element. It must not be forgotten too that phantasies forged in experience precipitate some of the events of external reality. What happens when a person perceives that an external reality threatens to approximate to a wish-fulfilling phantasy derived from a dangerous (e.g. murderous) wish is that the fantasy may be repressed or other defensive measures may be instituted.

Embryologists point to the far-flung later organic defects caused by small physical traumata in the "organizing tissue" of the human embryo—and, by analogy, psychoanalytic insight is that later functioning is determined, for good or ill, by what goes on in the early period of personality formation. The psychoanalytic idea of determinism is one which deserves greater consideration and, if taken seriously in conjunction with notions of the impact of external reality, cries out for protest at aspects of our current "mother-unfriendly, baby-unfriendly" society which among other things can be thought to produce a population with increased war-readiness.

There is a conflict of opinion as to whether or not it is appropriate to apply insights from the consulting room on a large scale, to the social processes outside. Some psychoanalysts think not and Ms Birkett quotes one. The psychoanalyst sees only a few cases. The patient brings only such facets as he chooses of external reality as perceived by him. It is inappropriate for the analyst to intrude to divert his attention to other issues he, the analyst, might find interesting. There is also the problem that, whereas in personal analysis a hypothesis can be tested by reference to a patient's reactions, it is not so feasible to test formulations made about social processes. On the other hand, there is the amazing example of Freud whose thinking had effects far beyond the consulting-room in which he actually observed only small numbers of patients.

Ms Birkett grants that those psychoanalysts who have developed group work do focus on the impact of current social forces, and she also mentions Elliott Jaques (1951) who analysed both factory cultures and how societies create a war mentality. There is also Isabel Menzies-Lyth's work (1988) on the processes hospitals evolve to defend young nurses against the anxieties of their work. Psychoanalysis in this country was also influential in the changing of the practice by which parents were refused access to sick children in hospital. In the field of criminology too, psychoanalysts have pointed to community as well as intra-psychic factors. Today, certain psychoanalysts are breaking new ground in combining the psychoanalytic viewpoint with infant observation and controlled experiment.

There is another whole area in which psychoanalytic insights are pursued about here-and-now interactions between communities and their members, i.e. therapeutic community work. This was originally evolved by psychoanalytically-trained psychiatrists in World War II in what was known as the Northfield Experiment. Responsible participation in the running of a democratic doctor/ patient community with observation of the tensions arising was offered as treatment for war casualties in preference to individual psychotherapy. Hinshelwood (1987a), Editor of this Journal, has written about psychological processes operating in a modern therapeutic community. Even so, as early as 1954 the American psychoanalyst Stanton in collaboration with his colleague Schwartz wrote about interactions between staff activity and variations in patient symptomatology in a mental hospital setting—work sadly not much taken up here where, as everyone knows, mental hospitals have been abolished rather than reformed on the lines suggested—with the result, of course, that numbers of ex-patients languish in prison or haunt the streets—a subject well worth study from the point of view of the effect of a society on its citizens.

In group and therapeutic community work psychoanalysts operate most closely alongside sociology, one of the disciplines which primarily concentrate on society's impact on individuals. Ms Birkett wondered if football hooligans might really "be pining for war". It is to the sociologists one must go for the study of this behaviour, and they would consider the phenomenon much more complex. There is difficulty in disciplines communicating with each other because of the specific terminologies they develop, but among sociologists who write about football violence Dunning (1988) shows some attitudes consonant with a psychoanalytic viewpoint.

Already in 1914 Ernest Jones had attempted to bridge the gap with sociologists. I am not able to speak authoritatively on the history of contacts between the two disciplines, but at different times psychoanalysts writing comprehensive works quote the findings of sociologists in relation to psychological reactions to disaster. One famous psychoanalyst at least, the American Erikson, has analysed the linkage between the social fabric and practices of societies and the type of citizen they characteristically produce.

In 1968 the psychoanalyst Foulkes collaborated with sociologists and others to put forward a view of the individual according much more influence to social forces than is commonly given. He sees the individual as having fluid personality boundaries and the unit as the community rather than the person. A few years ago certain psychoanalysts in this country came together to form an association for promoting understanding of our society. Others have been building on Foulkes' theoretical base and are shortly to publish their ideas. There is much to stimulate further thinking in this revolutionary psychoanalytic view about the extreme importance of social reality.

There have been some very left-wing psychoanalytic critics of the effects of Western society on its citizens, among them a Marxist, Kovel. Their views, in turn, have been criticized by the psychoanalyst Lasch (1978), who says

> The value of [Freud's] ideas for social theory lies in their radical challenge to received ideologies of every kind. We are still very far from having assimilated the implications of psycho-analysis for social and political theory ... Psycho-analysis really points to the need ...

to formulate ... a new vision of the good society and of democratic citizenship ... Freud's legacy represents a far more radical body of knowledge than most radicals have ever understood.

Ms Birkett's article dictates a retreat now from this broad sweep to consulting-room practice, to respond to her comments on Freud and Fairbairn. She assumes that Fairbairn (1950) in his article on war neuroses speaks for psychoanalysis as a whole, whereas psychoanalysis encompasses many differing viewpoints. Franz Alexander's exposé on the subject (1949) gives weight to her point that war casualties may have been through situations of horror and terror complicated by the loss of comrades and thus under much greater stress than peace-time imposes, and he explains how when psychological coping mechanisms have been stretched beyond capacity, people inevitably seek the comfort and safety of a childhood dependent type of adjustment. That means they regress to a dependency characterized by inability to consider a carer's needs; and shame and guilt over this perpetuate the regression. Fairbairn underestimates this when he regards the dependency of his servicemen patients as life-long. A metaphorical psychoanalytic way of referring to the regressed state, which Ms Birkett quotes is "a longing for the mother's breast"—an expression which emphasizes past/present continuity and the unity of mind and body. Regression is, incidentally, a general psychoanalytic concept, not an exclusively Kleinian one.

In treating such cases, any psychoanalyst known to me would—contrary to Ms Birkett's supposition—give ample opportunity in the first place for the abreaction of feelings about the traumatic precipitating incident, as no doubt Fairbairn did, though it is not what he stressed. It can only be that it is because of a preconception that Ms Birkett disbelieves Freud's statement in "A child is being beaten" that "emphasis on an early experience does not imply underestimation of later ones". It hardly needs stating that one of Freud's most momentous discoveries was how past experience, as perceived and fantasized by a person, lives on and, unconsciously, determines reactions to later experience. All psychoanalysts subscribe to this though more emphasis is placed on phantasy by the Kleinian group. It is not, however, a notion that always spontaneously occurs to patients so an extra effort, as Freud was indicating, may have to be made by the analyst to bring out the connection. There is debate today about the place of empathy as compared with historical insights in treatment, but experience suggests that both are necessary for symptom relief in a neurotic illness.

The legitimacy of the war institution has been taken for granted from time immemorial and Fairbairn was a man of his time—writing in 1942 when the country was in danger—in his blindness to the moral dilemmas involved in "a man's duty to serve his Country". Elliott Jaques later analysed the processes of self-idealization and projection whereby violent aggression by our soldiers is regarded as good, and the enemy non-human, and he pointed out how irresistibly powerful are the pressures to adopt these attitudes in war-time. The physical likeness of Fairbairn's sailor patient's father to the Chinaman he drowned no doubt breached these socially-inspired dehumanizing defences, but in addition it awakened the repressed guilt which normally slumbered on in his unconscious, over long-buried murderous wishes towards his loved/hated blustering father. Ms Birkett takes as oppositional factors which are synergistic—the influence of society/inner psychological factors; socially-inspired defence mechanisms/personal defence mechanisms; the influence of the past/of the present.

In her remarks on torture, Ms Birkett does not seem to appreciate that psychoanalysis does not set up to be a panacea. Psycho-dynamic assessment on psychoanalytic lines of the torture victim's psychology and circumstances, of the type of torture endured and its meaning for the patient could help to determine what kind of treatment might be best.

As already indicated, the literature on the subject of Psychoanalysis and War is more extensive than Ms Birkett realizes. Hanna Segal (1987, 1989) is the chief current spokesperson in this country; Hinshelwood (1986, 1987b) has contributed several articles and I too have written on the subject (Hunter-Brown, 1984).

The jumping-off point for later work is the correspondence between Einstein and Freud, "Why War?" (1933b). Einstein thought that unless mankind changes its way of thinking it will not survive. Both agreed that the source of ordinary people's enthusiasm for war must be a "basic lust for hatred and destruction". In support of this can be cited the ancient love of gladiatorial sports and the fascination for many in observing the Gulf War on television as a spectator sport.

Fornari (1966) says the French sociologist Bouthoul, who made a study of war, referred to a "deep-seated human bellicosity" as a mysteriously variable factor which at one time wanes to allow rational solutions, and at another time waxes to lead to bloodshed when it combines with power-hunger, revenge, the desire to redress injustices, and/or where there are conflicts of economic interest, ethnicity, religion, etc. to be resolved. Freud recognized the multiplicity of the issues and his letter still repays study. There is also the complication of what is now known as the "military–industrial complex".

Freud and later psychoanalysts have considered the significant "in-built", often unconscious, aggressivity in individual citizens to be increased by authoritarian upbringing, especially in the early formative period. Later analysts have also pointed to the contribution to aggressivity of failures in the early mother/child relationship. To this must be added all forms of assault on children, inhumanities towards them such as are involved in much of our current practice, for example, with regard to residential establishments for them, aspects of the treatment of offenders, and the bleak future and rootless homeless existence our society offers to numbers of its young. "Frontiers of war and peace are in each of us." By making war nations (and individuals) escape from dealing with their real internal difficulties.

Space does not permit of elaboration of the ideas of "large group" analysts' contribution to the psychology of war, which Ms Birkett mentioned, nor for enlarging on the paranoid projections and other defences as pointed out by Jaques and Fornari as intrinsic to creating a mentality which sanctions killing. Baker (1992) has demonstrated that in the Gulf War creating a false picture which eliminated the horrible realities of the "Turkey shoot" (using language which denies the humanity of the enemy) maintained public enthusiasm. Nor was invited public admiration of our "smart weapons" allowed to be clouded by the realization that the infant mortality rate in Iraq was subsequently tripled.

Ms Birkett raised the question of the competency of leaders. Freud stated that leaders should be "men of independence and reason, not open to intimidation and eager in pursuit of the truth"—

but he did not recommend they should undergo analysis. There have been some psychoanalytic studies of leaders. How leaders come to the fore is a matter for historians but one psychoanalyst has suggested a tendency for the leader to be one who is most in tune with the unconscious of his followers.

Ms Birkett ended with the hope that the very existence of nuclear weapons might be deterrent of war. Psychoanalysts have no easy answer to the problem of war prevention. Freud spoke of world government—ideal but probably Utopian, he said, recognizing the institutional powers of nations' war machines. He saw hope in "anything which encourages the growth of emotional ties among men". Like other groups, psychoanalysts encourage "thinking globally"—a matter which requires a momentous re-orientation. As one psychoanalyst put it, "Today civilised man no longer regards his planet as the centre of the universe, but still so regards his nation".

As regards hope through "deterrence", almost without exception psychoanalytic writers regard this as an illusion. They challenge the taboo against examining the psychology that underlies it, and name it as a policy of intimidation. They point out that in the past weapons accumulated have always been used. On our Tridents alone, our small island has the possibility of carrying weapons which could wreak well over thirty times the destruction produced by all participants in World War II. These weapons by their nature are weapons of offence and we continue to "improve" them. There are cogent reasons for modifying our policy, quite apart from the fact that it means that 25% of all our civil servants, and 45% of our research and development resources are involved in "defence" to the detriment of social and health provision which might otherwise contribute towards creating a content and peaceful populace.

Usually we are deterred from acting foolishly by contemplating the likely consequences of our behaviour, but in this it seems we are lulled into acquiescence by usage and by our need to deny anxieties too great to be borne—for doctors tell us they cannot cure the awful injuries nuclear weapons would inflict; scientists tell us the explosion of only a proportion of existing stocks would threaten mankind with extinction through "nuclear winter", and statisticians tell us that in the long run accident explosion is inevitable. We push these anxieties aside and, with our leaders, cling to the belief that "more is better".

The burden of Hanna Segal's message (1987) is that nations, like individuals who adopt the posture of threat, suspicion and manic self-aggrandisement as a means to achieve security rather than by creating friendly relationship in a context of appropriate self-assertion, are to be regarded as mad or psychopathic. She points out how the possession of such omnipotent destructive power stimulates in nuclear nations and their leaders a guilt-driven psychological need to find enemies to justify it, and stimulates in non-nuclear nations the desire to acquire it too.

I conclude (using words ascribed to Bettelheim):

> Ghetto thinking is not a crime ... it is a fatal mistake ... If we are not careful the white western world, which is already a minority of mankind, will wall itself up in its own ghetto by instruments of so-called deterrence. We all must enlarge the feeling of community beyond our group ... not because all men are basically good, but because violence is as natural to men as the tendency towards order.

CHAPTER SIXTEEN

Psychological defence and nuclear war

Robert D. Hinshelwood

Society is influenced by the unconscious aspects of the minds of the member individuals. This paper describes a psychoanalytic approach to some aspects of the social processes that give rise to the attitudes in Western society towards nuclear war and the nuclear threat. It is concluded that there are profound hidden factors that work against changing the current views on war and nuclear war, and that some peace groups are inadvertently recruited into maintaining the status quo.

People have a genuine fear of enemies, especially enemies powerful enough to annihilate us. Such fears may not simply subside in the absence of enemies. Human beings suffer particularly from such nightmares, and are prone to live them out in the actual world.

In this paper I take a psychoanalytic view of the social processes in which nuclear threat are embedded, and explore the possibility of the social system being structured as a psychological defence (Jaques, 1955). These unconscious psychodynamics of the social structures are important and, as I hope to show, make the position of some peace groups in the West highly problematic in a way that is not generally realised.

This approach may be difficult for those unfamiliar with a

psychotherapeutic mode of thinking. As a member of society, the psychotherapist is in the uncomfortable position of understanding some of the hidden unconscious issues, so he ought to have a role in passing on knowledge that may be helpful in removing the threat of nuclear war. Although uptake by the general public of psychodynamic understanding is extremely slow, conclusions about the psychological obstacles to averting the nuclear tragedy need to be aired.

The social system as a defence against anxiety

Elliot Jaques, a psychoanalyst, applied modern psychoanalytic ideas to studying the 'unconscious structure' of a manufacturing enterprise (Jaques, 1951). This famous study was followed by another one that showed how a nursing service in a London hospital was collectively organised as a psychological defence to protect the nurses, especially young students, from the pain of long shifts with suffering and dying patients (Menzies, 1960).

Jaques described the primitive psychic defences characteristic of the earliest phases of infancy: projection, introjection and identification. He showed they are extremely prevalent in social processes, and may be organised collectively by the individuals in the institution. Crucial is the fact that they are organised unconsciously by the individuals. To clarify this Jaques speaks of "the phantasy social form and content of an institution" which is unconsciously adhered to by the members and contrasts this with the "explicit or agreed and accepted functions" (Jaques, 1955).

One of Jaques' preliminary illustrations is the phantasy social structuring of a nation at war (Jaques, 1955). Consciously the structure is that of two opposing armies, each backed and supported by its community. However, unconsciously, the citizens of each side project all the bad qualities into the enemy. Thus the enemy becomes the embodiment of evil, based often on the shameful side of themselves—like the Nazi's persecution of the Jews who were supposed to be engaged in a conspiracy to dominate the world. This exaggerated evil of the external enemy means that the individuals in the home populace can support each other as exaggeratedly good.

Aggression is commonly regarded as bad, akin to hatred and cruelty, and is much easier to infer in an enemy (even if terrifying) than to acknowledge in oneself. But, in facing an aggressive enemy, another form of aggression can be accepted—brave, self-sacrificing, nobly countering evil. It comes to be socially regarded as good. Murder and all kinds of barbarities are sanctioned in the pursuit of national defence as 'good aggression', which combats the evil projected into the enemy. This 'good aggression' is introjected[1] by the citizens, in contrast to their own hatred that has been projected into the enemy. 'Good aggression' is, in turn, projected into their own soldiers. The soldiers thus introject from the populace the projected 'good aggression' and can feel untroubled by the normal pangs of conscience that aggression arouses. It is thus transformed into doing one's duty, or even especial exploits of bravery. The soldiers actually identify with the projection and become the nation's aggression. What is achieved is a "redistribution of the bad ... impulses in the phantasy relations obtaining among the members of society" (Jaques, 1955). The psychological state of the individual soldier is thus modified to create a sense of improbable security and guilt-free heroism through the introjected support from the increased comradeship, and at the same time a lifting of moral sanctions from his otherwise troubled conscience.

The point I wish to emphasise from Jaques' work is the way the unconscious adaptation of social institutions and processes renders areas of experience unconscious. These are areas of horror, only dreamed about. In the nuclear war debate this appears in the apparent complacency to the annihilating threat that we face. This is the experience which is psychologically 'defended against' by the socially organised defence system.

The experience

Experiencing the fears incompletely (Pentz, 1984) is not because of governmental prohibition, but because they feed into our preference to evade the worst fears most of the time.

The nuclear threat is special in human psychological life as it touches on the most elemental and primitive of experiences. Kovel has detailed much of the psychology of the nuclear threat— "Paranoia creates enemies out of inner need" (Kovel, 1983)—while the Kleinian School of Psychoanalysis has made a particular study of the varieties and intensity of human aggression and the defences against them (Segal, 1979). Melanie Klein herself lays great stress on the important level of the personality that is deeply preoccupied with thoughts of persecution and personality that is deeply preoccupied with thoughts of persecution and annihilation (Klein, 1946) and which derive from the earliest stages of infancy. She also emphasised the particular importance that the defences of projection, introjection and identification have in preserving mental composure in the infant and in the social adult.

The nuclear threat represents the manifestation nearest to reality of everyone's worst fears. It appears as the quite omnipotent destructiveness for which there can never be enough reparation to put things right again. Irreparable annihilation is a bedrock unconscious phantasy of all of us. In some sense or other, we all have an itch to press the button. There is no-one who has not wanted to obliterate people he dislikes or with whom he has furious arguments. At times we have all wished to annihilate even our nearest and dearest, and have developed bitterly destructive thoughts towards our own culture and country.

There is also the awful emotional experience that one will go up in it too, in reality. We have all of us at some level experienced such disastrous internal states that we feel collapsed, destroyed, obliterated, our own minds or selves gone to pieces. The experience of going to pieces emotionally in an explosive personal disaster, of being stirred by such a powerful anger that there is a threat to retaining personal civilised control, must be known to each of us. It is again very close to the bedrock of human experience.

The fact that the nuclear threat so nearly replicates in reality our worst phantasies gives it a special place in human psychology. It is true that the possibility of omnipotent destruction is not new. The saturation bombing at the end of the last World War, chemical warfare in the First World War, and the scourge of mediaeval epidemics of plague are all reality manifestations which touch on these same worst fears. However, nuclear war is of another degree since we have to conceive of a situation after the war in which there is no-one left to conceive of it or us.

We each have methods of coping with a desire for immortality, by means of institutionalised religion, family descendants, or physical or academic achievements. But none of these will remain, so unlike death in ordinary war, we know there will be no-one left to glorify the war and the sacrifice or to keep us and our achievements in their hearts. Death is normally a living event for the survivors but in nuclear war even one's death is obliterated.

Freud realised the place that fears of annihilation had in the human mind when he succeeded in understanding the mind of a paranoid schizophrenic whose core experience was a 'world-destruction' phantasy (Freud, 1911a). Glover trenchantly added immediately after the Second World War:

> No doubt the discharge of atomic bombs does not differ in principle from snowballing. There has been no change in fighting methods since Cain threw the first stone with intent to kill. Nevertheless the actual and potential destructiveness of the atomic bomb plays straight into the hands of the Unconscious. The most cursory study of dream-life and the phantasies of the insane shows that the ideas of world-destruction are latent in the unconscious mind. And ... the atomic bomb ... is well adapted to the more bloodthirsty phantasies with which man is secretly preoccupied. [Glover, 1946]

Fornari reflects extensively on this propensity of the human mind (Fornari, 1975). Humphrey also noted the frantic human fascination to advance into the holocaust, and referred to it as the 'Strangelove syndrome' (Humphrey, 1982).

Klein describes these 'secret preoccupations' in terms of the infant's experience at the outset of life. He is beset by horrendous phantasies, and impulses to perform them—happily frustrated by the infant's own powerlessness. The adult, less happily, is in a position to realise his worst fears. To grasp the infant's experience Klein finds helpful "Winnicott's emphasis on the unintegration of the early ego. I would also say that the early ego largely lacks cohesion, and a tendency towards integration alternates with a tendency towards disintegration, a falling to bits" (Klein, 1946). The experience of this 'primary anxiety of being annihilated' is the birth-right of the human infant, and is the bedrock on which personal development anxiously proceeds. Some of Klein's followers have taken great interest in a detailed understanding of phantasies of fragmentation and annihilation (Bick, 1968; Meltzer, 1975; Turquet, 1975).

The initial phantasy of an annihilating destruction is the crucial psychological experience. The dynamics start here. The rest is the interplay of defensive manoeuvres to escape the experience.

The defences

Omnipotent destruction, annihilation and despair are the emotional experiences to be defended against. Different people have, of course, their own individual defensive manoeuvres. We know now, however, that people adopt defences for two reasons: firstly, to protect themselves against experiences they cannot bear; and secondly, because they are embedded in a social system which provides defensiveness within its institutions. We must be interested in the second of these since without dealing with the collective defensiveness involved in war, and in the nuclear threat in particular, the individual defensiveness cannot be addressed.

As members of a democracy we are required to identify in certain ways. Although we do not have to conform to a single allegiance, there are sanctioned identities of protagonist and opposition. Democratic life is founded on the social idea of opposition. The most important defence manifested in our culture is the externalisation of our inner conflicts into the world outside ourselves and in particular into the political world. Internal states of destructiveness can be attributed to external objects. Perhaps it is salutary to observe activities in Parliament. There the verbal hostilities, rudeness and cheap attempts to get one up on each other combine with a severe degree of infantile behaviour to express in the highest forum of the land our most childish selves.

It is a customary attitude in many people to reject politics as if it need not happen at all, as if we could do without all these aggressive and immature politicians. The attitude of the apolitical liberal (as Bernard Crick calls him) is a self-rejection, since it is a rejection of our immature selves. It is a denial of our own infantile aggression and grandiosity. This side of one's own personality can be split from the rest and disowned, and projected into our elected representatives. We are enhanced in denying our immature selves by denying that our political representatives also represent our emotional and shabbily aggressive sides.

But more than this, our aggressiveness has much worse forms and these are attributed to (projected into) those with whom we have no collective identity. Enemy nations are a much needed receptacle for the experiencing of very evil destructiveness.

Another way of dealing with shame and guilt of our

aggressiveness is to glorify it and reach after a stereotyped form of masculinity. Robertson comments on this as "male weakness disguised as strength" (Robertson, 1984).

The parts

The national community can be regarded as consisting of three parts: the general population (the majority), the peace groups and the armed forces. This partition requires another nation identified as an enemy or a potential enemy, which is probably structured in the same way. To a degree there is psychodynamic co-operation between these parts as well as psychodynamic tension. In addition, there is psychological linking with the needed out-group, the enemy nation, a mutuality of projections that both need to make. I shall consider these divisions as four groups with a characteristic pattern of inter-group relations and describe these from the viewpoint of their defensive nature. In these descriptions I lean heavily on Jaques' outline sketch (Jaques, 1915).

The general population

The general population attributes evil aggressiveness to the enemy. In so doing they also mobilise a form of aggressiveness which feels 'good' in that it is opposed to the aggressiveness of the enemy. Thus there is a splitting of aggressiveness into good and bad components with a projection of the bad outside ourselves altogether and into the enemy. The good aggressiveness is not destructive and is retained within and identified with. Aggressiveness is also projected into the population by the enemy and is introjected, but is identified as the good non-destructive aggressiveness. Guilt is dealt with primarily by the repeated introjection of each other's assertions about the good nature of the aggressiveness.

The armed forces

The population does not necessarily retain the good aggressiveness for themselves. Most will project it into their armed forces, and identify with the servicemen. Some, however, will introject it and identify themselves with it by becoming servicemen. The forces, in turn, direct it towards the enemy, and the servicemen act out the good aggression of the population. The introjection by the military carries with it a quality derived from the scale of the projection from a whole nation. Thus the serviceman feels he contains the aggressiveness of the whole community, and may feel himself to be very powerful indeed, an illusory state which can lead to acts of special bravery. The small soldier with enormous power is typified in the myth of David and Goliath. In turn, the serviceman is supported in his view of his own aggression as non-destructive by introjecting the whole population's view. This greatly helps him to ward off any guilt over his aggressive acts. When it is sanctioned in such a massive way the population takes the place of his own conscience. The massiveness of the population 'inside him' makes him 'swell' with pride and bravery.

Dixon points out that the disposal of guilt is enhanced by the "vilification of the human", by which he means the requirement that the servicemen will suppress the normal responses of compassion and concern (Dixon, 1976). Dixon, like Robertson, links this with a hypertrophied and distorted idea of tough masculinity.

The fact that it is the military who do the acts contributes to the relief from guilt in the general population.

The peace groups

Another dynamic is at play to reduce guilt. The populace, in mobilising their aggressiveness, appear to lose some of their capacities for care and compassion. Where do their caring feelings go? Typically caring is projected into another group. Perhaps in earlier times it was into the church, but now it is into the supporters of the peace groups. They introject it, while also projecting their own aggressiveness into both the enemy and their own general population (and armed forces). The peace groups then represent the whole population's revulsion against war and are the receptacle for their guilt; and they are often persecuted as a token punishment (e.g. conscientious objectors in the First World War). For the social defence system, it is essential that the peace groups are a minority and weak—weak in the sense of sentimental and therefore slushy and unrealistic. The majority is seen as right. The denigrated 'caring' peace groups do not therefore threaten the mobilised aggressiveness which can then be guiltlessly idealised.

The peace groups introject these attributes with the same swelling pride and maybe sense of martyrdom. But in the process, they have themselves also denied the existence of large parts of their personalities by projecting their own aggressiveness into the general population. As a result they may seem both large (huge demonstrations) but weak and ineffective because they lack the assertiveness and punch that comes from 'good aggression'. They often espouse 'non-violent' political tactics, and may tolerate persecution as if guilty, a common fate of minority groups that society uses as receptacles for projections (Jaques, 1955). Some members of peace groups deal with the guilt in a characteristically masochistic way; by allowing themselves to be persecuted they can claim to put the majority of the population in the wrong and to discredit their violent aggression. They thus project guilt back into the population. In this instance the population do not, of course, introject the sense of guilt but gain confidence by viewing the submissiveness of these members of the peace groups as further evidence of the projected weakness and admission of guilt.

The illusion of survival

In a sense, all wars are 'holy' wars, because they depend on a projective arrangement of morally toned aggressiveness. Care and compassion are debased into sentimentality. The idealisation of the good aggressiveness is a most important element. Gathered together, the multiple projections of all the members of the population accumulate to give a sense of enormous power of the 'good aggression'. This can be inflated to omnipotence, and so create an illusion of being a match even for the horrendous destructiveness of the nightmare made real. This idealisation is indeed to give grounds for hope in ultimate survival, but it is hope grounded in a psychological illusion and not in realistic assessment.

The ability to retreat from the despair of unleashed aggression resides in the ability to repair its effects and to rescue survivors. Because the real capacity to care and protect has been debased, realistic hopes and protective measures cannot be properly mobilised. Illusory attitudes about survival are expressed in miserable symbolic gestures of providing shelters and post-war services and governmental organisation.

This illusory rallying behind unrealistic hope is seen by the peace groups as the weak point in the attitude of the general population. However, the provision for a post-holocaust future is made largely irrelevant by other dynamics. Most frequent is the denial that nuclear war could actually happen. The view may also be expressed that 'if the bomb does drop, I hope I will be right underneath it', which is denial by an illusory belief in instantaneous death.

The threat of nuclear war has not materialised over a prolonged period in terms of individual life-span. The four decades in which 'the bomb' has not been used is a reassurance to some people. There is also the advantage at the level of the unconscious that an obliterating destructiveness has been contained. This mitigates anxiety about the outbreak of the internal obliteration and destructiveness. Externalising the threat thus becomes reassuring internally. To retain this internal reassurance it is necessary for the external threat to continue so that it can go on giving the reassurance that it has never happened and therefore will not happen.

The illusion of survival based on omnipotence and the dependence on physical external reassurance militate strongly against the permanent disposal of the threat.

Hope and despair

Survival from the point of view of the peace groups is a different matter. Reacting to government propaganda on civil defence, some peace groups embrace a total view of the holocaust, without any survival chances. The complete loss of hope that this represents is counterpoised to the chirpy masculinism associated with the armed forces. This separation of hope and despair is a further dynamic within the social structure. Under the impact of these polarising projective mechanisms, one part of the nation experiences the despair for the whole while another part is released in an illusory state to pursue their grisly jobs.

The separation of these emotional responses, both of which in isolation are unrealistic, has consequences. The preaching of a passive doom may be transiently attractive to a frightened population, but in the long run it is immobilising of effective effort. Richards has noted more realistic responses in groups of students facing a post-nuclear future (Richards, 1984). Extracted from the public structuring of responses to the nuclear threat, these groups showed a less defeatist attack on the dour prospect, and could begin to plan some sort of appropriate resurgence of small scale social forms.

In contrast the military attitudes threaten a casual onrush towards the holocaust on the unrealistic basis that preparations for survival have been made.

The terrestrial boundary

The development of another boundary in the structural arrangements of the projective system follows from the possibility of really projecting warfare into outer space. Inflated rhetoric about 'star wars' is currently at a peak, based on the sense that the most awful thing is being given another twist to make it more awful. However, I suspect that there is an unconscious component in our society which makes for another anxiety in the imagined star wars. In Western culture outer space has been a childhood playground for phantasy and adventure in comics, television and films. It has been imaginatively populated by evil influences and sub- or -super-human monsters. Much of our nightmare world is placed beyond normal reach amongst the stars. However, the planned development of the nuclear threat into space brings this externalised threat into contact with the internal world. It suggests the imminent breakdown of the defensive function of externalisation and brings the nuclear threat right back into one's internal world again.

Conclusions

I have tried to detail the psychodynamics of individuals in a collective unconscious system typical of a nation at war or preparing for it. I have also tried to emphasise certain aspects which are unique to the nuclear threat. The importance of these dynamics is that, being unconscious, they are a serious hindrance to the normal methods of overcoming social problems.

The inter-group dynamics of society are as important as the individual dynamics, as very often the individual is not free to escape from the introjected attitudes he is required to adopt in his place in society. This is typified by the now often mentioned phenomenon of top generals who have promoted the cold war and the nuclear attitude, but who adopt quite different sets of attitudes soon after their retirement. We can understand this as the effect on them of amassed projections of illusory good aggressiveness only while they were in the armed forces.

These kinds of inter-group phenomena are of major importance. For instance it is possible that the activities of some peace groups merely feed into the overall dynamic pattern which supports the continuance of the cold war and its risks.

The inter-group dynamics are driven by a defensive function needed to evade the experiencing of the common threat. The long-term amelioration of the problem requires a reduced need to evade the anxiety, and hence less emotional defensiveness and less recourse to the polarising projections of war. The curious situation arises (which perhaps psychotherapists alone understand) that the more people can picture the nature of the nuclear threat in all its horrific aspects, the more the threat will retreat.

Robert Jay Lifton actively promotes the idea that one effective way for psychotherapists to go about contributing to reduce the nuclear threat is to raise social consciousness of the fear that we all have about it (Lifton, 1985).

If political activity of the traditional kind will not succeed and we resort to becoming 'psychotherapists of society', we clearly have more to do than raise awareness of the fears and impulses in our own patients. We have to consider the possibility of working on a larger scale. The social containment of anxiety is a little-understood feature of society, even by psychotherapists, and we have to consider the daunting prospect of changing the dynamic system.

Note

1. Introjection refers to a psychological experience of acquiring something internal from outside the individual, cognitive or emotive. Supportive

or reassuring comments from another person can be retained and remembered subsequently, with the accompanying sense of warmth and security as if the support continues to be actively given internally. Of course critical attitudes from others may give rise internally to uncomfortable self-criticism. This process produces, amongst other things, the conscience or super-ego.

CHAPTER SEVENTEEN

Silence is the real crime[1]

Hanna Segal

When we look soberly, however hard it is to do so at the moment, at the political situation and the threat of nuclear warfare, we observe a phenomenon that is more like a surrealist scenario, an unbearable nightmare or a psychosis, than a sane world. The Hiroshima bomb killed at one go 140,000 people and that does not include the many thousands who died from the after effects or the zombie-like existence of the survivors so vividly described by R. J. Lifton in his studies (1982). "But today, on average, each major city in the northern hemisphere is targeted by the equivalent of 2,000 Hiroshima bombs" (Barnaby, 1983).

The nuclear arsenal of either Russia or America is enough to blow up the world many times over. And still they both continue to develop and stockpile nuclear weapons and contend that this is needed for security. The foreseeable effects of what is genteelly known as nuclear exchange between Russia and America are well studied and documented by scientists. The medical evidence is that there will be no meaningful survival. There is growing scientific evidence that the exploding of only part of that arsenal will bring about a nuclear winter which will engulf all the northern hemisphere, if not the whole planet. These facts are constantly put before the public. Nevertheless the urgency of the threat to human survival does not seem to have led to a concerted effort to stop what is happening. Indeed, the way things are going, it seems likely that a nuclear war may be an inevitable consequence.

Many take the view, especially in governmental circles, that the threat to the human race posed by nuclear weapons is minimised by mutual deterrence that is maintained by remaining vigilant, well-armed, and technologically active. In a world of changing technology, this means constant research and upgrading of weapons and more and more powerful and destructive systems: the nuclear arms race. At the moment we are seeing this extended into space: Star Wars, a method of trying to prevent one's opponent having a deterrent capacity, one could say. I believe, contrary to the prevailing governmental view, that the arms race and the theory of deterrence that supports and justifies it is actually dangerous. Psychoanalytic understanding can help us to see that the theory of deterrence and its current practice may actually lead to our destruction. It is this argument I want to develop and explain in this paper as part of a plea to psychoanalysts to participate urgently in active efforts to halt what I consider a mad process.

The theory of deterrence as propounded by governments implies that it is the existence of nuclear weapons that has insured peace so far and will do so in the future. "They are too terrible", it is said, "nobody would be mad enough to use them". And yet the papers made available in England under the Thirty-Year Rule reveal that in 1954 the allies seriously considered dropping atomic bombs on China (*The Guardian*, 9.1.85). The report of a military conference of the Chiefs of Staff from the U.S., Britain, France, Australia and New Zealand says: "Should war with China be precipitated by Chinese Communist aggression in South-East Asia, air attack should be launched immediately, aimed at military targets. In the selection of these targets political considerations cannot be ignored. To achieve the maximum and lasting effect, nuclear as well as conventional weapons should be used from the outset." (*The Guardian*, 8.1.85). No papers are available to know whether or not the USSR may have been planning in the same way.

The idea of deterrence is to be stronger so as to frighten the enemy—to deter him from aggression. As the 1950 U.S. National Security Document NSC 68 states: "The only deterrent we can present to the Kremlin is evidence we give that we may make any of the critical points in the world which we cannot hold the occasion for a global war of annihilation". But the enemy's reasoning is likely to be the same. Hence, the doctrine inevitable leads to escalating anxiety and to the arms race. The nuclear arms race is the heir to the nuclear deterrence. The 'defensive' preparations to counter aggression in which both sides in an arms race engage must create unstable fear. The sort of thing that takes place has been described in a chilling statement by a former U.S. Secretary of Defence, Robert MacNamara. Commenting in 1982 about the defence policy of the 1960s he said: "... [by 1962] the advantage in the US warhead inventory was so great *vis-à-vis* the Soviets that the Air Force was saying that they felt we had a first-strike capability and could, and should, continue to have one. If the Air Force thought that, imagine what the Soviets thought ..." and "... Read again the memo to President Kennedy. It scares me today to even read the damn thing. What that means is the Air Force supported the development of US forces sufficiently large to destroy so much of the Soviet nuclear force, by a first strike, that there would not be enough left to cause us any concern if they shot at us. My God! If the Soviets thought that was our objective, how would you expect them to react? The way they reacted was by substantially expanding their strategic nuclear weapons programme." (His implication is—we were rather lucky; they might have reacted by a pre-emptive strike.) Preparing for war on both sides promotes the likelihood of a pre-emptive strike out of fear and the equilibrium of a system of mutual deterrence is inherently unstable. Hatred leads to fear and fear to hatred in an ever-increasing vicious circle. We are like lemmings, pursuing a path to racial suicide, blind to what we are doing.

Psychoanalysis is very familiar with vicious circles of hatred and fear. It teaches us that in an individual, destructive and self-destructive drives can only be modified when the individual can get some insight into his motives and visualise the consequences to others and to himself of his action. But we know that powerful defences operate against such insights. I suggest that there is some evidence that such resistances to knowing are active in our public life. For instance, there is a reluctance to visualise the actual consequences of a nuclear war. We hear now that the use of nuclear weapons can be strategic or minimal. At the same time, there is some evidence that the governments do not clearly visualise the consequences of nuclear war. The civil defence plans, at least in England, are a case in point. When the British Medical Association was asked by the government to prepare a report on civil defence, the report said that there could be no meaningful preparation, since after a nuclear blast, there would be no communications, probably no doctors or nurses and no edible food. The British Government's response was to try to suppress this report. Again, in November 1984, SANA (Scientists Against Nuclear Arms) organised scientific seminars, attended by prominent scientists, about the theory of a nuclear winter. They invited, amongst others, representatives of the Home Office. The Home Office spokesman replied that they knew nothing about the theory of nuclear winter and were not interested in the invitation. So governments both envisage a nuclear war and deny the reality of what it would entail.

This attitude involves the operation of denial. Close to denial, but not identical to it, is the turning of a blind eye. I think the mechanism here is of a particular form of splitting (described by Freud as disavowal, operating in perversions). In this split we retain intellectual knowledge of the reality, but divest it of emotional meaning. An example in public life is the fact that various opinion polls have revealed that the vast majority of people think that nuclear war is inevitable, and that probably there will be no survival. And yet the same vast majority live their lives in that shadow without taking active steps to change policy.

We wish to deny the consequences of our actions to others and to ourselves, and to deny any aggressive impulses or actions on our own part. Increases in armaments are often kept secret. Here the British Cabinet papers of the fifties are again revealing. When Attlee started manufacturing the A bomb it was in secret, not only from Parliament, but even from members of his own Cabinet. Similarly, when the Churchill government undertook the manufacturing of the H-bomb, they avoided the substantial opposition they anticipated. The Cabinet Committee responsible disguised the extent of the atomic programme by hiding the cost under 'other current expenditure' and 'extra-mural research'. Similarly, neither the public nor Parliament was ever informed of the contemplated use of atomic bombs against China, which I mentioned earlier. The hallowed word is security, but the secrecy, as those Cabinet notes make clear, is hardly motivated by having to hide from the enemy. Sooner or later the powers know all about one another's research. A note prepared for the Cabinet Committee said that the publicity could damage the West's defence interests, not because the Russians might learn something new, but because of the effect on public opinion. In dictatorial regimes like the USSR, this secrecy is built into the regime.

When our own aggressiveness can be disguised and hidden from us 'for security reasons', projective mechanisms and subsequent paranoia are increased. The enemy is presented as the devil. Mrs Thatcher speaks of the Russians as our hereditary enemy, yet since the Crimean War in 1854 the Russians have been Britain's allies in two world wars. President Reagan speaks of the Russians as the evil empire.

The reactions to the shooting of the Korean airliner in 1984 illustrates the same splitting and projection. Ronald Reagan, in an interview with Robert Scheer, said: "We have a different regard for life than those monsters do. They are godless. It is this theological defect that gives them less regard for humanity or human beings". By contrast, when a couple of years before, the Israelis shot down a civilian Libyan plane in exactly the same circumstances, both the American and British governments defended it as unavoidably necessary to protect secret military installations. I suppose the Russians cried 'inhuman beasts' at that time. Gradually each side creates a picture of the others as bloodthirsty, evil monsters beyond the pale. To hide our own aggressive desires we have to project the evil into an enemy—real or imaginary—he must appear an inhuman monster.

In genocide another element is added—that of contempt. The victim of genocide must be presented as not only inhuman, but as subhuman. As far back as the Middle Ages some crusaders used to roast and eat Arabs as a demonstration that Arabs were not to be seen as human. The Nazis called the Jews 'Untermensch'—subhuman. The American soldiers called the Vietnamese 'Gooks'. In the last war the Japanese called the Americans 'white devils'—inhuman monsters. But when they exercised utmost cruelty by practising vivisection on their prisoners, they called them 'logs'—totally unhuman, not even animal. To maintain a sufficient degree of paranoia and to deny the consequences to ourselves, we may have to dehumanise ourselves. In McNamara's memorandum to President Kennedy, he states that the Air Force considers the loss of 50 million American lives, in case of a Russian counter-strike to the first strike, to be acceptable.

This kind of functioning has been described in the individual as a regression from the depressive position, characterised by a capacity to recognise one's own aggression, and to experience guilt and mourning, and a capacity both to function in reality and to make reparation. The regression is to the paranoid/schizoid position, characterised by the operation of denial, splitting and projection. I am speaking here of mechanisms familiar in the individual (Klein, 1946, 1948b). It could be argued that we cannot transfer such knowledge directly to large group behaviour. Nevertheless, such mechanisms can be seen in group behaviour. Fornari (1975) has described wars as a paranoid defence against depressive anxiety. Indeed, in groups such mechanisms may be increased.

Psychoanalytic insight can throw important light on group behaviour. Co-operative groups were, as Freud pointed out in 'Civilisation and its Discontents' (1930a), formed not only to combat forces of nature, but also to combat psychological dangers—primarily to bind the destructiveness of man against man. He commented that we can love one another in a group provided there are outsiders whom we can hate. Subsequently, a school of psychoanalytical thinking about the behaviour of groups elaborated the related idea that groups also bind and contain psychotic phantasies, anxieties and defences (Bion, 1952; Jaques, 1965; Menzies, 1970).

Groups can have features which, if present and acted on in an individual, would qualify him as mad or psychotic. Groups are usually narcissistic, self idealising, paranoid in relation to other groups. Conflict within the group and guilt about aggression can be dealt with by projection on to an outside group. In our private lives we have to contend with a superego which puts a check on destructiveness. If we vest the individual superego in a joint group superego, we can apparently guiltlessly perpetrate horrors which we couldn't bear in our individual existence. I think that the degree of dehumanisation we encounter in such group practices as genocide, we would see in an individual only in the psychotic or the criminal psychopath. When such mechanisms get out of hand, the groups, instead of containing psychotic functioning, put it into practice and we get such irrational behaviour as wars and genocide. A perfect example of such irrational war was the 1914–1918 war. Lloyd George said: "We muddled into it". According to numbers of historians the arms race was a significant, if not the most important factor, in this 'muddle' (Taylor, 1963).

According to Bion, a group may have the features of a 'work group' which is reality oriented, and features of a 'basic assumption group'. When the work group predominates we get a reality-oriented attitude (like Freud's idea that we form groups to combat the forces of nature). It also realistically contains and modifies the psychotic elements (basic assumption). But in situations of excessive anxiety, the basic assumption type of group dominates. And the group can then behave in a destructive and self-destructive way which, in an individual, would be psychotic. Russell (1940) speaks of the loyalty to the state as having positive and negative motives: "There is an element which is connected with love of home and family". But he says later: "No other organisation arouses anything like the loyalty aroused by the national state. And the chief activity of the state is the preparation for large-scale homicide. It is loyalty to this organisation for death that causes man to endure the totalitarian state and to risk the destruction of home and children and our whole civilisation." Groups can hold views which in an individual could be named mad. A particularly worrying example of this group phenomenon in our time are the views of the Born Again Christians. They actually look forward to a nuclear war as Armageddon, which will cleanse the earth from evil, represented by Soviet Russia. The magazine Family Weekly noted that many believe that the social order is collapsing, with Armageddon just around the corner. However, the approach of Armageddon should not be a cause for fear, but for real hope! Why? Because Armageddon is God's war to cleanse the earth of all wickedness, paving the way for a bright, prosperous new order! The Bible explains that the righteous "will possess the earth, and they will indeed find their exquisite delight in the abundance of peace" (Psalm 37:1 1). With bad conditions forever gone, every day of life then will be a delight. Not even sickness or death will mar the happiness of the people. God will "wipe out every tear from their eyes, and death will be no more, neither will mourning nor outcry nor pain be any more" (Revelations 21:4, cited in *Circular* from Jehovah's Witnesses, 1982).

It is astonishing that some of the leaders of the Western world seem at least partly to share those religious views:

> I do not know how many future generations we can count on before the Lord returns. [James Watt, US Secretary of State for the Interior, Franklin, 1982]

> Jerry, I sometimes believe we're heading very fast for Armageddon right now. [President Reagan, Franklin, 1982]

> I have read the Book of Revelation and, yes, I believe the world is going to end-by an act of God, I hope—but every day I think that time is running out ... I think of World War II and how long it took to prepare for it, to convince people that rearmament for war is needed. I fear we will not be ready. I think time is running out ... but I have faith. [Caspar Weinberger, US Secretary of Defence; Interview, *New York Times*, 23 August 1982]

A report in the British newspaper, *The Guardian*, estimates that 35,000,000 Americans are registered as Born Again Christians. I am not implying here that 35 million Americans, are mad. I don't know how many Mohammedans believe that if they die in a Holy War they will go straight to heaven. As individuals they are not all mad. But it is in the nature of groups that they can maintain corporately such mad beliefs.

In this situation leaders are very important. We like to trust them. That's part of feeling safe in a group. But according to Bion, when the basic assumption, a psychotic constellation of impulses, phantasies and defences, dominates, the group throws up leaders which best represent that psychotic element. Hitler would be the outstanding example. There is also some evidence that Stalin was openly psychotic towards the end of his life, etc.

As I see it, we now live in a world situation producing great anxiety and defences against it, which, because of the very existence of atomic weapons and the arms race, are massively increased. For the first time humanity has in reality the power of complete annihilation and self annihilation. Glover wrote in 1933: "The first promise of the atomic age is that it can make some of our nightmares come true. The capacity so painfully acquired by normal man to distinguish between sleep, hallucination, delusion and the objective reality of wakened life has for the first time in history been seriously weakened." In this not quite sane situation, the lure of omnipotence is increased and so is the lure of death. I speak of the lure of death because, in my view, beliefs such as are held by Born Again Christians, and similar groups, reveal almost nakedly the death instinct—the welcoming of Armageddon, idealised as the will of God and a prelude to eternal bliss. Universal death is seen as universal salvation—the aspect of Nirvana of the death instinct, as described by Freud. In this situation of a reactivation of the death instinct, and seeing its possible final embodiment in the prospect of atomic war, we are, I believe pushed into what I would call the world of the schizophrenic.

I think the existence of atomic weapons mobilises and actualises this world of the schizophrenic. The obliteration of boundaries between reality and phantasy, as described by Glover, characterises psychosis. Omnipotence has become real, but only omnipotent destruction. We can, at the push of a button, annihilate the world. In this world of primitive omnipotence, the problem is not of death wishes and a fear of death which pertain to the depressive and Oedipal world, it is governed by wishes for annihilation of the self and the world, and the terrors associated with them.

Lifton (1982) makes the point, very convincing to me, that atomic annihilation destroys the possibility of symbolic survival. In natural death or even in conventional war, men die, or at least those who have acquired some maturity die, with some conviction of symbolic survival in their children, grandchildren, in their work or in the civilisation itself of which they were part. Coming to terms with the prospect of one's own personal death is a necessary step in maturation and in giving full meaning to life (Jaques, 1965; Segal, 1952, 1958). The existence of nuclear weapons and the prospect of nuclear war makes difficult a growing acceptance of death and symbolic survival. The prospect of death in atomic warfare leaves an unimaginable void and produces terror of a different kind. Those of us who work with psychotics get an inkling of this kind of terror. In normal development, as Freud has described, and Klein elaborated further, Eros, the life forces, succeed in integrating and taming destructive and self destructive drives and convert them into life-promoting aggression.

In the depths of our unconscious, however, such unintegrated wishes and terrors still exist. We are all only partly sane and such circumstances as prevail now mobilise the most primitive parts of ourselves. Einstein had said that with the advent of atomic power, everything has changed except our way of thinking. And in a way he is, of course, right. It has not changed it for the better. We have not come to realise that the advent of the atomic weapons made meaningless the idea of a just war, or the defence of civic values, since the war would destroy all values. It has not changed our thinking in the direction of realising that our national, racial, religious or political narcissisms are not only paltry, but lethal, and that our concern should be with the survival of the human race. But, I am afraid that the atomic bomb may have changed our thinking for the worse.

Confronted with the real terror of annihilation, our schizoid defences are increased denial 'It won't happen, or it won't be that bad'—the turning of a blind eye, splitting and projection are increased. There is also a regression to part object relationships, which exclude empathy, compassion and concern. The distortion of language, present in all wars, has reached an Orwellian degree of absurdity in the terms used to describe nuclear warfare—Nukespeak. The code signal for the dropping of the bomb on Hiroshima was 'Baby is Born'. The bomb itself was called 'Little Boy'. The bomb thrown on Nagasaki was called 'Fat Man'. Recently, nuclear has become 'Nuke'. All these words cover up the utter destructiveness of what is being done and make it sound manageable, unaggressive, even cute. At the height of the Falklands conflict some youngsters in England wore T-shirts showing 'Nuke Buenos Aires'. I doubt if those same youngsters would wear a badge saying 'Annihilate several million people'. To 'Nuke' sounds so innocent. Even 'nuclear exchange', often discussed, hides the lethal nature of the exchange.

The worst linguistic deception is perhaps the word deterrence itself. Over the years it has completely changed its meaning. The first idea of deterrence was that the Americans had the A bomb and could use it to deter Russia from invading Europe. Soon, of course, the Russians had the bomb as well, and deterrence changed its meaning. It became, to deter the other party from the use of nuclear weapons. This seemed to make some sense. Since the bomb was dropped by a country possessing the bomb on a country which did not, it made some kind of sense to think that if the big powers were both armed, each would deter the other from the nuclear initiative. Even at the time, the reasoning was not very sound on how to prevent other countries acquiring nuclear weapons, how to maintain a balance of terror as a basis for co-existence, since such balance of terror would inevitably increase the paranoia. With the increasing arms race, the system came to be known as MAD (Mutual Assured Destruction).

Then in the last few years, deterrence changed its meaning again. It became, more like the original meaning, threatening the use of atomic weapons should Russia be in any conflict with her neighbours seen as a threat to the U.S.A. This change in America became more explicit in the 1960s and 70s. That's when we started hearing that nuclear war could be won—that we must start to think of 'a rational nuclear war'. "The U.S. must possess the ability to wage nuclear war rationally" (A U.S. Defence Advisor, 1982). Again, distortions of language are used to hide a change from a purely defensive to an aggressive warfare. The notion of a 'flexible response' was introduced; another attractive phrase invented to cover this change from a defensive to an aggressive posture. Flexible response means that in the case of a conventional conflict between Russia and her neighbours, so-called strategic nuclear weapons would be used. In 1981, in an interview in the *Daily Telegraph*, Mr Weinberger, U.S. Defence Secretary, said: "The simple fact of the matter is that, unfortunate and awful as it would be for the world, it is possible that with nuclear weapons, there can be some use of them in a limited, or in connection with what is up to that time a war solely within the European theatre." The confused English does not disguise the meaning. But how limited is limited? 'Little Boy' dropped on Hiroshima had a yield of about 13 kilotons, but the modern Polaris has a yield of 60 kilotons; the Cruise Missile of 200 kilotons. How many Hiroshimas for a little strategic limited war in Europe. Unsurprisingly, the Europeans didn't relish the idea.

The term Strategic Defence Initiative (SDI), to describe the latest escalation of the arms race, sounds fine. It is defensive, not offensive. But it conceals the fact that a fool-proof defence would put the side which had it in an incontestable first strike position. In fact, Henry Kissinger argues that if America could be fully protected by the Strategic Defence Initiative "that would be in the European interest, because it would increase our willingness to use nuclear weapons in Europe's defence" (Kissinger in an interview for Stern Magazine). Such a stand would inevitably lead the Russians in turn to increase their offensive arsenal—a new hotting up of the arms race. The alternative term 'Star Wars' is even more misleading. It has a heroic science fiction sound. It conjures up the picture of a war amongst the stars—not affecting the earth.

All this Nukespeak is a distortion of language to disguise from ourselves and others both the full horror of a nuclear war and our own part in making it possible or more likely. Everything is presented as defensive by both super powers. One's own destructive wishes and activities are always blamed on the others. Fragmentation, characteristic of this schizophrenic process, has increased with the nuclear arms race. In particular, there is a fragmentation of responsibility—with a resulting lack of clear accountability. One consequence is that the military industrial complex increasingly acquires its own dynamic. There is a view that dropping of the bomb on Hiroshima, and particularly on Nagasaki when Japan was already disintegrating, was pushed by the military wishing to test a new weapon. According to the Oxford Research Group (1986), the nuclear weapons policy is "at best a post rationalisation for the development of the weapon systems whose raison d'être has become institutionalised".

This is particularly so in the case of nuclear weapons which take up to twenty years to develop. The Government is not accountable, as it has inherited tentative decisions on research taken years ago which have now acquired their own momentum. The contracts the Europeans are making now for the SDI will be hard to reverse, should the government's policy change. They contain provision for quite swingeing compensation in the event of cancellation. The expenditure on nuclear weapons apparently is not accounted for in any way. For instance, the development of the Chevaline Warhead for Polaris was carried on through four changes of government and completion in the early 1980s with no public debate, and the first mention of Chevaline in Parliament was by Defence Secretary Pym in 1980. The overall estimated cost of the programme was then £1,000 million. It had originally been estimated at £7.5 million. According to the Oxford Research Group, in the West, the least degree of accountability to Parliament, or even to government, is in Great Britain. But their research in five countries comes to the conclusion that the situation is very similar in other countries. We could be led to believe that the position is different in Soviet Russia and that the Politburo has absolute power. But according to the Oxford Research Group, the situation there is practically the same. Galbraith, in a number of his works, shows the structural similarities of the capitalist and Soviet system:

> Q: Does the technological structure have a similar existence in both public and private corporations? A: Oh, yes. And in both, it requires independence. As I have said, the technological structure cannot suffer the uninformed intrusion of either stockholders or politicians. [Galbraith & Salinger, 1981]

So we have a near autonomous existence of continuing increase and proliferation of nuclear weapons.

There is also fragmentation and lack of accountability in the provisions for using nuclear weapons. In an extremely important American book, *The Command and Control of Nuclear Forces*, Paul Bracken (1984) describes such fragmentation of command centres, that should an atomic war happen, and should there be survivors, it would be impossible to trace who had started it. This fragmentation is also in evidence in a minor way in non-nuclear conflicts now. Who gave the order to sink the Belgrano—and on what information? The Government says the commanders in the field must decide. The commanders say they had Government orders. Similarly, the Russians could never trace satisfactorily who bears responsibility for the shooting of the Korean plane.

Another aspect of fragmentation and lack of accountability is evidenced in the spread of nuclear weapons, which I think now concerns America and Russia. The split-off fragments of their nuclear know-how and material are now spread throughout the world and out of their control. Any of those fragments may start a general flare up.

The growth of technology is also used for a typically schizoid dehumanisation and mechanisation. There is a kind of prevailing depersonalisation and de-realisation. Pushing a button to annihilate parts of the world we have never seen is a mechanised split off activity. Bracken contends that the war is likely to happen through our machines getting out of control. Everything is so automated that over-sensitive machines could start an unstoppable nuclear exchange. The MIT computer expert, Joseph Weizenbaum, comes to the similar conclusion: that modern big computers are so complicated that no expert can see through and control them. The whole nuclear early warning system is based on these machines—perhaps the worst danger if the paranoid international tensions reach a high level. Since one effect of nuclear explosion is a disturbance in communication systems, it might not be in the powers of governments to stop an escalation even if they wish to. But the fact that we can even think that 'machines will start the war, not us' shows the extent of the denial of our responsibility. We seem to live in a peculiar combination of helplessness and terror and omnipotence—the helplessness and omnipotence increasing each in a vicious circle. This helplessness which lies at the root of our apathy is partly inevitable. We are faced with a horrifyingly threatening danger. But partly it is self-induced and becomes a self-fulfilling prophecy. Confronted with the terror of the powers of destructiveness, we divest ourselves from our responsibilities by denial, projection and fragmentation.

The responsibility is fragmented and projected further and further away—into governments, army, scientists, and finally, into machines beyond human control. We don't only project into our so-called enemies. We also divest ourselves from our responsibilities by projecting them into governments. They in turn can't bear such responsibility and they project into us, the people, public opinion, etc., as well as fragmenting their responsibility, as described above. When we project into governments, we become truly helpless. We are in their hands. Then we can either become paranoid about the government's or Reagan's doing, or Thatcher's, or the Kremlin's. Or, we idealise our governments and leave the responsibilities in their hands—they are the experts. And then we make ourselves truly helpless. And the governments offer us the escape of megalomania. We like to feel big and powerful and think we can frighten our enemy. But we forget how dangerous a frightened enemy can be. (McNamara)

If all that is a result of unbound, split-off, and denied operation of what Freud called the death instinct, does it make it hopeless? I do not think so. In the individual analyses of patients we find that the hopeless situations are due not solely to the power of the instincts, but largely to the vicious circles between impulses and defences. In normal development, self-preservation and love (Eros) can integrate the death instinct and turn it into useful life-promoting aggression. But in situations of acute anxiety, vicious circles between the death instincts and the defences against it preclude such integration.

The fateful question for the human species seems to me to be whether and to what extent their cultural development will succeed in mastering the disturbance of their communal life by the human instinct of aggression and self-destruction. It may be that in this respect precisely the present time deserves a special interest. Men have gained control over the forces of nature to such an extent that with their help they would have no difficulty in exterminating one another to the last man. They know this, and hence comes a large part of their current unrest, their unhappiness and their mood of anxiety. And now it is to be expected that the other of the two 'Heavenly Powers', eternal Eros, will make an effort to assert himself in the struggle with his equally immortal adversary. But who can foresee with what success and with what result? (Freud, 1930a, p. 145).

This was written in 1930 (with the last sentence added in 1931). It is more than ever applicable today. We are at a cross-roads. We must try to find means to mobilise out life forces against the destructive powers. To do that we must confront those powers and dangers without denial, hoping that the realisation of what we are about to do to ourselves will mobilise our life forces and our reality sense.

What role can we, as analysts, play in this tragic drama? I think first we must look into ourselves and beware of turning a blind eye to reality. We are like other humans with the same destructive and self-destructive drives. We use the same defences. We are prone to the same denials and, moreover, we can hide behind the shield of psychoanalytic neutrality. We know that, as psychoanalysts, we should be neutral and, for instance, not take part in political debates as psychoanalysts, whatever our own political convictions, which we can pursue as individuals. But there are situations in which such an attitude can also become a shield of denial. To be acquainted with facts and recognise psychic facts, which we of all people know something about, and to have the courage to try to state them clearly, is in fact the psychoanalytic stand. We must face our fears and mobilise our forces against destruction. And we must be heard.

There has been a change in the nature of the movement opposed to the nuclear arms race. Today it is largely led by informed opinion. I do not mean to imply that all informed opinion is necessarily part of that movement, but that in the forefront of the movement opposing nuclear weapons are doctors, scientists, historians, teachers, lawyers —all those used to looking objectively at facts. There are some signs that the clear message is beginning to get through a little. We belong with them. We are also scientists—looking at psychic facts. We must add our voice clearly to their voices.

Secondly; I think we have a specific contribution to make. We are cognisant with the psychic mechanisms of denial, projection, magic thinking, etc. We should be able to contribute something to the overcoming of apathy and self-deception in ourselves and others. When the Nazi phenomenon was staring us in the face, the psychoanalytic community outside Germany was largely silent. This must not be repeated. Nadejda Mandelstam said: "Silence is the real crime against humanity" (1971).

We psychoanalysts who believe in the power of words and the therapeutic effect of verbalising truth must not be silent.

Postscript

Perestroika, The Gulf War and 11 September 2002 [2001]

September 11 2002 [2001] was a major trauma, which had powerful repercussions, particularly for the Western world. Why was this so when we consider that there had been other human disasters in the world quite recently, costing hundreds of thousands of lives—in Bosnia, Rwanda and other places? Of course, the massive attack was an enormous assault on the Western feeling of security, like the destruction of one's family and home but the trauma of a terrorist attack has an additional factor. The crushing realisation that there is someone out there who actually hates you to the point of annihilation and the bewilderment it causes. 'Why me?' One of President Bush's first reactions was to cry out, "Why us? We are good people." But there is another factor specific to the attack of

September 11th and that is the symbolism of the Twin Towers and the Pentagon. 'We are all powerful with our weapons, finance, hi-tech—we can dominate you completely.' And the suicide bombers sent an equally omnipotent statement: 'I with my little pen knife can puncture your high-flying balloons and annihilate you.' Thus we are pushed into a world of terror vs. terror, disintegration and confusion. It awakened our most primitive fears for ourselves, the group we belong to and for the world. It is the deepest fear of a disturbed infant and a schizophrenic. I said that bewilderment is an important element in it. When I saw it happening I participated in it. What has happened to us? And yet soon after the immediate shock I had another feeling. I felt something very familiar. It seemed to me like 'Chronicles of a Death Foretold'.

This is one of the reasons for this Postscript. This need not have been a bolt out of the blue. I want to show in this Postscript that the psychoanalytic approach did, in fact, predict with great accuracy the almost inevitability of the Gulf War and showed the dangers that followed from our reaction to it. I do not claim that we were Cassandra-like prophets predicting disasters but we were able to detect certain trends in the development of our socio-political group functioning and the dangers that they implied. I also want to emphasise in this Postscript the dangers of not learning from experience. Not learning from experience is an important component of psychotic functioning. People who don't know their history are bound to repeat it. But it is not only a matter of remembering but of understanding. We are only too apt to remember our grudges. But learning from experience is linked with understanding it and the psychoanalytic approach can throw some important understanding on our experience. My 1985 paper was an inaugural paper of International Psychoanalysts Against Nuclear Weapons and since then numerous papers have appeared on the international scene, trying to follow and understand the developing patterns. Because the pattern has changed since 1985.

I shall give here a brief overview of my paper 'From Hiroshima to the Gulf War and After' which summarises some of our views.

The MAD system had been undermined by perestroika. The paranoid structure could no longer be maintained. We lost the enemy. Perestroika was a time of hope, a possibility of change of attitude. But it was also a time of possible new dangers and a search for a new enemy. Giving evidence to the House Services Committee in December 1990, Edward Heath said:

> Having got rid of the Cold War, we are now discussing ways in which NATO can be urged to rush to another part of the world in which there looks like being a problem, and saying, 'Right, you must just put it right; we don't like those people; or they don't behave as we do; and so on; and so we are going to deal with it'.

NATO went in search of a new enemy to justify its continued military power.

George Kennan was shocked to discover, when he was visiting Western capitals, that despite the disappearance of the supposed Soviet threat, our apparent reason for keeping a nuclear arsenal, the Western countries could not even conceive of nuclear disarmament, a world without the atom bomb. It was, he said, like an addiction. And though apparently much had changed with perestroika, one thing had not changed. Nuclear fire-power was constantly increasing, in so-called modernisation.

So what was going on? We are familiar with those moments of hope clinically when a paranoid patient begins to give up his delusions, or when an addict begins to give up the drug and get better. The improvement is genuine. But as they get better they have to face reality. With the diminishing of omnipotence they have to face their dependence, their feelings of helplessness, and the fact that they are ill. With the withdrawal of projections they have to face their own destructiveness, their inner conflicts and guilt: they have to face their internal realities. Moreover, they often have to face very real losses and damage brought about by their illness, in external reality. And formidable manic defences can be mobilised in defence against this depressive pain, with a revival of megalomania and, in its wake, a return of paranoia. Similarly, in the social domain, when we stopped believing in the Evil Empire we had to turn to our internal problems. We had to face our social problems: economic decline, unemployment. And, in particular, we had to face the waste of our resources on an unnecessary arms race, the guilt about the Third World and about unnecessary wars. The guilt and shame of Vietnam had to be wiped out.

Faced with that possibility of confronting our inner realities, we turned to manic defences: triumphalism. Perestroika was claimed to be the triumph of our superior system and power. Our nuclear mentality did not change. The megalomaniac search for power, noticed by Heath, and the addiction to the bomb, noted by Kennan, was bound to create new enemies to replace Soviet Russia. Firstly, because in fact it creates new enemies; and, secondly, because we need a new Evil Empire to justify our arrogant aggression and project into a new Evil Empire. In some ways the danger was increased by the proliferation of nuclear weapons after the collapse of the Soviet Union and the intensification of war by proxy. Afghanistan is a good example. Numerous schools of terrorism were spread around the world by both but more so by America, the USSR being very much in decline.

I and my colleagues of the IPANW, in a number of mostly unpublished papers presented to various audiences, warned about the dangers inherent in the post-perestroika situation. But numbness and apathy had set in. Anti-nuclear war organisations lost much of their membership. Public meetings were poorly attended. There was a feeling of great relief and a wish to believe that all was well now—and increasing denial of the dangers that were still there. Specifically, we warned that unless attitudes to the whole problem changed we were in danger of finding a new enemy. We did not think of Saddam Hussein, who at that time was the pet of both East and West, busily being armed by them; but in some ways he was very appropriate, since he was in a similar position. He too had lost an enemy, Iran, and probably had to face inner socio-economic tensions. And then the Gulf War confirmed our predictions: not, perhaps, our worst predictions of a nuclear escalation, but certainly the prediction of an unnecessary and devastating war.

Was that war well based and necessary? What were the reasons given to us? They were dubious. The first casualty, not only of war, but of preparation for war, is the truth. The reasons given were phoney. That Iraq had broken international law by invading Kuwait was one. But it had been breaking international law by invading Iran for years with the West's support. Another was that we went to war for the defence of human rights because of the terrorist Hussein government. But we did not raise an eyebrow at his genocide of Kurds. Nukespeak reigned.

Another reason given was for our legitimate interests in oil. That is a bit nearer the truth. In the Fifties, for instance, Selwyn Lloyd reported: "We agreed that at all costs these oil fields must be kept in Western hands". But even that is not entirely correct. The American concern was not so much the accessibility or price of oil as the financial dependence on the Gulf States.

None of the supposed causes of the War are convincing if one looks at them rationally. So what were the real reasons? Actually, I think I have grounds for believing that the deepest causes had unconscious psychological roots. I think that war was the inevitable result of the mental constellation established after perestroika. We needed an enemy to project evil onto and we wanted a new Evil Empire. And Saddam Hussein provided an ideal enemy. He challenged our triumphalism and this was intolerable. Our power and our righteousness had to be re-established.

The Gulf War was an unmitigated human disaster. Hundreds of thousands of victims and the devastation of the whole area. And except for protecting our rights in Kuwait it achieved nothing. Saddam Hussein is still in power and Iraq still subject to daily bombing. Triumphalism became naked. The bombardment from the sky of a retreating, demoralised army (mainly Kurds forced into it) and then bulldozing the survivors was described as 'a Turkey Shoot'. And yet, it was presented as a great and bloodless victory. Have we learned anything from this experience? Not much. Listening to some of President Bush's and Bin Laden's broadcasts I hear an echo of the exchanges between Bush Senior and Saddam Hussein. Kissinger said about Hussein, "We knew he was a bastard but we thought he was *our* bastard". We also supported Bin Laden and other Islamic fundamentalists because we thought they were "our bastards" against Soviet Russia, etc., etc. Kissinger also said, "We shall bomb Cambodia into the Stone Age. We did and got Pol Pot". We have not learned that terror leads to counter-terror.

After the Gulf War the denial was monumental. A year after the war was hardly talked about. I heard an American student saying that in the Gulf War there were only six casualties. But behind this monumental denial a nefarious change of pattern was happening. The military authorities had learned something from the Gulf War —namely, that from the sky they can destroy enemies without incurring any casualties. This was the beginning of a myth about American invincibility. This change of pattern is best summarised by General Powell's statement, "American soldiers will not be pawns in the conflict of global interests". If he had meant *human beings* are not to be made pawns in global fights for power it would have been a most beautiful statement but that wasn't what was meant. What was meant was "we have such powers in the sky that we can do the work with bombs from on high and we shall remain invulnerable".

This is what was symbolised by the Twin Towers and the Pentagon building and revealed the tremendous anxiety and guilt, which underpinned the need for such grandiosity.

I think the 11 September 2001 bombing was highly symbolic. I think we have been precipitated into a world of fragmentation and at points total disintegration and psychotic terror. Also, into total confusion—who are our friends? Who are our enemies? From what quarter do we expect aggression? Old enemies are now our friends, Soviet Russia and the Northern Alliance fundamentalist groups that used to be supported by the USSR. Our ancient friends could be enemies—Chechnya, for example. And we wonder if it is all outside or whether there are enemies on the inside. And the same confusion can be seen in the Arab world.

The spreading fragments of a collapsing empire are felt all over the world and imbued with evil like the plague. This is the most primitive terror in our personal development—not ordinary death but some vision of personal disintegration imbued with hostility. Of course, the situation is made much worse when God comes into the equation. The point I made in my 1985 paper about fundamentalist Christians longing for Armageddon is now matched by the Islamic fundamentalists. Our sanity is threatened by a delusional inner world of omnipotence and absolute evil and sainthood. Unfortunately, we also have to contend with God Mammon.

'Terrorism' is a broad term. I think there are great differences between State terrorism and the terrorism of rebels. There are differences even between the secular terrorism of, say, the Palestinians and the terrorism of religious fanatics. But I have concentrated more on what insane premises they have in common. All terrorism is murderous and suicidal. The dread of annihilation, which is part of all of us, is the dread of our own death drives with their aim of disrupting, dispersing and annihilating life. Our primary defence is to project it outside and to kill it there. But it doesn't work. We cannot annihilate all evil and terror without destroying ourselves because it's a part of us.

Even a 'crusade against terrorism' to obtain freedom and democracy is as dangerous and illusory as other fundamentalist beliefs that we attain Paradise if we destroy the evil that we attribute to others.

The real battle is between insanity based on mutual projections and sanity based on truth. Some individuals, say mass murderers, succumb to madness but they are a very tiny minority. The vast majority of us find other ways to deal with our psychotic parts. How is it that terrorism of whatever kind can get such massive support? I think part of the problem is that we submit to the tyranny of our own groups. If we project too much into our group we surrender our own experiences and the group tyrannises us and we follow like blind sheep led to the slaughter. This does not mean that we should insulate ourselves and enjoy some superior ivory tower of our insights. We are all members of some group or other and share responsibility for what 'our group' does. Even when we are passive and feel detached our apathy abandons the group to its fate. But speaking our minds takes courage because groups do not like outspoken dissenters. We are told, "ours is not to reason why, ours is to do [to kill] and die". But we have minds of our own. We still have choices. We could say, "ours *is* to reason why, ours is to live and strive". And I think that silence is still the real crime.

Note

1. This paper was first given in Hamburg in 1985, in the wake of the IPA Congress, at the inaugural meeting of the International Psychoanalysts Against Nuclear Weapons and published in 1987 in the *International Review of Psychoanalysis*, 14, 3–12.

THE AFTERMATH OF WAR

Introduction

Jean Knox

The papers in this section address the impact, both short and long-term, that terror and war have, not only on the individuals and communities who are their victims, but also on their descendants. They describe the range and depth of the psychological devastation wrought by the extremes of cruelty experienced under torture, in wartime or exile and during the Holocaust. A common theme is the need for a therapeutic approach in which non-verbal communication plays as significant a part as interpretation.

Garwood movingly describes and analyses the intense guilt felt by survivors of the Holocaust, with its multiple traumas of powerlessness, annihilation anxiety, object loss, and torture. He suggests that the essential psychic process underlying survivor guilt is self blame which is a defensive omnipotent phantasy. The success of therapy partly depends on the therapist's capacity to tolerate, contain, and work through his or her painful countertransference responses to the patient's account of intolerable experience. Hart describes the disruptions of external and internal reality and the distortion of the normal mourning process that results from the multiple traumas of exile. She suggests that the therapist needs to be sensitive to the symbolic value of traditional mourning practices.

There is a dark edge to Papadopoulos' suggestion that human destructiveness is tragically more ordinary than we care to admit and in his view that, when terror and violence are unleashed in a community, faith in humanity is lost along with all the other losses. He uses the metaphor of thawing to describe a healing process which must be allowed to proceed at its own pace and in its own way, rather than having a standard therapeutic framework imposed on it.

Fonagy describes the impact of trauma across generations through his work with the grandchild of a Holocaust survivor. He demonstrates that the transmission of specific traumatic ideas across generations may arise from an infant's vulnerability to dissociative states created by a parent whose own trauma makes their caregiving frightened or frightening. He suggests that a therapist's playful engagement with feelings and beliefs may be more effective than a classical interpretative stance.

Finally, a note of hope for a traumatized society, as well as for the individuals in it, is introduced by Kapur in his exploration of the reparative impulse in Northern Ireland through his work with the Trauma and Recovery team after the Omagh bomb. He gives examples which suggest that there is a growing wish in Northern Ireland to reconstruct what has been destroyed and to develop intrapsychic and interpersonal relationships characterized by personal responsibility and concern rather than hatred and revenge.

CHAPTER EIGHTEEN

Destructiveness, atrocities and healing: epistemological and clinical reflections

Renos K. Papadopoulos

Destructiveness, in its various forms and variations, has occupied a central place in both psychoanalysis and analytical psychology. In the main, psycho-analysis seems to have approached destructiveness through the notion of 'aggressive impulses', drives or instincts, whereas analytical psychology seems to have placed its emphasis on the notions of 'shadow' and 'the problem of evil' in its treatment of the same subject. Both schools have accepted that destructiveness is one of the most fundamental issues in considering human nature.

However, any consideration of destructiveness and violence is inevitably influenced (consciously or unconsciously) by a host of other factors, from philosophical views, cultural and theological positions as well as moral and ethical values, to the pragmatics of the socio-economic, political and historical realities; that is why, in its totality, destructiveness is a multi-faceted and multi-dimensional phenomenon which cannot and should not be limited to the realm of any single discipline. Yet, because it is such an emotive issue, it tends to cloud even further its complexity. Therefore, it is imperative that we focus our attention on the very way we approach destructiveness before we embark on any further elaboration. In other words, I would argue that it is essential that we reflect on the epistemology which we imperceptibly employ in approaching the subject of destructiveness.

Epistemological concerns

Regardless of how one defines destructiveness (that is, in terms of 'aggression' or 'the evil', etc.), there are three over-arching factors that seem to interweave within the way we conceptualise it. The first has to do with the position in which we locate ourselves during the process of discussing destructiveness, the second refers to the way we approach destructiveness (implicitly or explicitly) either as a personal characteristic or a collective phenomenon, and the third factor concerns our ideas about the origin and aetiology of destructiveness. As with any logical and philosophical pursuit, one has to ask the question: 'who' is the person who is addressing the topic of destructiveness and 'under what circumstances', 'within which context' and 'for what purpose' is this pursuit taking place? In answering these questions, what emerges is that our very position and identity as analysts (that is, as mental health professionals) affect the way we approach destructiveness.

At first glance, one would claim that there is nothing unusual in the idea that society recruits mental health professionals to assist with understanding and explaining destructiveness by providing them with psychological insights about this phenomenon. Viewed from this perspective, mental health professionals are mere commentators who supply, mainly on demand, their particular expert opinion. This type of assistance is based on the formula which is used widely in society and which I have called 'the Societal Discourse of the Expert' (Papadopoulos, 1998b). This discourse governs the rules and regulations, the expectations and obligations, the positions, identities and relationships of everybody involved in the totality of the sets of actions and interactions, belief systems and networks, which are activated whenever we turn to experts for help in areas where specialist expertise is needed. The Societal Discourse of the Expert creates a certain type of inter-dependence among its actors which, at best, facilitates smooth and easier living conditions and, at worst, fosters exploitation and manipulation (that is, authoritarianism, on the side of the expert, and impotence, on the side of the consumer). In the context of destructiveness, the Societal Discourse of the Expert develops particularly intricate ramifications which should make us re-examine the idea that what is happening is simply a recruitment of professionals to explain an area 'where specialist expertise is needed'.

On beginning to examine this further, it is important to observe that as members of the mental *health* profession we are *de facto* located on the side of health and, perforce, against non-health or pathology. This means that the lenses we use in approaching any issue are coloured by this oppositionality. Whatever phenomenon we address, this dichotomous narrative is active and forms a certain predisposition which is unavoidable, regardless of whether we are aware of it or not. This means that when, for example, we look at human pain and suffering we cannot but formulate our observations and theories (whatever these may be) within this narrative of polarity, and therefore the idea of pathology or health will stain, inevitably, any conceptualisation of these phenomena (albeit in a crude or a subtle way). Similarly, in examining the very same phenomena, other professionals will view them through their own lenses; for example, theologians will be predisposed to formulate their comments in the context of the language of good and evil and sociologists in terms of societal considerations. Thus, whenever we address destructiveness, as mental health professionals, we are bound to locate it in the context of the pathology-health polarity. Moreover, in so far as destructiveness is something that is humanly abhorrent, it will invariably end up being pathologised; that is, destructiveness will not be associated with health and, thus, will be located on the pathology end of the polarity.

Elsewhere (Papadopoulos & Hildebrand, 1997), I compared the mental health professional's narratives of destructiveness with those of divorce; both are widespread phenomena which demand our attention and understanding. With reference to divorce, society seems to have achieved a rather remarkable feat, by avoiding its pathologisation: until not long ago, we used to talk about divorce using terms such as 'broken homes' which implied that there is something psychologically wrong with people who get divorced. Thus, our narratives used to suggest that the divorced partners were 'unable to form relationships'. However, in so far as the phenomenon of divorce is so wide-spread, society has changed its narratives in an appropriate way and we now talk about 'one-parent families' and, with reference to the divorced partners, we talk about 'incompatibilities' and emphasise the 'effects of circumstances', etc. In other words, 'we have managed to normalise the experience of divorce without minimising its disruptive effects' (Papadopoulos & Hildebrand, 1997, p. 208) or the pain involved.

However, society seems to have failed to do something comparable with reference to destructiveness and violence. Destructiveness is an equally wide-spread phenomenon affecting most of us, in its various shapes and forms, and yet we tend to find it difficult to get a proper grip on it. By simply condemning it, we do not get closer to the phenomenon and thus we cannot begin to understand it. We seem to get caught up in a debilitating conundrum: on the one hand, we cannot afford to 'normalise' destructiveness while, on the other hand, we cannot delve more deeply into it in order to understand it more fully, unless we adopt a less judgmental stance. This impossible situation has multifarious repercussions; one of them is exemplified by our attitudes towards the outbreak of new wars. After each eruption of violent hostilities or war we believe that we shall never forget it, that we shall learn from the horrible experience and thus avoid any future repetitions. Yet, when the next outbreak occurs we react with remarkable dismay as if we did not expect it to happen. 'It seems that there is a protective function in human beings which enables us to 'forget' painful memories of war and react with the wrath of naïve ignorance when conflict recurs. It is as if humanity needs to keep cleansing itself from the horrors of war by constantly 'forgetting' them and thus renewing its virginal innocence' (*ibid.*, p. 208).

A simple explanation of this complex phenomenon may be that, as human beings, we cannot afford to be neutral about destructiveness; inevitably, moral considerations influence our perception and judgement of destructiveness and violence. This means that there will always be an epistemological confusion (in mixing theoretical with moral dimensions) whenever we approach the subject of destructiveness.

Limitations of a linear-causal epistemology of destructiveness

Thus, in so far as destructiveness is a multi-faceted phenomenon, it is indeed impossible to develop one clear and mono-dimensional theoretical understanding of it. Moreover, as we have seen, an epistemological confusion prevents us from having a clear perspective on destructiveness due to our position as mental health professionals with all the resulting predispositions (societal and theoretical). Nevertheless, destructiveness, being such an important facet of our lives, imposes pressing demands on us to develop a clear understanding of it. It is then that we seem to resort to an implicit methodology which is the predominant one that we use in our lives: this is the approach that understands this phenomenon by means of reducing it to one or several clear causes. For example, we think that we 'understand' anger when we believe that we have identified what has 'caused' someone to be angry. This process is based on a linear epistemology according to which causes have clear effects which, in turn, become causes for other effects. In this way, for example in a family, when we approach an angry father, a nagging mother and a disruptive son, we tend to order them in a causal and linear way, trying to discover 'the' original reason which causes the rest of the chain to unfold; then, depending on our own perspective as observers, we order these three phenomena in a sequence of causality. Our understanding therefore of a situation becomes equal with our 'discovery' of 'what has caused it'. Jung repeatedly warned us against the limitations and even dangers of a causal-reductive epistemology especially when applied to our understanding of human nature. The difficulty with this kind of epistemology is that, although it is used quite appropriately with reference to many facets of our lives, it has severe limitations when applied to complex and multi-dimensional phenomena, particularly in the realm of human relations, because these do not follow a neat sequence of causality; instead, one incident or behaviour influences the other in an inexorable circularity which maintains the totality of the pattern. This is why systemic family therapists have used the term 'circular epistemology' to refer to the approach that appreciates that all elements of a system influence each other in such a way that the distinct pattern of the system is maintained.

Applying these considerations to destructiveness, we can see how a causal-reductive approach to understanding is obviously inadequate. However, such an approach is appealing both to our ordinary human 'rationality' as well as our psychological need to locate one clear cause, which we can then blame for being responsible for the destructiveness. This process is the basis of scapegoating, according to which blame is placed on someone else, thus making us feel pure and free from the mess of destructiveness. Moreover, a causal-reductive approach to destructiveness forces us to commit another epistemological error—that of ignoring the role of the observer in the process of observation. Analytical psychology, as well as modern systemic and ecological approaches, helps us to understand that not only are the phenomena we observe interrelated among themselves, but also we, as observers, are part of the same larger system. Yet it is psychologically comforting to place ourselves in the position of 'objective observers' and 'detached scientists' when we deal with the painful chaos of destructiveness.

Psychologising and pathologising destructiveness

Returning to the position that mental health professionals assume in relation to destructiveness, we can now understand more fully why it is appealing to be assigned the privileged position of 'objective commentators'. Society faces a painful paradox because, on the one hand, the phenomenon of destructiveness itself, being widespread and affecting most of us, demands to be comprehended, and on the other hand, what professionals seem to offer (with their 'neat' theories) does not provide any satisfactory explanation. It is within the context of this disturbing dilemma that society recruits mental health professionals to find a way out; thus, it could be argued that what mental health professionals tend to provide may not be, after all, an understanding of the phenomenon of destructiveness but an anaesthetisation of the pain derived from the incomprehensibility of it. Within the cloud of the inherent epistemological confusion and the anguish emanating from the unintelligibility of this complex phenomenon, the theories mental health experts advance in attempting to understand destructiveness may ultimately amount to being not much more than ornate psychologisations and pathologisations which are intended to ease the resulting distress. Thus, unwittingly, I would argue that we are used by society, as experts, to explain away the disturbing complexity of destructiveness and replace it with sanitised theories. Under the pressure of these circumstances, we tend to employ causal-reductive approaches which isolate destructiveness and treat it as if we were investigating something exotic, out there, which has nothing to do with us and our own nature. Once we slip into this position, then inevitably our identity as mental health professionals imposes on our observations the additional constraints that we have already identified, that is, the pathology–health polarity; this results in us combining the causal-reductive approach within the oppositional narrative of pathology and destructiveness which then together produce an inevitable psychologisation and pathologisation of destructiveness. By no means do I wish to suggest or imply in any way that destructiveness is 'normal' or accept-able. But is placing it on the 'normal'–'abnormal' polarity the only way out? Is psychologising and pathologising destructiveness the only possible way to deal with it? Perhaps the first step towards such a deeper understanding would be for us to appreciate the fact that we are indeed trapped and imprisoned by and within these constraints wherein the pathology narrative occupies a key position.

Two examples can illustrate this process. The first is the case of the recent war in Bosnia when western journalists, stunned by the incomprehensibility and ferocity of the conflict and the lack of any obvious 'causes', went out of their way to explain it away in terms of 'historical' reasons. In brief, it was argued that ancient animosity among the different ethnic groups was covered up by the Tito regime and once that collapsed, the hostilities broke out. Then, mental health professionals came to add authenticity to this causal-reductive explanation by translating it into psychological language; consequently, the 'covering up' was equated with the intra-psychic process of 'repression' and the whole 'explanation' of the war was thus based in a pathological context.

Yet historical evidence shows that there was never ethnic purity in that region (Malcolm, 1994) and therefore the emphasis on the 'repression' interpretation is suspect. In contrast, no historical explanation was advanced in the case of the Gulf War where the emphasis was on the denomination of one leader which was used as the justification for the war; obediently, mental health professionals followed the predominant narrative imposed by society and went on explaining away the pathological traits of Saddam Hussain. What I am trying to convey here is that a paradox exists that prevents us from developing a deeper understanding and appreciation of the multi-faceted complexities of destructiveness and violence. If we could afford to avoid moralising, without ignoring the moral dimension, and equally avoid psychologising, without ignoring the psychological dimensions, we could perhaps begin to contemplate that, after all, destructiveness may be a tragic facet of the human condition.

The tragedy of destructiveness

Returning to the three overarching factors, we now see that:

(a) Our position as mental health professionals is coloured by the Societal Discourse of the Expert and we are thus entrapped within the dichotomous narrative of oppositionality (pathology–health);

(b) As mental health professionals, we seem to be predisposed to approaching destructiveness as a personal (and indeed an intra-psychic) phenomenon, especially as a result of employing (mostly in an imperceptible way) the comforting but debilitating linear-causal epistemology; and

(c) In terms of aetiology, we would be divided according to the party lines of our analytical perspectives. This division would be based on the debate which can be expressed roughly as follows: is aggression an innate quality or drive or it is a reaction to external circumstances? We know that, as analysts, we do not seem to have a good track record when it comes to addressing wider social issues and this may be the result of our internal over-involvement with this debate. By being preoccupied with our own internal theoretical arguments we seem to have missed glaring external factors such as environmental pressures, socio-political realities, and historical legacies. Spasmodic expressions of concern about social issues appear not only to have little effect but they also exemplify the fact that we do not have, as yet, any approaches which could join together in a seamless way our theory, clinical practice and social concerns as citizens which may then provide us with coherent responses to societal expressions of destructiveness and violence.

As a consequence of the resulting epistemological confusion, narratives about destructiveness and war seem to occupy a paradoxical position in the western world; usually they are formulated as referring to either distant and irrelevant phenomena or to noble and heroic events. Stories of pain, terror, and atrocities are told as if they belonged to the past or as if they provide us with abstract moral lessons. This could be the reason why, when new conflicts erupt, we tend to react with some degree of confusion. In this manner, we seem destined not to learn from history but react with horror every time new armed conflict and war rear their head.

Destructiveness may be a tragic facet of our human condition: it is difficult to find any other word to describe it more appropriately, especially if we connect it with the original meaning of the word. It is well known that 'tragedy' comes from '*tragos*' (goat) as it was connected with the rituals performed by men dressed as goats in ancient Greek ceremonies. However, it may be less known that '*tragos*' is an onomatopoeic word which comes from '*trogo*' (to eat) and '*traganizo*' (to crunch). Thus, goats with their voracious appetite crunch anything in sight regardless of whether it is good or bad for them. Indeed there is something tragic in this potential self-destructiveness involved in the goat munching away at everything indiscriminately. Equally, impulsiveness and lack of discrimination are key characteristics of destructiveness. By emphasising the tragic aspect of destructiveness, we bypass the impossible questions as to whether it is inevitable or not, innate or reactive, personal or collective. By acknowledging the tragic element of destructiveness, we accept that as human beings, we are part of the tragedy of destructiveness and our task then becomes the endeavour to locate ourselves as individuals in a meaningful way within it rather than explain it away.

Ordinariness and the ecology of violence

One of the consequences of perceiving destructiveness as a tragic aspect of being human is that our position has the possibility of being shifted and, consequently, the arrogance of the 'detached expert' can be replaced by compassion. From this new perspective, we may admit that destructiveness has always been part of our society. According to Heraclitus, "war is the father of all things": conflict and strife, oppositionality and destructiveness are part of life and, in addition to their obvious negative effects, they may also have a positive function. Therefore, we do not need to be fixed in a position from which we simply condemn destructiveness and need to distance ourselves from it. Usually, we tend to ascribe all kinds of bizarre and conspiratorial theories behind manifestations of destructiveness in order to distance ourselves from these allegedly inhuman phenomena. Yet, tragically, they may be much more 'ordinary' than we would like to admit; by this I do not mean that destructiveness is 'normal' (but it certainly should not be characterised as 'abnormal' either). Lamentably, in the final analysis, violence could be seen as being much more of an 'ordinary' and human response that we would like to accept, and this realisation makes us feel most uncomfortable. Accepting the ordinariness of destructiveness does not support any argument that it is an innate or a necessary phenomenon; it merely acknowledges that given the conditions in society and the vicissitudes of our existence, this phenomenon is fairly common and ordinary.

This new perspective allows us to move away from the impossible dilemma that was posed above, that is, how to avoid pathologising destructiveness without 'normalising' it, which would imply condoning it. The way out is to create a new narrative within which the emphasis is on the 'ordinariness' of destructiveness rather than its evaluation as either 'normal' or 'pathological'.

Hannah Arendt's famous expression "the banality of evil" aptly conveys precisely this recognition, that is, violent and destructive acts may often be tragically more ordinary than we care to admit. It is indeed very threatening for us to accept that acts of destructiveness can be human and are committed by ordinary people; instead, we seem to be compelled to attribute inhuman and diabolical motivation to them.

In his novel *Captain Corelli's Mandolin*, Louis de Bernières, in a most sensitive way, expresses his thoughts about the ordinariness of destructiveness. In describing the situation when soldiers, after a period of anxious inactivity, experience action; he writes:

> We found that there is a wild excitement when the tension of waiting is done with, and that sometimes it transforms itself into a kind of demented sadism once an action is commenced. You cannot always blame the soldiers for their atrocities, because I can tell you

from experience that they are the natural consequences of the inferno of relief that comes from not having to think any more. Atrocities are sometimes nothing less than the vengeance of the tormented. [de Bernières, 1995, p. 61]

The author does not judge or blindly condemn violence in an outright and dismissive fashion but, in a remarkably brave way, attempts to understand it. He characterises violence as a 'natural consequence'; not as good or bad, not as pathological or normal. Although he is not advancing a psychological theory and he is not using specialist language, his expression "natural consequences" implies very clearly that atrocities, the actions themselves, are part of a bigger whole and one cannot simply focus exclusively on them ignoring the rest. "Atrocities are sometimes nothing more than the vengeance of the tormented" means also that the soldiers themselves are brutalised and placed, unmercifully, within a cycle of violence which they did not instigate and which had begun before them. Violent acts are not committed, necessarily, by perverted individuals but by ordinary people who are caught up in tragic circumstances; most human beings are capable of violence. This narrative emphasises what could be called 'the ecology of violence' rather than individual motivation. Moreover, this perspective locates us not as detached observers but makes us acknowledge that violence is also part of us, part of our lives. According to Jung, of course, destructiveness is part of our shadow.

We cannot deny the fact that our psychological and social worlds contain 'shadow' and violent elements. However, as human beings, we have the capacity and resilience to be creative and constructive, especially when we are fully aware of our own shadow and destructive elements. The way Jung accounts for these 'tragic circumstances' is by means of the archetypal shadow which, when it is activated in a particularly strong and gripping way, inevitably interconnects the wider collective with the personal (and indeed, intra-psychic) dimension; under these conditions, it is very unlikely that individuals will be able to resist this archetypal 'radiation' and to maintain their own personal integrity. Thus, destructiveness reigns supreme and the archetype overwhelms all personal individualities. It is, indeed, frightening to acknowledge that, essentially, this phenomenon is 'ordinary', despite its devastating effects.

Archetypal fascination

However, the power of the archetype is manifested not only when it overwhelms individuals but also when it fascinates them. This phenomenon is equally common and ordinary. Destructiveness and violence are endemic in our society today. Violence sells and it strongly influences our art, literature, film, theatre and even fashion and design; so much so, that nowadays it is appropriate to refer to 'designer violence'. Destructiveness is chic, cool and hip. There is an ever increasing ingenuity in how to present violence in most artistic forms. At any given time, most films in any big city in the world are full of violent scenes. In a poem entitled 'Reyerta' ('The Fight'), Federico García Lorca described a fight with most vivid descriptions of horrible and violent acts, all in an incredibly poetic way: referring to the killing of the hero of the poem he writes that he "rolls down the slope dead, his body laden with lilies and a pomegranate on his brow. Now he rides a cross of fire on the highway to death ..." This lyric language is used to describe a ghastly piece of excruciating violence when a person was knifed to death by "clasp-knives, rendered beautiful with enemy's blood", which "glinted like fishes" (Lorca, 1960, pp. 37–38). The dilemma is that, on the one hand, we cannot ignore the fascination and attraction destructiveness exerts on people and, instead, concentrate only on condemning it, because such an emphasis is not likely to produce many changes. However, on the other hand, it is not easy to acknowledge this fascination, and it is not comfortable to address these dark aspects of destructiveness. Nevertheless, we know that violence can have an exhilarating and even 'liberating' effect on the individual. This happens for at least four reasons:

(a) In the act of violence, the individual does not need to think; this is what de Bernières (1995) described—there is a "relief that comes from not having to think any more" but, at the same time, this relief is an "inferno". The 'not thinking' here does not refer exclusively to the cognitive thinking or the Jungian 'thinking' function; instead, it would be more apt to relate it to Bion's idea of the 'capacity to think' which, for him, is the ability to create a space to reflect when one is overwhelmed by pressing impulses. Thus, not having space to reflect provides a tragic kind of 'relief' in so far as the person eradicates the pain caused by difficult considerations and by the awareness of inner contradictions and conflicts.

(b) Gripped by a destructive archetype, people achieve a false 'wholeness' in so far as they are dominated by 'acting out' behaviour. Although 'acting out' is frowned upon in psychoanalysis and analytical psychology, we fail to appreciate the attraction it may have because it mobilises the totality of the personality to act in unison. In acting out there is no division between thoughts, feelings and actions: all become one and action flows. This is tragically similar to the coveted aim of many spiritual practices which, after many years of hard and disciplined training, aspire to achieve moments or a state of being where action flows and inner divisions are abolished. By no means do I suggest that Zen meditation and impulsive acts of destructiveness are the same; however, it is imperative that we appreciate that they have some striking similarities.

(c) Destructiveness can have a certain kind of chilling purity which is extremely seductive. This is difficult to convey, but it can be approximated once we connect it with the process of archetypal possession where one polarity, in its extreme form and devoid of personal content, dominates the individual. This has a numinous quality because, regardless of the content of the archetype itself, the fact remains that it is a distilled form of an image in its pure state and it has an unmistakable and most refreshing authenticity. Any purity exerts a powerful attraction and makes people wish to continue the connection with it. Under these conditions, people offer themselves to protect this purity from any threat of contamination and this is the tragic background from which acts of atrocities can be committed in the name of defending and indeed 'cleansing' the perceived source of purity. In other words, if a group of people identify with a collective within the context of archetypal possession, they will be willing to sacrifice themselves in order to guard this purity and, in doing so, they will be in a position to do just anything to prevent its pollution. This complex dynamic is close to the 'Luciferian light' of evil which may attract certain people under these circumstances.

(d) Individual identity is subsumed by a wider collective identity. Ordinarily, within the context of personal identity people are burdened by a variety of conflicts and inner struggles; they feel refreshed when they shed (at least temporarily) this identity by connecting with wider forms of identity. Society has special sanctioned times, places and conditions where this happens automatically, such as in sports competitions when a person becomes a fan, abandoning personal history and identity and joining with the crowd of supporters of a team; there is an exhilarating and liberating effect when a person becomes one speck of the sea of the 'red' or 'green' colour of their team. There are numerous such sanctioned settings where this process of emphasising and connecting with the collective aspects of our identity happens in an innocuous and even growthful and useful way: professional association, community activities, family events, etc. are just a few of the many examples. However, under certain conditions when acts of destructiveness are played out on the societal plane, people become polarised and, as Jung put it, 'willy-nilly' a collective identity is imposed on them (Jung, 1928). The tragedy is that there are some paradoxical 'benefits' of this imposition of a collective and a cancellation (however temporary) of the personal identity (Papadopoulos, 1997). Both victim and oppressor, or victim and saviour glow in the righteousness of their 'cause'. It is self-evident that a victim will feel self-righteous because, being an actual recipient of brutalisation, he or she does not need to get in touch with any personal shadow material; after all, these people are not responsible for the calamity that had befallen them and therefore they deserve our support, sympathy, love and eternal care. Although it may be less obvious why the 'oppressor' may feel liberated, it becomes clearer when we remember that perpetrators of violence rarely consider themselves as such; instead, they see themselves as serving 'selflessly' their cause, they defend the purity of their collective (as outlined above). There is no need to develop the idea that the 'saviour' feels liberated and infatuated by the role that is assigned to him or her as the inflationary and hubristic dimensions of this position are fairly clear.

Towards an ecology of destructiveness

A serious appreciation of all these considerations leads to an approach which emphasises the 'ecology of destructiveness' rather than isolated explanations and simplifications. Not only are the various roles that destructiveness imposes on people (victims, survivors, saviours, oppressors, observers, critics, etc.) interconnected among themselves within archetypal scenarios, but the epistemological method which we assume with regard to this issue demands (as we have seen) an ecological approach; within such an approach we are enabled to appreciate how we cannot be detached observers or commentators, how destructiveness is tragically more 'ordinary' than we care to admit and that it has dark and shadow attractions.

The ecological perspective can also provide the safest possible framework to examine the psychological states which victims and survivors of destructiveness experience.

Traumatic experiences

Psychological literature has many worthy accounts of the nature and meaning of the traumatic experiences engendered by severe brutalising war situations, but this is not the appropriate place to review them and comment on them; instead, I wish to concentrate on some observations which emerge out of an ecological approach to destructiveness and which are based on my work with survivors of violence and disasters in various settings.

To begin with, the very identity of a person is not limited within the strict boundaries of an individual organism or, even less, an intra-psychic location. This means that survivors of atrocities lose much more than their identifiable personal material possessions and human relationships. Accepting that the identified aspects of our individuality (name, gender, nationality, profession, various group affiliations, etc.) are based on a complex mosaic of what could be called an "identity substratum" (Papadopoulos, 1997), under these difficult conditions individuals are likely to lose a great deal more which is less evident. This mosaic substratum consists of many elements which form a coherent whole but which we tend to take for granted as we are less aware of their presence and their significance; these include such elements as the reality of belonging to a certain language group, of getting used to certain sounds, to a particular geographical landscape and milieu, the fact that we are surrounded by particular types of architectural designs, etc.

Ordinarily, we do not think about these elements because they are quite basic and we take them for granted. However, "in their totality they form a background mosaic upon which the more tangible aspects of our identity are based" (p. 15). These losses also need to be accounted for as part of the traumatic experience and the seriousness of their implications should be considered.

Moreover, there are two other aspects of our identity that we lose as victims under these conditions. When a neighbour attacks a neighbour and kills members of his family and destroys his home, the victim does not lose only the family members and his house or even the friendship of the neighbour but he also loses what is usually referred to as 'faith in humanity'. This is not an abstract faith or irrelevant ideology; without it a person "can no longer trust that human values such as friendship, loyalty, respect, decency, love can possibly exist" (Papadopoulos, 1997, p. 13), and this kind of loss has far reaching implications because it affects the very identity of the individual. The narratives of people I have been working with convey very clearly the frightening impact this loss has for people, especially because they are less aware of its presence and its importance in the first place.

The second type of loss that people in these tragic situations invariably experience is connected with the first one and has to do with our capacity to predict life. Ordinarily, we seem to trust ourselves to judge the source of danger and we take the necessary precautions; however, under these catastrophic and unpredictable conditions, we are faced with the fact that we are unable to predict the source of our calamity and therefore we cannot defend ourselves. This interferes with our trust in "reading life" (Papadopoulos, 1997, p. 14) and can have severe implications because it affects not only our personal identity but our very position within our socio-ecology.

Overall, if we understand these reactions as normal reactions to abnormal circumstances we do not need any pathological polarities to help us understand them. Moreover, we appreciate that this "disintegration of the identity substratum" (Papadopoulos, 1997, p. 14) may be a temporary response, part of a needed 'frozenness', variations of which we, as helpers, are also likely to experience under the intensity of our close proximity with this kind of pain. By adopting the narrative of 'frozenness' rather than pathologising terms such as 'dissociation', 'regression' etc., we appreciate that this is a human and 'ordinary' reaction; moreover, we realise that similarly with the actual process of physical thawing, each object requires its own tempo, intensity, distance from the source of heat and overall conditions for successful thawing. "Thawing is a delicate process which may damage the frozen item if not used appropriately" (Papadopoulos, 1997, p. 15).

Therapeutic interventions

Although it would be impossible and indeed inappropriate to discuss in detail the range and types of therapeutic interventions I have been using in the context of this kind of work (see Papadopoulos, 1996, 1997, 1998a,b, in press; Papadopoulos & Hildebrand, 1997), nevertheless I shall endeavour to outline the basic principles which have emerged as useful in this work with survivors of violence and disaster. These principles govern the following three distinct but interrelated aspects of the therapeutic interventions:

(a) initial contact and overall framework;
(b) boundaries and conduct, and
(c) aims and techniques.

(a) Initial contact and overall framework

To begin with, it is of paramount importance to consider the very basis of the connection between the survivors and the professionals. It is necessary to remember that if we were to allow things to take their ordinary course, these people would contact us only if they were diagnosed (regardless by whom or through whichever procedure) as needing assistance from a mental health professional. The most likely diagnosis with this kind of case is 'Post Traumatic Stress Disorder' (PTSD) which is the special 'disorder' specified by the Diagnostic and Statistical Manual of the American Psychiatric Association (DSM-IV) (Spitzer & Williams, 1994); although this diagnosis is fairly controversial (Friedman & Jaranson, 1992; Marsella *et al.*, 1996), it is still widely used. This means that the two preconditions for any professional meeting would be the formulation of their suffering and pain within the mental health paradigm (that is, as a psychiatric 'disorder') and the location of the contact between 'therapist' and 'patient' within the context of a mental health referral network; according to the latter, the contact between the 'patient' and the 'therapist' is mediated by the referral network and the therapist is expected to report to somebody about the progress of therapy. Thus, invariably, the initial contact is likely to dictate the specific nature of the overall therapeutic framework within which the survivors and their helpers are located; this means that the relationship between the survivor and therapist is likely to be framed within the pathologising narratives and thus subjected to all the other complex implications which were discussed above.

Mindful of all this, I have endeavoured to establish contact with survivors in a way which would avoid the usual mental health referral network. Unfortunately, this route is not available to most therapists who work exclusively within the context of traditional settings. The cardinal rule for me has been to create ways of legitimising a connection with survivors which would not be based on the traditional patient-therapist 'contract'. An example of creating such an alternative context is the case of my work with a group of Bosnian ex-camp prisoners who were freed by the Red Cross, as 'medical evacuees', in the early stages of the war and brought for medical treatment to a hospital in the UK. The hospital authorities then requested 'psychological assistance' from the Tavistock Clinic, where I work, for this group of 18 men. Vigilant of the details of the conditions of the initial contact, I realised that I had an opportunity to bypass the traditional therapeutic contract, emphasising my respect for the fact that the men themselves had not requested this kind of assistance, I was able to negotiate with the authorities a new role for myself which I argued was more appropriate under the circumstances. According to this new role, I positioned myself as a general helper in the ward applying my therapeutic insights and skills in ways that did not fix me as a therapist expected to offer each one of them therapeutic sessions as such. This meant that I was able to relate to patients and staff in an open way, spending unstructured time with them and assisting with anything that I was capable of doing (from making cups of tea to cleaning, from translating between Serbo-Croat and English to liaising between them and the various authorities).

My identity as a mental health professional, and more specifically as a psychologist and therapist was not concealed. The men, in any case, did not wish to see a therapist as they did not feel that they had any mental health problem or disorder. Everybody was fully aware of my professional identity and preferred my stance of not following a traditional role and not requiring them to see me at set times, under set conditions. They felt comfortable with the fact that it was not imposed on them to see a therapist. Within this context, my aim was to maximise the therapeutic impact of my ordinary contact with them. More specifically, I would attempt to introduce therapeutic dimensions into our ordinary conversations and, for example, remind them of their painful losses and their disorientation as we would talk about everyday issues.

Moreover, I would appreciate their reserved stance as appropriate and not treat it as 'resistance', as a therapist would normally do. In a respectful and discreet way, my interpretations would aim to normalise their experiences (that is, as 'normal reactions to abnormal circumstances') within a framework which emphasised the tragic but not pathological dimensions. Overall, I endeavoured to include two dimensions in my responses to them: the first would address their concerns in a therapeutic way, and the second would place their concerns in the framework of their recent life events and experiences, thus providing a normalising context for them. Similar to all therapeutic situations, I would make every effort to convey these dimensions, mindful of their timing and formulation (in terms of using the appropriate language at the appropriate time). In this way, without denying my specialist expertise as a therapist, I would utilise it within a normative framework, trying to avoid psychologising and pathologising their tragic predicament.

The basic principle of this approach is similar to the idea of 'barefoot' professionals in the Maoist revolution in China where professionals, mainly medical doctors, were expected to abandon their established work settings and go to the countryside where they would live among ordinary people and utilise their knowledge and skills in ways which would be more fitting and effective. The emphasis was on the creative adaptation of professional practice applied to different and deprived settings.

Gradually, as they got to know me better, the men would approach me and ask to have some private time with me. I allowed this to happen, again not imposing any therapeutic style or expectations in our conversations apart from vigilantly watching how to maximise the therapeutic impact of our contact. In other words, I did not impose any therapeutic schema, such as debriefing, abreaction, catharsis, re-living previous trauma, developing coping skills. Respecting that they themselves were 'in charge', I did not direct their conversations in any way but allowed them to talk to me about anything they wanted following their own pace.

(b) Boundaries and conduct

Specific boundaries are essential in any inter-action where therapeutic benefits are expected. No therapy can possibly occur outside the sanctioned time, space and special conditions which define the therapeutic temenos. Therapeutic frames (however they may be defined) provide the essential conditions to contain all the confusion, feelings, fantasies and impulses that are generated by the intensity of the work, which are indispensable for any positive therapeutic outcome. The need for clear therapeutic boundaries was more needed in this kind of work where the excruciatingly painful experiences of the medical evacuees, in addition to their deep deprivation, created an almost unbearable intensity which could be likened to an "archetypal radiation" (Papadopoulos, 1998a). Thus, moving outside the traditional therapeutic frame was a pretty hazardous exercise. Nevertheless, once one is aware of these issues, it is relatively easy to re-create therapeutic boundaries in the context of new therapeutic settings.

More specifically, with reference to time, the boundary I imposed was to be available to them only within the context of one afternoon a week. However, accepting that the nature of the work required more flexibility (especially at the beginning), I was prepared to remain in the ward from early in the afternoon to late at night, but never after midnight or on any other day. With reference to space, I was prepared to speak to them anywhere within the hospital complex but not outside it; wearing my usual work attire (which always includes a jacket and a tie) and carrying my work desk diary, I was able to re-create the therapeutic temenos with these 'props' wherever I went with them. However, the most difficult area to re-create appropriate therapeutic boundaries was the way I conducted myself with them. Being in touch with their deep deprivation (from material things to human warmth), it was difficult to restrain myself and not offer them gifts. Outside the framework of formal psychotherapy, the 'ordinary' thing to do would have been to take them token presents; such expressions of care and affection are part of both their and my cultures, especially in times of need. Yet, throughout, I restrained myself from offering them any material gifts because I was fully aware that such action would have altered irrevocably the therapeutic connection; besides, no amount of presents could have possibly eradicated the fundamental and multiple deprivation of their being. Tragically, many other workers, overwhelmed by their spontaneous impulse to respond with human generosity and without the awareness of the importance of therapeutic boundaries, kept offering gifts to these men and kept transgressing professional boundaries by taking them out for weekends. Invariably, most of these relationships ended acrimoniously with tragic and at times even violent confrontations.

(c) Aims and techniques

Following on from the above, it could be said that the aim of the specific therapeutic intervention that I was able to develop with this group of 18 Bosnian medical evacuees was to provide a maximum possible "therapeutic presence" (Papadopoulos, 1996, 1997). This meant that I was in a specific relationship with them which, although it was clearly within a professional context, did not follow the traditional psychotherapeutic framework. They used to call me 'mister doctor' and we addressed each other in the polite plural form of 'you'. If they were asked to clarify their relationship to me, most probably they would say that I was a special friend who also had some professional competence; I would strongly doubt that any of them would have characterise me as his 'therapist'. The closest comparable example to this unique therapeutic relationship would be how one relates to a friend or a relative who is also a professional, in times of need; under these conditions, the 'client' would be in control of the situation and would filter whatever the professional friend said.

However, what were my therapeutic aims, if I avoided entering into a traditional therapeutic relationship? The answer to this question relates to the conceptualisation of their condition in non-pathological terms, which was advanced earlier. Put simply, my aim was to 'thaw' the frozenness which had developed appropriately as a healthy response in order to minimise the disintegration of their identity substratum. In order to do this, it was necessary that new ways of experiencing their condition, outside the pathological polarity, were developed. In other words, the predominant narrative which accounts for these kinds of circumstances renders the experience as pathological; this narrative is interwoven by society, by experts and by the people themselves. In order to clarify the point, I wish to offer the example of President Nelson Mandela. Nobody ever thought of offering him therapy for Post Traumatic Stress Disorder after his release from prison, following twenty-seven years' incarceration. Such an idea would indeed be absurd, laughable and insulting to the dignity and stature of the man, because he had a clear sense of meaning and purpose for what he did. Thus, his lengthy suffering was clearly located within the context of personal and collective narratives in such a way that rendered it heroic rather than pathological. Therefore, it is the meaning attributed to the experience that matters rather than the external event itself. As psychotherapists, and particularly Jungians, we are well aware of this phenomenon. It is the specific type of meaning attributed to an event or an experience that matters most because it is this that determines whether a person will perceive himself or herself as needing psychotherapeutic assistance. However, the meaning does not emerge on its own outside the parameters of narratives that join the personal and collective realms. Consequently, my aim was to facilitate the emergence of narratives within which the experiences of these men would have the opportunity of being 'normalised' without ignoring the evil nature of the deeds that had been perpetrated against them.

With reference to destructiveness, it was argued above that "the way out is to create a new narrative within which the emphasis is on the 'ordinariness' of destructiveness rather than its evaluation as either 'normal' or 'pathological'" (p. 462). Now, with reference to the consequences of destructiveness, we arrive at a similar aim. Translated into practice, the special 'therapeutic presence' has an advantage over other types of therapeutic frames because its very base is rooted into a normalising narrative. Instead of imposing on the medical evacuees techniques from traditional therapeutic frames (for example, debriefing or emphasis on coping skills), the attention here was on empowering them to develop their own new narratives within which their experiences would acquire different meaning. In this context, what they needed was the presence of a helpful person who would also be well aware of the multiplicity of traps and possibilities inherent in therapeutic interactions (that is, the varieties of the transference/countertransference matrix). In essence, what they needed was the experience of what I called "therapeutic witnessing" (Papadopoulos, 1996, 1997). By this I mean that what the therapeutic presence was providing was an actual human witness who could facilitate (with minimal intervention) the thawing and re-connection of the various parts of their personal and collective narratives. The 'witnessing' of their testimony (cf. Felman & Laub, 1992) was not always verbal.

> Respecting that certain experiences had to be shared in silence without even needing to be spoken about (due to their unspeakable horror and inhumanity), there were times when our shared silence was honouring the unutterable. There was a shared understanding that we knew what we were silent about and why. At other times, when referring to certain inhuman experiences, the very use of language would somehow attempt to re-establish the humanity of the person in the light of those inhuman experiences. For example, in narrating to me an episode where for days on end they had lived in filthy conditions, soiled by their own excrement, one of the ex-prisoners could not even get himself to utter the words 'human excrement' (or any other similar word); instead, he went through a tortuous route implying the word but without actually naming it. This could be appreciated as a way through which he was restoring his own human dignity even whilst narrating an inhuman experience. [Papadopoulos, 1997, p. 18]

Thus, ultimately, the healing of these painful experiences due to atrocities may not lie in devising sophisticated therapeutic techniques but in returning to more 'traditional' forms of healing based on assisting people to develop appropriate narratives. The healing effect of story-telling, in its multiple variations, has always been a well-known phenomenon.

Jungian connections

Although this kind of work seems different from most analytical practices of a one-to-one structure in private or hospital consulting rooms, I would argue that the basic principles underlying them are remarkably similar. Moreover, I would suggest that Jungian insights can usefully inform and indeed enrich such approaches, as has definitely happened in my own work with survivors in various contexts and settings. Some of these Jungian insights include the following:

Jung's emphasis on the importance of the analytical vessel provides a distinctive perspective within which to appreciate "the therapeutic frame as an indispensable container of the powerful interactions of the analytic process" (Papadopoulos, 1998a). Jung's alchemical metaphor of psychotherapy offers an apt illustration of the importance of a "strong and clear vessel within which difficult and potentially disruptive material can be contained" (*ibid.*). Re-inventing fitting attributes of a strong container is not impossible in any new situation, as long as we are not seduced by the novelty of the situation. A strong therapeutic vessel can enable the appropriate emotional proximity to the survivors and their experiences, in a way that would render any therapeutic work safe. Moreover, Jung's openness in employing creative ways of applying therapeutic processes is well known. He eschewed established therapeutic styles and was always looking for novel applications. More specifically, one of his particular sensitivities was the awareness of the limitations of our psychotherapeutic practices, due to their Eurocentric nature. Jung was one of the first European psychologists to draw our attention to this type of limitation and as analytical psychologists we are in a position to develop further this awareness (cf. Samuels, 1993; Gambini, 1997; Papadopoulos, 1997, in press b).

The ordinary nature of human suffering is another central aspect of the Jungian approach. His conceptualisation of psychological problems and his efforts to avoid pathologising them emphasised this perspective. Characteristically, he argued that "behind a neurosis there is so often concealed all the natural and necessary suffering the patient has been unwilling to bear" (Jung 1943, para. 185). In this way, it could be said that Jung's efforts were directed towards making human suffering more accessible to people. One way in which he articulated this concern was to emphasise the relevance for the individual to develop his or her 'personal myth'. The Jungian idea of a personal myth implies the articulation of a personal narrative which accounts for the uniqueness of the individual within the context of collective narratives. This is precisely what I was endeavouring to achieve with my 'therapeutic presence' and 'therapeutic witnessing'.

Appreciating these phenomena as essentially archetypal experiences exerting powerful fascination, the therapist locates himself or herself in a humble way in front of them, aware that they may overwhelm his or her personality with their 'archetypal radiation'. This fascination is exerted at many different levels. It "ranges from the fascination with meeting the people who had gone through such powerful experiences, to the content and the events they relate to; from the overwhelmingly heroic feeling which imbues all the workers, to the variety of emotional reactions one has in these situations" (Papadopoulos, 1998a). However, this fascination extends to darker aspects of the human psyche in most complex ways. "Shadow elements emerge and threaten to engulf the personality; destructive images acquire obsessive fascination. There are real dangers that therapeutic work in these situations becomes a vehicle for unconscious mutual fuelling and re-activation of these images. Extreme polarisation of perceptions, ideas, personalities and situations threatens with its indiscriminate destructiveness" (*ibid.*). Under these distressing conditions, it is no wonder that the 'frozenness' emerges to save the individual from complete disintegration. In this way, it could be said that what we are dealing with here are special types of defences of the self.

Several analytical psychologists (for example, Fordham, 1974; Kalsched, 1996; Proner, 1986; Redfearn, 1992; Schwartz-Salant, 1989; Sidoli, 1993) dealt in various ways with the particular types of defences which are aimed at protecting the very core of the self. However, most of them follow the approach according to which predispositions which were developed in earlier stages of one's life are largely responsible for the emergence of these kinds of defences. Nevertheless, experiences in working with survivors of violence and disaster show that such defences may appear in individuals without such early experiences; the disintegrating power of the traumatic events may, tragically, be sufficient in recreating such defences in any individual regardless of his or her earlier history. This is an important phenomenon which will require further investigation.

Finally, Jung did not shy away from acknowledging that some psychological phenomena are indeed connected with actual evil. Without entering into any discussion on this facet of the Jungian approach, it would suffice to be reminded that this dimension is most relevant in this kind of work. Unless we respect the complexity of the multi-faceted nature of destructiveness, in working with survivors of atrocities we are likely to fall into tragic positions from which we will end up psychologising evil and pathologising human suffering.

CHAPTER NINETEEN

Omagh: the beginning of the reparative impulse?

Raman Kapur

Omagh: the beginning of group reparation

The pain of mourning experienced in the depressive position and the reparative drives developed to restore the loved internal and external objects, are the basis of creativity and sublimation. These reparative activities are directed towards both the object and the self. They are done partly because of concern for and guilt towards the object, and the wish to restore, preserve and give it eternal life; and partly in the interest of self-preservation, now more realistically orientated. The infant's longing to recreate his lost objects gives him the impulse to put together what has been torn asunder, to reconstruct what has been destroyed, to recreate and to create. At the same time, his wish to spare his objects leads him to sublimate his impulses when they are felt to be destructive. [Segal, 1964]

Group processes fundamentally influence how we feel, think, and behave towards others. Systems theory (Agazarian, 1994) has taught us that individuals and small-group processes are not immune from the emotional beliefs and values in wider social system. And so to Northern Ireland. This is a society that has been exposed to trauma for nearly thirty years, yet little has occurred within the province to repair the destructive effects of murderous acts replacing the normal activity of everyday human relations. It is indeed remarkable that for all that has been written about Northern Ireland (e.g. Cairns, 1996; Curren et al., 1990) no-one has written about or developed psycho-social interventions to repair the terrible wounds of the past. My thesis is that the tragedy of Omagh represents a watershed in Northern Ireland's state of mind, in that for the first time substantial work began immediately after it, in the establishment of a team of dedicated professionals to address the psychological wounds of those traumatised. Up to this point, in areas affected by the troubles, it had been a struggle to get recognised the need for substantial work to deal with trauma. This watershed is reflected in other aspects of Northern Ireland society, where the talk is more of a dialogue and discourse rather than psychic retreats into self-made islands where the enemy is feared and group processes fragment into the pursuit of individual survival.

What follows in this paper is:

- the application of Kleinian theory to an understanding of Northern Ireland society as a group process
- the description of activities within this societal group that signal the onset of the reparative impulse
- a description of my work in Omagh conducting support groups for the 'trauma and recovery team' working with those affected by the bomb.

Northern Ireland: a Kleinian analysis

Elsewhere, a colleague and I have written (Campbell & Kapur, 1997; Kapur & Campbell, 2001) on how Kleinian psychoanalytic theory can be used to understand societal and individual object relations in this troubled society. I will review here the societal dimension and how this theoretical framework can illuminate key underlying processes.

In our first paper (1997) on this subject, several dysfunctional types of object relations were identified, namely: the hard man; no surrender; and the omnipresence of distrust.

The hard-man concept describes the rigid structure of the internal world where destructive narcissism (Rosenfeld, 1987b) is idealised. This is similar to Bion's (1961) concept of the psychotic personality, where the pleasure is gained through sadism and the predominant currency in relationships is superiority and triumph over others.

The 'no surrender' state of mind is characterised by excessively critical and inflexible representations of such a state of mind.

Finally, the depth of suspicion is manifested through a preoccupation with 'imminent annihilation'—an 'attack before being attacked' is the motto of such states of mind, with individuals remaining on a high state of alert, or "persecutory anxiety" (Klein, 1946).

Onset of the reparative impulse

Writers in the area of trauma have developed different phases of post-disaster responses which all lead towards the recognition, working through, and recovery of trauma. Kubler-Ross (1969) first developed the idea that people progress through distinct coping stages on learning of their loss or bereavement—from denial to rage/distress, and then resolution. Horowitz (1979) has developed a more clinically and empirically elaborated model, where he describes phases of distress, working-through and assimilation. It is this working-through phase that is of particular interest here. This paper is arguing that Northern Ireland society as a large group has, until recently, remained in the distress and denial phase of the troubles, and is only now beginning to wake up to the level of destruction it has inflicted on itself. I will quote directly from three writers to highlight my point.

> In an ideal social world, individuals would be able to talk freely about the events that occupy their thoughts. If social constraints are erected, such that people feel inhibited about talking about a meaningful personal upheaval, the disparity between talking and thinking should increase. That is, people will think about the crisis much more than they talk about it. During this period of social inhibition, we should see increased health problems, signs of interpersonal conflict and higher rates of depression, anxiety and sleep problems. As rates of both talking about and thinking about

> the event approach zero, these psychological and health difficulties should abate. [Pennebaker & Harber, 1993, p. 131]

> People need a 'safe base' for normal social and biological development. Traumatisation occurs when both internal and external resources are inadequate to cope with the external threat. Uncontrollable disruptions or distortions of attachment bonds precede the development of post-traumatic stress syndromes. People seek increased attachment in the face of external danger. Adults, as well as children, may develop strong emotional ties with people who intermittently harass, beat and threaten them. The persistence of these attachment bonds leads to confusion of pain and love. [Van de Kolk & Hart, 1989, p. 404]

> Moreover, it is also common for victims of trauma to be reluctant to talk about their experiences for several reasons. First, they fear that the mental health profession will not understand what they have 'gone through' since 'they were not there' and therefore cannot understand 'what it was like'. Second, upon becoming symptomatic, especially with episodes of involuntary, unbidden intrusive imagery, the person typically fears he is 'going crazy'. Such anxiety may innovate entrance into treatment, but it is more typical for the person to isolate himself, avoid talking about his inner concerns, and perhaps, engage in self-medication with alcohol or drugs. [Wilson, 1989, p. 198]

Northern Ireland boasts some interesting statistics which point to the possibility that dysfunctional intrapsychic and interpersonal relationships may be significantly associated with a society that is frozen in a constant post-traumatic state:

- highest rate of local traffic accidents in Europe
- highest rate of heart attacks in the UK
- poor diet, leading to high rates of strokes and related cancers
- high academic attainment, with lowest number of children in the UK achieving any formal qualification on leaving school
- highest rate of professional misconduct in soccer in the UK
- one of the highest rates of child sexual abuse in the UK

Could these and other indicators be representative of a society that has denied the impact of trauma and so acted out its internal distress through different styles of psychopathology?

What follows is a description of two themes that emerged from my work in conducting support groups for the Trauma and Recovery Team in Omagh. These support groups consisted of mental health and social care professionals, an art therapist and a counsellor who presented their individual work with their clients. I will use some of this material to illustrate wider group processes within Northern Ireland, which I believe now are only beginning to be addressed. As with the previous description, I will use Kleinian object relations theory to understand further my observations.

Rage

On Saturday afternoon, 15 August 1998, at 3.10 pm, a car-bomb exploded in the small market town of Omagh, Northern Ireland. The explosion led to the deaths of twenty-nine men, women and children, and two unborn babies. Over 370 people were injured and were admitted to hospital, or attended for treatment as a result of the explosion as a result of the explosion, with sixty-nine being significantly injured or seriously injured. Many other people witnessed the carnage, and Northern Ireland came to a standstill. How can we be part of such human destructiveness? And what are we going to do about it?

I will detail below the emotional reactions of the event that I believe represents how the troubled mind of Northern Ireland is struggling with its response to trauma. For a long time, this response has been muted. In everyday language, the common themes would be 'Whatever you say, say nothing', where there is an implicit acceptance of the safety and value of silence. It is not safe to talk, and if you do your emotional and physical life could be in danger. However, several years into the peace process, I believe there is a wish to achieve a more peaceful state of mind through people thinking about an idea that talking is a good thing to do. The spontaneous creation of the Trauma and Recovery Team, I believe, represented an unconscious desire by society to say that it is now time to talk.

> Group functioning is often basically influenced and disrupted by psychotic phenomena. Freud said that we form groups for two

reasons: one, to 'combat the forces of nature'; and the other, to bind 'man's destructiveness to man'! groups typically deal with this destructiveness by splitting, the group itself being identified and held together by brotherly love, and collective love of an ideal, whilst destructiveness is directed outward towards some other groups. We love one another dearly, says Freud, if we have someone to hate. Generally we tend to project into another group parts of ourselves which we cannot deal with individually, and, since it is the most disturbed, psychotic parts of ourselves which we find hardest to deal with, those tend to be primarily projected into groups. [Segal, 1995, p. 145]

Someone closely affected by the bomb repeatedly presented, in the support groups by different members of the team who had made contact with him, as seething with anger and hatred. Typically, there would be a representation of someone who was holding the moral ground, with 'right' on his side, with members of the team being perceived as well-intentioned fools who could not really understand the depth of his personal loss. This theme of self-righteousness was communicated with an air of 'holy truth' which could not be questioned. If any questioning took place, a moral crime would be committed and the perpetrator punished by exposure to the media as a well-intentioned 'buffoon' or someone who stupidly and cruelly drew attention to issues that were not relevant to this person's moral crusade.

Using my terminology previously cited in this paper, the takeover of group processes by a moralistic and violent state of mind would be characteristic of a hard man who despises his own vulnerability, idealises aggressive object relations, and intimidates others to prevent any thinking about his difficulties. In Northern Ireland society this model of human relations is rife, and in my view represents a society still in denial of its own capacity for destructiveness. The courage to reflect quietly on the personal responsibility for human destructiveness and to give up the massive projective processes, would put society either into the depressive position (Segal, 1964) of reparative guilt, or plunge it further into destructive persecutory guilt (paranoid-schizoid position) which could be managed only by intrapsychic implosions or a redoubling of explosive psychotic projections. For this person to say 'It's me, this is all to do with my inadequacy, my loss' would represent such a "catastrophic change" (Grinberg et al., 1985) as fundamentally to question psychic structures that have never been resolved for at least the thirty years of the Troubles. However, my view is that Omagh is changing these primitive states of mind by providing, for the first time, the "talking" therapy (Pennebaker & Harber, 1993) that society now deems to be crucial for recovery. This watershed development as a pro-active measure to prevent the further fossilisation of traumatic states, means that people with angry and hateful states of mind have an opportunity to think about becoming more peaceful.

A description of a reported interchange illustrates the point. A member of the support group told how this person burst into his office, looked him straight in the eye, and said "What are you going to do to get me some justice?". There followed a tirade of verbal abuse, in the face of which the staff member felt impotent, inadequate, and at moments almost responsible for this person suffering his loss. At this juncture, the staff-member felt it was his lack of skills and understanding in working with trauma that accounted for his inadequacy, rather than what was being put into him. Also, the staff-member was encouraged by the group to consider another way of relating to this person which could be something like "I know you feel everyone is to blame for your loss, me included, and I think this is the only way you know of to let everyone know how badly you feel." This alternative to a therapeutic collapse began to open up, albeit slowly, an opportunity for this person to consider an idea that maybe it was something going on within himself that could help understand his hatred and anger. This opportunity to be introspective, rather than continue a projective process, if grasped, will lead to a resolution of issues rather than a perpetuation of rage.

In Northern Ireland society I have found that individuals with such intense rage often take up a leadership role. Segal again writes,

> Groups under the sway of psychotic mechanisms tend to select or to tolerate leaders who represent their pathology, for instance Hitler or Khomeini. But not only do those groups choose unbalanced leaders. They also affect them. The groups thrust omnipotence on their leaders, and push them further into megalomania. There is a dangerous interaction between a disturbed group and a disturbed leader, each increasing the other's pathology. [Segal, 1995, p. 196]

Violent object relationships are idealised and perpetuated by a recycling of perverse self-esteem measures aimed at maintaining a 'feel-good' factor. Time and time again, Northern Ireland society has produced political leaders who gain the addictive media limelight by the excited expression of violence. As stated earlier, the incidence of child sexual abuse is particularly high in Northern Ireland. Could this in any way represent the perversions that creep into everyday group processes where violence and rage is unwittingly rewarded?

When we analyse further this group process, there also emerges the strong presence of basic-assumption dependency group functioning in this society (Bion, 1961). The group believes that the 'raging bull' leader can be totally depended upon, with the lure of charisma promising approval from 'Big Ian' (a reference to Dr Ian Paisley) whereby individual resources and abilities are projected into the 'leader of the gang'. This dysfunctional group process can also be observed in professional circles, where the delusion of elitism is propagated through the idealisation of the leader. Of course, this process occurs in many other societies. But my thesis, borne out by my anecdotal observations, is that this is more frequent in Northern Ireland society.

So is this changing? In conducting the support groups for the Trauma team, the clear multi-disciplinary focus, with an attempt to flatten the hierarchy, is unusual; serious attempts have been made to value each individual's contribution and to minimise the idea that all truth rests in the leader. Knowledge and ability have been recognised as residing in the group, rather than in the 'Big Manager' or the 'Big Psychotherapist'. Of course, this requires skill on behalf of the leader, because, as Segal points out,

> ... there can be a dangerous parasitic relationship whereby the leader needs the idealisation for their own sources of self-esteem. [Segal, 1995, p. 197]

This movement towards more 'work group' (Bion, 1961) functioning, involving the interpersonal engagement of the whole group (Yalom, 1985), leading to more depressive-position (Segal, 1964) functioning, is slowly becoming more evident in Northern Ireland society. Political leaders are now referring more to 'thought' and 'patience', rather than explosive rage, as a way of resolving difficulties. In Omagh, significant members of the local Health and Social Care Trust took the initiative and proactively established a 'reparative group' consisting of professionals dedicated to dealing with the effects of the trauma. This is in contrast to the previous thirty years during which the mourning of loss was denied, and 'We just had to get on with it'.

To illustrate a change of basic-assumption dependency group to a basic-assumption work group, I will describe a group discussion.

In this discussion, there was an issue about where the expertise lay in finding a psychological treatment to help a particular patient affected by the bomb. The group gazed at me, and I remained quiet—a common phenomenon in supervision groups elsewhere. This was then followed by an idea that I may not know what was going on, and thus my silence. At this point, there was an idealisation of a cognitive-behavioural approach. I, as a Clinical Psychologist, felt attracted to this neat model to explain the complexity of the problem and thus retain my status in the group as an expert. In Northern Ireland I believe there is an idealisation of experts to deal with complex human situations/tragedies to avoid the messy struggles before an answer is found. The pull on me was massive, particularly as somewhere I felt hugely inadequate, trying to begin this reparative process. I wanted to do more, and in the car, driving home to Belfast, I often felt I wanted to turn back and give the group a 'gold medal' and instantly make them feel better.

The group paused. I waited. And then someone—an experienced mental health professional—came up with an idea that helped us understand the patient under discussion. I rapidly felt the pressure releasing from me and was delighted to 'feel the authority' going back into the group. Of course, what I had to give up was my narcissism and the wish to be idealised. While this is a common phenomenon in supervision groups, I believe that this hierarchical model of understanding problems is particularly prevalent here.

Narcissism

Traumatically stressful life events can alter the form and quality of identity in the life-cycle. It is common for the victim to experience a

> loss of cohesion and continuity in the self after the trauma. There is almost always a form of narcissistic injury to the sense of integrity and cohesiveness of the self as experienced subjectively by the person. [Wilson, 1989, p. 214]
>
> Some traumatised people remain preoccupied with the trauma t the expense of other life experiences and continue to re-create it in some form for themselves or for others. Clinically these people are observed to have a vague sense of apprehension, emptiness, boredom and anxiety when not involved in activities reminiscent of the trauma. [Van de Kolk, 1989, p. 399]

Traumatic events attack the core of self-identity and at the same time can accentuate psychotic (Bion, 1961) aspects of the personality which can become addicted to destructive processes. Here the media attention can become the narcissistic limelight for those traumatised by the bomb to recover a feeling of well-being and self-worth whereby they become the representation of emotional suffering. This aspect of the traumatic event is most difficult to explore clinically because of the perversion of sources of self-esteem—the tragedy and suffering of the event. In adopting Bion's conceptualisation of psychopathology, individuals can demonstrate a mercurial and fragile relationship with others which appears powerful and excited (Fairbairn, 1954) when issues surrounding the tragedy are narcissistically displayed.

A patient suffered terrible physical wounds in the blast. Being close to the bomb, she suffered first- and second-degree burns and other physical injuries. In the discussions within the support group, there was tremendous empathy and concern for her plight, yet also a growing irritation as to how others, with similar, worse, or lesser injuries were not receiving the same attention. The wounds of this particular patient were both physical and narcissistic. Clinically, this mobilised previously-dormant psychotic processes, which demanded emotional attention to her plight. Otherwise people would quickly be accused of being uncaring. Manic defences (Segal, 1995) were also evident, whereby excitement was gained through controlling and triumphant experiences over others. 'I'm in charge and I have the worst injuries.' Others affected by the bomb would feel peripherised by the attention given to this patient.

The reaction in the support group to this 'injured state of mind' reflected the internal world of this patient. On presentation, there would be an intense interest in the patient because of the high profile of this particular casualty from the bomb. In discussing the case, the support-worker found it difficult to maintain boundaries, as the staff-member often had to respond to the immediate demands of the patient, or be accused of neglect and of not really caring. This particular patient had also lost 'loved ones'. But there was little or no space to talk about this loss, and on many occasions the staff found themselves containing the 'dead parts' of families, as these could not be tolerated by those directly affected by the bomb. The bomb had exploded many disturbing parts of people which were being projected into the Team, who were being asked to contain human destructiveness, yet were also struggling to give some meaning to events which would lead to resolution. For such severely injured states of mind, staff were left feeling trapped by being asked to perform therapeutic miracles to take away from the patient the physical pain she was enduring; they were forced to contain the murderous rage against those who perpetrated the atrocity; and, in turn, the murderous rage stirred up in the casualties and the families. To take away any source of attention that the injury gave to the individual patient was like robbing them of all they had left.

However, movements did occur when staff felt able to put down boundaries and explore issues that helped the patient think about a resolution of issues. After much patience, the staff-member was allowed by a patient to talk about how the media attention, while exciting, also gave her something to think about rather than the mourning of loved ones and accepting the loss of a 'normal life' which her injuries did not allow her to pursue. This depressive-positioning work did occur, but only after much patience and thought on the part of the staff-member, who created an atmosphere of 'being emotionally available when you are ready to talk', rather than rushing in with good intentions to prove therapeutic worth in the face of such human tragedy.

In exploring this dynamic within the overall group processes, we found emerging a pattern of a potential contest for the worst injury, as this would bring potential media attention. In Northern Ireland, there has emerged the delicate issue of the victims of the Troubles. Considerable media and political attention has now been dedicated to alleviating the suffering of the victims. Victim groups have been developing over the last five-to-ten years, to highlight the issue of those affected. With this development there has also appeared a feeling of 'moral righteousness' with the "unthinkable thought" (Grinberg *et al.*, 1985) to question this righteousness. Could this be used as yet another narcissistic source of self-esteem, where the real victims may never get the help they need?

This manic flight into a 'fight–flight' group atmosphere proved very difficult to explore in the support group. Any preliminary exploration by the therapeutic worker around the truth value of the statement left the worker with a subjective feeling of having committed yet another moral crime. Projective processes (Main, 1957) are rife, with each individual accusing the other of immorality, yet also unwittingly using this moral perch as a source of narcissistic wellbeing. This style of relating is similar to what Ostell (1992) has called "absolutist thinking", in which a categorical and evaluative style of thinking arises from a belief in the rightness of certain values, goals and behaviours.

As Ostell and Oakland (1999) have recently described, when the demands of absolutist people are not met, their characteristic emotion is anger and the offending party is typically blamed and criticised.

Within the Northern Ireland group as a whole, I think there are signals of more work group (Bion, 1961) functioning, whereby there is a possibility that people can achieve their feelings of worth and satisfaction from everyday ordinary intimacy, where there does not have to be a traumatic event to give people a feeling of wellbeing. For example, there is more of an interesting urban and rural regeneration projects, designed to improve the social fabric of Northern Ireland, where people can feel good because of having a better life, rather than having an identity linked to violence. A pluralism of political parties is emerging wherein strongly-held views are talked about rather than 'acted out', which is evidence of movement to symbol formation in the depressive position rather than the concreteness of actually going out and killing someone. However, this group addiction to the headlines, and being in a group situation where there is pre-oedipal rivalry for 'mother's' attention, is difficult to break down. This is a new idea for ordinary people in Northern Ireland, the fear being that individuals and groups could lose their 'special place' in the eye of the world. This involves excited mental states (Fairbairn, 1954) which inevitably produce disappointing experiences being re-channelled into a group psychology that values mutual and positive human relations as a way of building a less narcissistically driven society.

Conclusion

Healthy group functioning is characterised by work group functioning (Bion, 1961), maximal interpersonal engagement (Yalom, 1985), a positive group matrix (Foulkes, 1964), and positive and creative object relations (Schedlinger, 1982) whereby individuals experience a group atmosphere of mutuality and reciprocity, with a minimum of hierarchical relationships. A traumatised group cannot demonstrate these processes until considerable efforts have taken place proactively to establish therapeutic processes that help dissolve psychotic denial and allow the emotional injuries to be healed. My thesis is that Omagh is leading the way in Northern Ireland society as the first spontaneous attempt to set up a group formally, immediately after the event, to create a container (Bion, 1961) to detoxify the psychotic content of a society that has been severely traumatised. Other sociological events, such as the publication of a report on how the victims of the troubles can be helped (Bloomfield Report, 1998), the creation of a more diverse and multi-cultural society (the author of this paper is the first ethnic minority Chief Executive of a public sector organisation) along with important political movements towards dialogue—all represent attempts to put in place psychological mechanisms that can provide constructive, rather than destructive, experiences.

The arrival of American colleagues from the American Group Psychotherapy Association, who now conduct an annual group psychotherapy conference, along with formal links with the Tavistock Centre, provide all members of the community with an opportunity to establish groups which foster positive object relations, rather than a return to primitive and projective group processes. This not only dilutes away from insularity, but gives people in Northern Ireland an idea that there are good experiences from the outside that can be 'taken in' to improve society.

The examples I have taken from the support groups illustrate the complexity of the therapeutic task in trying to develop intrapsychic and interpersonal relationships that are characterised by personal responsibility and concern, rather than hatred and revenge. I believe the will to repair is slowly awakening in Northern Ireland society where there is a wish to reconstruct what has been destroyed, and so create a better emotional life for the whole society, Catholic, Protestant, and other ethnic minorities that are now forming part of a pluralistic society.

CHAPTER TWENTY

The transgenerational transmission of holocaust trauma: lessons learned from the analysis of an adolescent with obsessive compulsive disorder

Peter Fonagy

Some relevant psychoanalytic contributions

Freud, in 'Totem and Taboo', made a remarkable assertion. He wrote: "We may safely assume that no generation is able to conceal *any* of its more important mental processes from its successor" (Freud, 1913a, p. 159). A number of outstanding psychoanalytic clinicians, writing almost two decades ago, made major contributions applying Freud's radical insight, to cases of children of victims of the holocaust.[1] Three key contributions are selected as they make a compelling case for traumatic reactions in the *children* of survivors, mediated by the impact of holocaust trauma on the early emotional environment provided by the survivors for their offspring.

Judith S. Kestenberg's innovative investigation of the effect of the holocaust on the second generation led to her description of the *transgenerational* transposition of trauma (Kestenberg, 1982). Kestenberg's patient, Rachel, appeared to live in the reality of her father's past, withdrawing from all social contacts, hiding like her father, who escaped by concealing himself outside the concentration camp. She is noted to have developed an insusceptibility to bodily and affective signals, retreating into narcissistic grandiosity which could withstand and survive torture and persecution. Kestenberg recognises that what is at work in second generation victims is *not* covered by the concept of identification; that it is tantamount to the patient's *immersion* in another reality and integrally involves the patient's body. The mechanism of 'transposition', according to Kestenberg, *resurrects* the murdered objects whom the caregiver (the survivor) cannot adequately mourn. The objects are re-created in the mind of the second generation survivor at the cost of extinguishing the *psychic centre* of her *own* life. Of course Kestenberg's observations overlap with those of Heidi Faimberg (1987) concerning the 'telescoping' of generations which is readily observed in victims of trauma.

Ilse Grubrich-Simitis (1984, 1981) further advanced our understanding. She focused on the impact of the extermination camp conditions on the ego's capacity to use metaphor, and the related capacity to structure past, present and future time. She pointed out that ego impairment of this kind may evoke a 'timeless concretism' in psychic functioning (p. 303) which manifests in the second generation. The immense anxieties of the traumatised victims, for which no intra-psychic defence is adequate, find expression in their effect upon the primary object relationships of the second generation. Building on the work of Masud Khan (1963), Grubrich-Simitis cogently links the mother's inability to promote her infant's early ego needs, to a vulnerability in the infant to later trauma. James Herzog (1982) evocatively described the psychological environment created by such traumatised parents as "a world beyond metaphor" (p. 114). In her 1984 paper, Grubrich-Simitis writes, considerably ahead of the revival of the intersubjective tradition in psychoanalysis, that a phase of *"joint acceptance of the Holocaust reality"* (p. 317) must be experienced by patient and analyst if the ultimate harmlessness of fantasies is to be accepted by the patient.

The third contribution from the early 1980s is that of Howard B. Levine (1982). In agreement with Judith Kestenberg, Levine recognised that children of survivors appropriately experience themselves as the target of persecution since the eliminationist anti-Semitism of Nazi ideology included them as the yet unborn carriers of Jewish genes. Levine points to the ways in which holocaust trauma undermines parenting capacity in the survivor: Depression, poor control of affect including guilt and aggression, unrealistic parental expectations, over-protectiveness, and the undermining of individuation, and so on. Levine's formulation of the "child of survivors complex" is that the syndrome is *neither exclusive* to such children, *nor* necessarily present in *all* of them but is, nonetheless, likely to manifest in problems of the separation-individuation process and the management of aggression. Children of survivors are poorly equipped to deal with the knowledge of the parental holocaust experience, and may find themselves identifying with parental character traits produced by that experience. Levine also stresses that what he describes may be generic to all extreme trauma, including severe sexual abuse, violence etc.

While all these suggestions are immensely illuminating, they do not fully explain the problems of third generation victims particularly at the level of psychoanalytic mechanisms. These are children of individuals onto whom trauma was transposed, who created murdered internal objects on the basis of their interactions with survivors, who were brought up in a "world beyond metaphor" but who themselves had no direct experience of trauma. Of course, we may simply assert the transgenerational continuity of these processes, but this would implicitly equate the actual trauma of the first generation of survivors with the manifestations of those experiences in the second and the third generation. In this paper it is suggested that additional constructs are needed to explain how *transmitted* trauma may impact on parent–infant (primary object) relationships, and in this context attachment theory may be of particular value.

Attachment theory

Attachment theory has been the black sheep of the psychoanalytic family. John Bowlby's early writings on the resolution trauma and loss (Bowlby, 1960) were the subject of severe criticisms from Anna Freud, Rene Spitz and Max Schur as well as others who considered it mechanistic, non-dynamic and based on thorough misunderstandings of psychoanalytic theory (Freud, 1960; Schur, 1960; Spitz, 1960). Opposition to his views provided one small area of common ground for the followers of Anna Freud and Melanie Klein (Grosskruth, 1986), and for decades Bowlby was a relatively isolated figure in psychoanalysis.

Attachment theory is, however, experiencing something of a psychoanalytic renaissance (e.g. Lichtenberg, 1995). This is perhaps due to the increasing ecumenicalism of psychoanalysis (e.g. Pine, 1990) or the general acceptance of an object relations perspective in the basic psychoanalytic model (Sandler & Sandler, 1998). According to attachment theory, the primary function of early object relationships is to provide the infant with a sense of security in environments which induce fear (Bowlby, 1969, 1973). Bowlby assumed that on the basis of the interactions between the infant and a caregiver, self-other representations develop (he termed these internal working models) which reflect the child's cumulative experience of sensitivity on the part of that caregiver. This aspect of infant–caregiver relationships is present in most psychoanalytic formulations and clearly overlaps with some current uses of Bion's containment concept (Bion, 1962b), Winnicott's holding environment (Winnicott, 1965), Kohut's suggestions concerning selfobjects (Kohut, 1971), and Sandler's concept of safety (Sandler, 1960). The child's confidence in the caregiver's capacity to appreciate his state of distress and to act upon this understanding is reflected in the security of the bond between infant and mother (Ainsworth *et al.*, 1978).

Research using Mary Main's Adult Attachment Interview may have also contributed to the increasing acceptance of attachment theory ideas. The AAI represents an attempt to assess current mental representations by adults of their childhood attachment experiences (Main *et al.*, 1985). Several studies, including one by our team in London, have demonstrated that in as many as 80% of cases, infant attachment classification can be predicted on the basis of adult attachment classification made before the birth of the child (Fonagy *et al.*, 1991b; Steele *et al.*, 1996). Parents with an insecure (incoherent) view of their childhood attachment experiences are highly likely to build an anxious attachment relationship with their infants (van IJzendoorn, 1995).

Attachment and dissociation

The relevance of attachment theory to the present context is clearer in the light of trans-generational studies which have shown that caregivers with unresolved experiences of mourning and trauma appear to cause disorganisation in their infants' attachment relationships. The interview reveals such 'lack of resolution' through apparently minor cognitive irregularities when either loss or trauma is discussed (slips of the tongue, confusions of past and present, confusions of identity, momentary lapses of reasoning, prolonged pauses or unexpected intrusions of the trauma into other contexts, etc.) (Main & Goldwyn, in preparation). Caregivers showing this pattern have infants who tend to manifest bizarre or 'disorganised' behaviour when reuniting with their caregiver following a brief period of separation—behaviours such as head banging, freezing, hitting, hiding, or collapsing. It is important to note that it is not trauma *per se*, but its lack of resolution, its unmetabolised character, that appears to be associated with disorganised infant attachment. Disorganised infant behaviour upon reunion may accompany avoidant, resistant or even secure attachment, just as lack of resolution of trauma can be found in dismissing, enmeshed (preoccupied/entangled) or secure-autonomous interviews. Remarkably, disorganised attachment behaviour in infancy manifests as rigid, controlling behaviour in middle childhood and sometimes quite severe psychological disturbance in adolescence (Lyons-Ruth, 1996). There is considerable evidence that infants manifesting some degree of disorganisation in infancy can become controlling, bossy children with their attachment figures even if their attachment classification was originally disorganised-secure (Cassidy & Marvin, 1992). Parents of such children report experiences of feeling controlled by their child (George & Solomon, 1996) and of seeing children as replicas of themselves (Solomon & George, 1996). Consistent with this pattern of externalisation, is the precocious caregiving behaviour manifested by many such children (West & George, in press).

Why should unresolved trauma in one generation be associated with disorganised attachment behaviour in the next? One persuasive theory, recently confirmed by direct observation (Schuengel, 1997), suggests that lack of resolution of trauma may be associated with parental *fear* in response to infant distress (Main & Hesse, 1990). Scheungel (1997) videotaped natural interactions between mothers and infants who manifested disorganised behaviour in the strange situation. Videotapes of the interactions were independently coded. The patterns indicated significantly more frightened, frightening or dissociated reactions were found in the behaviour of mothers whose infants manifested disorganised behaviour. It is assumed that the child perceives the parent as either frightened or frightening. As the parent's reaction is unpredictable, neither the strategy of avoidance or resistance is sufficient to allow the child to cope with these episodes. The child's working model governing the infant–caregiver relationship is incoherent and consequently the infant's behaviour in the strange situation is disorganised.

Psychoanalytic observations may help us in elaboration of this process. Acute trauma, such as even temporary separation in infancy, brings forth three biological responses: fight, flight and dissociation. These reactions are rarely prolonged in infancy if the child's emotional environment is sufficiently attuned and responsive. In the absence of responsiveness, the infant's flight or fight reaction may manifest as a behavioural defence of infancy as observed by Selma Fraiberg (1982). The infant may display a flight reaction and withdraw from the caregiver (Ainsworth's avoidant pattern) or manifest a rudimentary attempt to fight her (the resistant pattern). Whereas the former may be an adaptive pattern when faced with an intrusive caregiver, the latter might be helpful to the infant whose caregiver is only sporadically responsive (Belsky *et al.*, 1995). Neither of these strategies is available to the infant confronted by a caregiver who is overall responsive, yet at times absent—is frightened or frightening in response to the child's need for comfort. The infant's emotional expression perhaps triggers a temporary failure on the part of the caretaker to perceive the child as a person in his own right. The child comes to experience his own arousal as a danger signal for loss of emotional contact, accompanied by an intensification of the need for comforting. His best strategy may then be dissociation, the splitting of consciousness, absenting himself mentally from a situation from which he cannot escape (Liotti, 1995). Internal working models, based upon such interactions, may then contain a construction of a self representation that is threatening, even devilish, alternatively helpless or out of control, disintegrating, or defensively grandiose and all-powerful.

The behaviour of the infant in this situation gives clear indication of multiple, incoherently integrated structures, highly reminiscent of dissociative adult patients. Like dissociative adult patients they often show disorientation and look glazed, as if in a trance, express intense affects but are unable to relate their behaviour to current events. This lack of integration is clear in dissociated adult patients who may ask for attention, then reject offers of help, then express a sense of feeling dangerous, go on to accuse the therapist of having damaged them, then voice the hope that they are loved and so on—all sometimes within a matter of minutes. Of course, such reactions mostly follow trauma in later childhood or adolescence (Allen, 1995; Terr, 1994; van der Kolk, 1994). What is being claimed here is that dissociative response to trauma in adolescence or adulthood is *primed* by the presence of a dissociative core in the self-representation. In other words, *disorganised attachment creates a predisposition to a dissociative response.*

These ideas may help us understand 'the children of survivors syndrome'. Let us assume that some survivors of the holocaust, often manifesting no overt symptomatology, find the experience of child rearing at times an intolerable challenge. At moments interactions with their infants may have triggered memories accompanied by unbearable psychic pain from which they could only find refuge in states of dissociation. These may have been momentary experiences in a personality otherwise well-defended and apparently intact. Such moments of dissociation might, however, have been sufficient to create disorganisation in their infant's attachment behaviour. It is important to recall that disorganised attachment may frequently accompany otherwise secure internal working models. Other survivors, including those with profound post-traumatic disorganisation of character, may have led their child to be avoidant or resistant as well as disorganised. It is not mere insecurity of attachment which constitutes the child of survivor syndrome. It is the disorganisation which contains within it the seed for a dissociative response to later trauma, through its impact on the child's experience of internal reality. More specifically, self-states and associated mental representations which appear to trigger a frightened or frightening reaction from the caregiver will be marked in the child's mind as dangerous, and sensitise him to specific ideas associated with this reaction. The disorganisation of early attachment creates a potential for the child to experience these representations as part of concrete reality rather than psychic reality. This risk persists for the child of the child of the survivor, whether manifest psychopathology was evident in the parent or not, and may account for the apparent 'transmission' of specific memories and related affect across three generations.

Case presentation

Glen started his analysis in a profoundly dissociated state. For the most part he was mentally absent and totally inaccessible. Although he was fifteen, he had the appearance of a ten-year-old. He sat in a chair withdrawn, staring vacantly, there and yet not there, huddled in his tent-like coat far too big for him. Sometimes he hid his face in his hands, occasionally he looked at me through a gap he made between his fingers. Frequently, he totally failed to respond to what I said, or would respond after a long interval, ignoring other things I had said in between. I had a sense of immense hostility, of uncontained confusion verging on madness, and yet this did not seem to be what he was expressing. There were sessions when he was able to talk and at these times the infantile nature of his mental functioning was revealed in a stark and disturbing way.

His clinical diagnosis would have been obsessive-compulsive disorder (OCD). The diagnostic profile described Glen as "almost pre-psychotic" and painted a picture not usually considered suitable for psychoanalytic treatment. Such labels, however, cannot adequately convey the word and thought magic which had totally overtaken his life. His life was completely organised around rituals from the moment he got up and had to tidy his room, in a particular order, sometimes repeatedly if he felt he might have got the order wrong, all through the school day, and to the moment he got into bed when he had to place his pillows at certain angles to the room, to the sunset and to his body. On the surface, he wished to avoid "bad luck" but underneath was a dread of intrusive ideas, concretised as alien beings, spiders, and bacteria. He was terrorised by the delusional (almost hallucinatory) idea that the creature from the film *Alien* lived in the fireplace or in the garden.

His dissociative state was not restricted to the clinical setting: his referral was prompted by his parents observing him walking through the house in a kimono holding a candle, failing to respond to his parents' anxious inquiries as to what on earth he thought he was doing.

There appeared to be little in Glen's background that would easily justify his state of mind. His father was probably an authoritarian man who certainly lacked empathy but who was also rather concerned about his son. Mother also seemed to be a caring person but she tended to be depressed; she denied the pervasive nature of Glen's disturbance and described her relationship with Glen's father as deeply troubled. I knew that she had been in treatment with a colleague of mine following an earlier referral of the child to the Anna Freud Centre.

It was difficult to know how best to formulate Glen's difficulties; he seemed relatively bright and in some ways even talented, but totally isolated, and embattled in a constant struggle against a regressive pull in order to contain intense destructive fantasies. His symptoms had worsened rapidly before his referral for treatment and he and his parents were clearly terrified that he was going mad.

Once treatment began, I was quickly at a *total* loss about how to help Glen. Nothing seemed to work. I attempted to do interpretative work with little success. Not one of a wide variety of interpretations had any apparent effect and it was clear that I was not getting through to him. I became angry with him and found it quite hard to resist the temptation to give up on him. I blamed others, the diagnostic team for not screening him adequately, his parents for not recognising his difficulties, but above all him for remaining inaccessible and making me so helpless. After a year of treatment the frustration was almost intolerable and seeking consultation seemed the only solution.[2]

The consultation helped in making me aware of the presence of trauma somewhere in Glen's history. Second, the consultant recognised my anxiety about driving Glen mad which undoubtedly made me interpret more than was helpful. Third, the consultant supported me in my work with his paranoia, which turned out to require a radical change of approach. I abandoned some of my formal interpretative style with him; I became livelier, almost trying to cajole him out of his suspicious stance. I started making jokes and humoured him about his feelings of anger with me, his wish to kill me so I would stop bothering him "once and for all". I imitated his behaviour, showing him rather than telling him how he appeared to me. I chatted to him about my messy room and how I thought he disliked it but didn't want to say in case I might be offended. On a wet morning we talked about him being cross about getting wet, just so he could come and be bored by me for 50 minutes. On one occasion, when he mentioned a teacher of his who was bald and inadvertently glanced at me, I said how pleased he must feel that he had hair and I didn't, and how ridiculous he thought I looked.

This change of strategy began to bear fruit. Slowly he became visibly more relaxed, his posture changed, he took his coat off. He also opened up verbally and told me about important anxieties, particularly surrounding work. He shared with me, in a manner implying his wish for me to help, his worries about his homework, his wish to be appreciated by his teachers and the dread that he might disappoint them. I suggested that he must have been frightened all along about not coming up to my expectations, that he might feel just terrible were I to be disapproving, and were he to care even momentarily about what I thought and felt about him.

Glen started looking at me, and there were *fewer* periods of long silence. He began to talk about the thoughts and feelings he had had when he had been withdrawn. He had imagined that he was throwing knives into my body or just missing me, *loving* the feeling of control and torture. He gave me room to interpret that his worry about my power over him could be related to his wish to control and frighten me; that he wished to destroy people because he was so afraid of them. He was increasingly grateful for my interpretations and some days almost seemed pleased to see me. By the end of the first year, a therapeutic alliance had developed where I was seen as both useful and, on the whole, non-malevolent.

Over the next couple of years he made increasingly good use of the analysis and improved symptomatically in ways that both he and his parents clearly noticed. For example, the rituals almost completely ceased and no longer preoccupied him. His obsessional work patterns gave way to a far more relaxed but by no means disorganised attitude. The most remarkable change was at the level of his relationship with me. Even at moments of great anger and resentment, of which there were a fair few, I mostly felt in the presence of a young person rather than an *alien being*. Only in retrospect did I become aware of how dehumanised I had felt with Glen in the first period of his treatment.

There were several key points. The first was our recognition of the significance of his early period at school when he was regarded as a slow learner and offered remedial teaching. He had found the experience humiliating, not least because of the exceptionally high performance of his older brother and his "'friends'" thinly disguised mocking attitude. He was terrified that I wanted to exploit him: "You don't want to help me, you just want to research my problems". In the transference, I was the father/analyst ready to exploit and humiliate him. Reversing the transference, empathising with the wish to humiliate me, seemed to help.

Although I did not notice this at the time, the material we were working with had a special character. A choice had to be made between success and catastrophic failure. The world was for geniuses and retards, millionaires and beggars, masters and slaves. But where one ended up seemed arbitrary.

Importantly, I now think, our understanding of Glen's problems took a leap forward when some feelings concerning the holocaust indirectly entered the material. This was initiated by a school visit to the film 'Schindler's List' which he was seriously considering not going to. He was greatly disturbed by the film. Over a number of sessions he was once again silent. The dissociated, dream like states returned with somewhat of a vengeance. I told him that I knew from our past work together that he was suffering but I could not help him because he dared not let me. He accused me of being a torturer. I was surprised but I said (somewhat insensitively) that I wondered if he was not confusing me with a part of himself. He got angry. "You understand nothing! You are *not* Jewish!" I reflected that perhaps at the moment it felt safer for me not to understand and not to be Jewish because that protected me from the torturer part of him. He cried but between his sobs he explained that he did not understand, but felt that if people were as inhumane as the Nazis then really they should not be considered human. I said: "I think you are telling me that I don't understand what it feels like when you have thoughts which make you feel inhuman". He eventually disclosed, as I had suspected, that he had fantasised being the Camp Commandant in the film who was using Jewish workers for target practice. This quickly led to the elaboration of these fantasies and a shameful disclosure that he constantly fantasised about attacking people and killing them in painful ways.

It took us some time, but eventually we talked at some length about his fantasy of torturing me. He described the various ways he had thought of causing me pain, particularly enjoying the idea of my begging for mercy. Interestingly this was linked to his neurotic concern about his father's tendency to shut himself off in his study, particularly after playful teasing by his family. He feared his father might commit suicide and dreaded both being blamed and the horrible feelings of self-blame. Historical material emerged about his experience of his father's vulnerability and the fragility of his parents' marriage. Eventually it transpired that his concern was far greater about his mother's depression than his father's. It seemed that his mother terrified him by retiring to bed, sometimes as early as 6.00 p.m., leaving the children to look after themselves. His fears about my fragility suddenly made more sense to both of us and he told me how reassured he had been when he realised "that you can take a joke". His sadism out in the open, he became increasingly relaxed in the sessions, would sit slouched in the chair, would play games at my expense, mock my room, mimic my habits, comment on my baldness and my tendency to wear the same clothes all the time. In the transference I seemed to become a pre-depressed mother and he was visibly enjoying the experience of the revival of this relationship. Other clinicians working at the Centre noted the change in him: Unbeknown to me, he was walking down the stairs whistling.

About two years into the treatment he began to trust me with his sexual secrets. He masturbated to pictures of naked women. He felt deeply ashamed about this and wondered if I would refuse to see him after he disclosed his practices. His aggression deeply permeated his sexuality. The excitement of guns, pain in others and sexual pleasure appeared to be confused in his mind. My acceptance of these fantasies led to an immense sense of relief and he started thinking about asking girls out, although initially at least, he had little success.

Glen's analysis was completed in three and a half years. During this time anxieties about performance in exams, masturbation and other aspects of sexuality emerged as would be developmentally expected. His adaptation improved remarkably. His obsessional rituals either stopped or they no longer bothered him. His exam performance was well above average and he was offered places in a number of universities. He continued in psychotherapy for a further year, and I continue to receive bulletins of his progress.

Attachment, self-development and transgenerational trauma

The reader may be puzzled why this brief report of an analysis of a neurotic adolescent is included as part of a paper on an attachment theory approach to transgenerational trauma. There were some features of this case which I believe are critical to an understanding of both Glen's pathology and his remarkable improvement in psychoanalytic treatment. It should be pointed out that some of this information comes from my awareness of therapeutic work with Glen's mother who was also treated at the Anna Freud Centre many years before Glen by one of the most senior members of the Clinic.

Glen was one of three third generation holocaust survivors I have treated at the Anna Freud Centre and the model I shall outline fits all of them. Glen's mother was the daughter of a concentration camp survivor who came to England after the war. Both her mother's parents had been destroyed and only her mother and a younger brother had survived from a large family. Glen's grandmother almost never talked with her daughter about her camp experiences, although she mentioned the horrific episode of being separated from her own parents who were not selected for 'work' on their arrival in the camp. Glen's mother suspected that her mother, an attractive woman, had been sexually exploited in the camps and that her mother's shame and humiliation about this had led to the family's 'conspiracy of silence'.

Glen's birth coincided with the death of her father, a kindly man, considerably older than her mother. Her mother became psychotic after the loss, and she had felt very torn between offering support to her mother and looking after her new-born child. She recalled staring at the baby and wondering if it was worthwhile "to bring another human being into a world with so much suffering".

Glen's mother's development and pathology fit well with what we know about those in the "persistent shadow of the holocaust" (Moses, 1993), the fate of second generation survivors. Of special interest here is the possible impact of such transgenerational trauma upon her own parenting capacity. In the final part of this paper I would like to suggest an attachment theory formulation of transgenerational vulnerabilities associated with severe trauma, using Glen as an illustration. A key construct underpinning our thinking on this subject (Fonagy *et al.*, 1995) is that of mentalisation or reflective function. This is the generic human capacity to understand behaviour, not simply in terms of observable outcomes or physical constraints, but by postulating thoughts, feelings, desires and beliefs, taking what Dennett (1987) called the "intentional stance". We have shown that high reflective capacity in the caregiver, in narratives of childhood attachment relationships, predicts attachment security in infants, particularly if the caregiver reports a significant history of trauma or deprivation (Fonagy et al., 1991a, 1994). It also predicts the child's capacity to interpret the behaviour of others, in terms of beliefs and desires in middle childhood (Fonagy, 1997; Fonagy et al., 1997). An understanding of mental states does not spontaneously emerge from the observation of internal experience. Rather, the infant's observation of the self becomes meaningful in the context of the caregiver's reactions to his or her expressions of intentionality. The internalisation at the core of the child's self is a perception of the caregiver's perception of him as an intentional being (See Figure 1).

Winnicott (1967, p. 33) warned us that failing to find his or her current state mirrored, the child is likely to internalise the mother's actual state as part of his or her own self structure. The child incorporates into his or her nascent self-structure a representation of the other (Fonagy & Target, 1995). When confronted with a

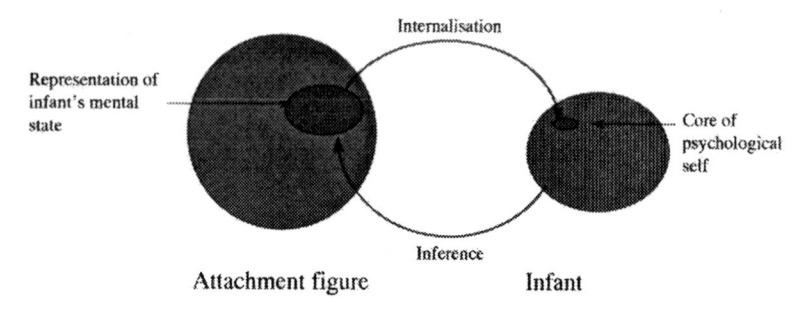

Figure 1. The birth of the psychological self. The infant 'discovers' his or her intentional state or subjectivity within the mind of the attachment figure who through a process of inference creates a representation of the child's mind and behaves in relation to the child in accordance with this representation. The infant perceives and internalises the caregiver's representation to form the core of his mentalising or psychological self.

frightened or frightening caregiver, the infant takes in as part of himself the mother's feeling of rage, hatred or fear, and her image of him as frightening or unmanageable (see Figure 2). This painful image must then be externalised for the child to achieve a bearable and coherent self-representation. The disorganised attachment behaviour of the infant, and its sequelae, bossy and controlling interactions with the parent, may be understood as a rudimentary attempt to blot out the unacceptable aspects of the self-representation. Later attempts at manipulating the behaviour of the other permits the externalisation of parts of the self and limits further intrusion into the self-representation (see Figure 3). A potential for dissociation is created by this lack of integration of the self, and is used to prevent further encroachment. Glen began the analysis in a dissociated state, with an overwhelming need to control his environment. My initial, regrettable reaction to Glen's distress, one of angry irritation, was a revival in the transference of the externalisation of his perception of his mother's reactions to him in infancy, which constituted the unbearable parts of his self-representation.

Dissociation is a converse of reflective function, or mentalisation.

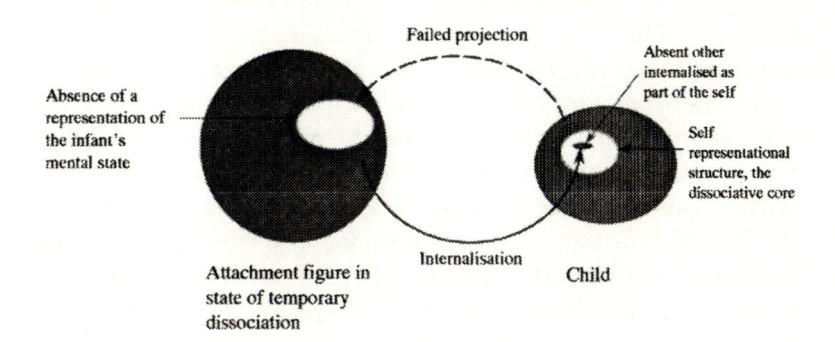

Figure 2. The birth of 'the alien' self. In infant-caregiver couples where the attachment figure is in a state of momentary dissociation when faced with the infant's distress no representation of the infant's mental state is present. The child is then unable to find himself as an intentional being in the caregiver's mind and internalises the absence of a representation into the self as well as the actual other which is alien to the self-representational structure.

```
      Alien self   Dissociative
                   self representation
                                          Externalisation
```

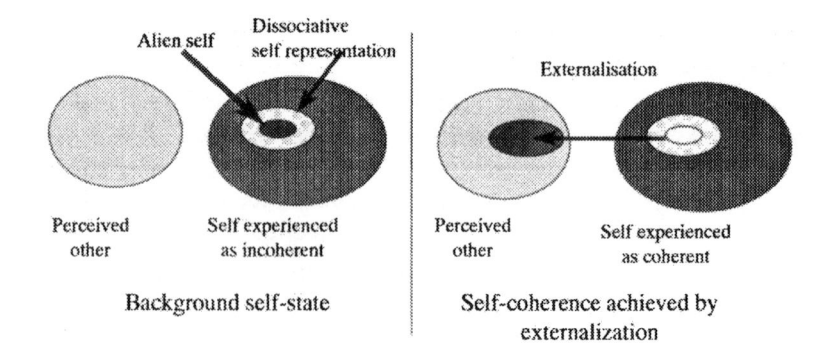

Perceived   Self experienced   Perceived   Self experienced
  other   as incoherent   other   as coherent

    Background self-state   Self-coherence achieved by
                                              externalization

Figure 3. A model of disorganisation of attachment beyond infancy. The individual whose self structure is at least in part dissociated, experiences the self as incoherent. In order to create a coherent self structure, he or she must manipulate the behaviour of a physically proximal other to achieve the illusion that the alien part of the self is actually outside rather than inside. The self can then be experienced as coherent.

The term dissociation refers to a disjunction between related mental contents (Ross *et al.*, 1989), which would normally be integrated into a singular subjectivity by mentalisation. The individual has awareness of the stimulus but is unable to become aware of that awareness. The individual has feelings and thoughts, but cannot represent these as feelings and thoughts. Without the ability to reflect, the normal meaning of experience is lost. Experiences of the self exist in limbo, separate from other aspects of mental function.

Glen had experienced no major trauma, yet the dissociative defence, which normally only extreme stress can create *de novo*, was, I believe, socially transmitted to him in infancy. From an attachment theory perspective then, it could be argued that Glen's attachment was on the whole dismissive but also over-controlling, as might be expected as the developmental sequel of disorganised attachment in infancy. We may speculate that as a consequence of the disorganisation of his attachment system, there was a vulnerable breach in his self-structure created by his lack of contact with his experience of himself. Hence his dramatic reaction to what were ultimately neurotic conflicts. We believe that the kind of catastrophic reaction which occurred, collapse of his personality, came about through a dysfunction in his self representation due to what were described as the profound psychological absences of his mother of infancy, the sequelae of her own infancy and unresolved traumata.

The dissociated core of the self is an absence, rather than genuine psychic content. It reflects a breach in the boundaries of the self, creating an openness in the self to colonisation by the mental states of the attachment figure. As Kestenberg (1982) demonstrated, this is not a process of identification as it is not a modification of the self-representation to match the established representation of the other. The dissociative core permits the *direct transmission of unconscious traumatic fantasy from mother or father to child*. Glen's material contained many ideas from the holocaust; he appeared to experience these as his own, notwithstanding the distance of two generations. We have noted the profound impact of the film *Schindler's List* on his fantasies, as well as his paranoid anxieties of persecution. Perhaps even more relevant, his thinking was permeated by specific images which we can trace to his grandmother's experiences, as probably imagined by his mother. In this category I would include: his cruel work regime, *used* to obliterate psychic reality; his terror of being mocked or humiliated by those he considered his friends; his preoccupation with baldness which was perhaps more than a transference manifestation to a bald analyst as of course his grandmother's head had been shaved; the arbitrary choices between life and death, success and failure may link to the fate of his *great*-grandparents. He would often say, with complete conviction, that what would happen to him in the day was going to be determined by some random event, such as marks on the Coke can which he would get from the school vending machine. Both he and his mother showed a frightened rejection of sexuality, and an assumption that sex meant exploitation and sadism. Many themes recurred in Glen's analysis that were also present in his mother's analysis, and could be linked to holocaust experiences.

As part of *her* therapy, Glen's mother expressly linked these and other concerns to her *own* mother's experience—her fear of being photographed, of losing her hair, of being tortured with knives, the terror associated with the thought of being mocked and humiliated by people she knew well, an almost total work inhibition, a terror of exploitation. The match of psychic material between Glen and his mother felt in excess of what could be accounted for by coincidence. Of course in Glen's mother these images figured in a very different neurotic constellation, they were not focused on castration and homosexual concerns, as were Glen's. Nor was she as clearly preoccupied with violent sadism. In our view, once these structures are introjected into the self, they become part of developmentally expectable neurotic constellations, the vicissitudes of sexual and destructive conflicts. This may account for a severe presentation which nevertheless appears to respond rapidly to analysis and, after a rocky start, yields good outcome.

The mechanism of transmission and the mechanism of change

The images of horror which are transposed into the self re-emerge in the minds of a subsequent generation, not by a process of magic or even a latter-day Lamarckian model of evolution (as Freud probably conceived). I believe that the specificity derives simply from the selectiveness of moments of non-responsiveness on the part of the caregiver. For example, during our exploration of Glen's fantasies of throwing knives at me, he told me of his terror of knives, which during his period of severe obsessionality he had had to keep locked away. He also had to check, repeatedly, that no knives had been left out at night, as someone could get up, accidentally knock a knife off the table, step on it with bare feet and cause serious injury. He mentioned, almost in passing, that his mother had not let him touch knives until he was at least 9 or 10 and on the one occasion when at the age of six he had picked up a knife, she had screamed and fainted. This had caused him to drop the knife and cut himself. Specific images of the child's mind as generated in the caregiver's construction of the child's mental states could trigger associations on the part of the caregiver, and generate dissociative episodes; the representational boundary between self and other in the child's mind becomes permeable, and the child's model of the caregiver's mental state enters the dissociative core self.

Grubrich-Simitis (1984) made a critical observation concerning second generation survivors: "The patients frequently regard what they have to say as thing-like. They appear not to regard it as something imagined or remembered, as something having sign character. The open-ended quality of fantasy life is missing. Instead the expressions have a peculiarly fixed and unalterable quality, which may at first sight strike one as psychotic" (p. 302). Grubrich-Simitis links this to "the realisation of a psychotic universe" in the extermination camp, which brings about a breakdown of inner reality. I believe this formulation, somewhat modified, may be extended to the third generation. Glen's mind, as we have seen, provided a kind of wax mould for his mother's representations of traumatic experiences. And once these representations had been created they acquired a reality and force indistinguishable from that of externally perceived events. His near-delusional beliefs, which many including myself erroneously considered pre-psychotic whilst recognised by him as ideas, were just as powerful as events in the physical world. Developmentally, in these areas at least, he functioned at the level of a two year old, experiencing his mind as if it were a recording, device with an exact correspondence between internal states and external reality. We have used the term *psychic equivalence* (Fonagy & Target, 1996; Target & Fonagy, 1996) to denote this mode of mental functioning which Grubrich-Simitis refers to as "concrete" (as opposed to metaphoric).

The pervasiveness of the concrete, psychic equivalence mode of subjectivity would be hard to over-estimate in the initial phase of Glen's analysis. It is also important to note that what emerged as an effective technique was a deliberately, and perhaps provocatively, playful stance to confront this dead structure. Although there was clearly warmth and humour and many other non-specific features of this approach, perhaps most significant was the demand on Glen's ego. The analyst made real that which Glen was determined to dissociate, in a desperate attempt to deny its immediacy. Glen's analyst forced Glen to play with the ideas of humiliation, torture, annihilation and exploitation. Glen's tendency had been to regress to a mode of mental functioning where ideas can have no implication for the world outside (the *pretend mode* of the normal two-year-old child). Gradually, and through close contact with the analyst's mind, which could hold together Glen's terrifying perspective of equivalence and his desperate need to dissociate internal states from reality, an integration of the equivalence and pretend modes gave rise to a psychic reality in which feelings and ideas were known as internal and yet in close relationship with what was outside. Klauber (1987) wrote that "transference not only helps the patient to discriminate but also to imagine" (p. 44).

Klauber was probably addressing the same phenomenon which Grubrich-Simitis described and we have attempted to place within a developmental perspective. Glen could not possibly express his aggressive thoughts until he could learn to imagine, or more specifically, until he could understand that what he was doing was imagining. The change in therapeutic style recommended by the consultant to the case was of course powerfully advocated by Bowlby (1988) himself as well as other clinicians in the attachment theory tradition (Hopkins, 1984).

The model of therapeutic change which seems most relevant to Glen's improvement are the ideas of Thomas Ogden on potential space (Ogden, 1985, 1986, 1989). The therapist's task appears to be analogous to that of the parent who creates a 'frame' for pretend play (e.g. Mayes & Cohen, 1993; Vygotsky, 1967)—except in this case it is thoughts and feelings that can become once again accessible through the creation of a transitional area. Within the dissociative state, ideas are unmentalised representations, or more accurately the dissociative state of separation between internal and external reality may be conceived of as a defence against the experienced equivalence between what is internal and what is external. Glen's analysis and perhaps that of other dissociating traumatised patients was about working with precursors of mentalised ideas. The task could be conceived as one of elaborating Glen's concrete models into intentional ones. The analyst's task was one of integrating or bridging Glen's pretend or dissociated mode of functioning where little of importance felt real with moments when words and ideas could carry unbelievable potency and destructiveness. With highly traumatised patients, this can indeed seem like an awesome task. With Glen, the process appeared to be relatively straightforward. The analyst worked by entering Glen's pretend world trying to make it real while at the same time avoiding entanglement, which arises out of the equation of thoughts and reality.

An essential component of this process is the attachment relationship that is established between patient and therapist. Importantly, attachment, as has been suggested, is closely linked to interpersonal understanding (Fonagy *et al.*, 1995). The therapist's understanding of the patient's latent (non-conscious) intentionality recreates certain structural aspects of the infant-caregiver relationship. It revives a situation where the patient attempts to find 'his mental state' in the words and gestures of the therapist, much like not yet self-aware infants searches for their intentionality in the actions of the mother (Fonagy *et al.*, 1991a). The establishment of an attachment relationship, I believe, is a precondition for the kind of rehabilitative change that is required by dissociative traumatised patients. It should not surprise us then that individuals with secure attachment classifications, whose minds are presumably more open to accommodate mental states in the other, tend to make better therapists (Dozier, 1994).

Qualifications and conclusions

Perhaps at this stage some qualifications are in order. It should be acknowledged that the argument whereby the dissociated state of the mother creates a vulnerability for a similar state in the child, which in its turn could create an exceptional receptivity to specific interpersonal representations entailed in the traumatic experiences of a prior generation, is not only highly speculative but can only be supported by rather scanty clinical data. For example, Glen's pathology may well have been the consequence of disturbances in his relationship experiences within his own generation. An adequate account of his pathology might be given in terms of his problematic relationship with his father and his therapeutic experiences with an alternative male figure which might have acted as a kind of corrective emotional experience (Alexander & French, 1946). Where the more traditional account of Glen's neurosis appears to fall short of satisfying at least the present writer, is in the striking co-occurrence of a very severe presentation, the apparent absence of major environmental deprivations and the relatively rapid response to a somewhat modified psychotherapeutic approach to his treatment. Of course it is always possible to argue that trauma and deprivation was present in Glen's own childhood, but this remained hidden from the analyst and other clinicians. Alternatively, a psychosocial account may be entirely replaced with an explanation in terms of genetic vulnerability. At least in the present writer's experience, neither of these scenarios is consistent with a rapid response to psychoanalytic psychotherapeutic intervention. Thus while the evidence for this elaborate theory of

Glen's disturbance is admittedly somewhat thin, the clinical puzzle he presented is sufficiently intriguing to merit a certain amount of speculation, along lines which others might find useful and add their experiences should these be consistent or inconsistent with the present formulations. From a research perspective, much needs to be learned about the caregiving behaviour of second generation victims of major trauma. While the impact of trauma on caregiving is relatively well established (e.g. Liotti, 1992, 1995; Schuengel, 1997), we do not know enough about the caregiving which the second generation of victims are offered. Yet, it is clear that stability of attachment classification may often be maintained across three generations (Benoit & Parker, 1994). Ongoing studies in Israel and Germany by Avi Sagi and the Grossmans exploring the impact of the holocaust on the second and third generation may indeed provide exactly such useful data.

Why did holocaust experiences have such a uniquely traumatising impact, not only (we can assume) on every immediate victim but also on generations to follow? Perhaps the answer lies in some of the mechanisms which understanding the third generation has helped us identify. Every infant experiences occasional failures of parental attunement (Tronick, 1989). Even the best parents will sometimes fail to reflect the infant's intentionality in moments of distress, and will then briefly undermine his feeling of being human, with a subjectivity, thoughts and feelings which are normally turned into a meaningful psychic reality with the help of the caregiver. Each person is instead, at moments, treated as inhuman, leaving a dissociative area in the self, however small and normally inactive. It is this infantile experience that is activated by the conditions of the holocaust. The holocaust involved a society which appeared to be (and to remain) civilised, turning on a group within it and stripping them of all humanity, dignity and safety. People who could have been expected to treat their compatriots as fellow human beings with intentionality, suddenly began to treat the Jews with hatred and a systematic brutality previously unimaginable even between enemy peoples or between humans and animals. The same people continued to behave in a normal way in other relationships.

It is in this duality that perhaps the cruellest aspect of the trauma lies. Mindless persecution destroys our deepest rooted and most cherished expectations about human behaviour, that it is regulated by a mutual recognition of mental states. The genocide occurred within countries, rather than through external attack, the victims were tortured and degraded by fellow members of a community, people *like* the victims. Just as child abuse is particularly damaging when perpetrated by a family member, so we may expect persecution to be annihilating when it is carried out by people whom we might otherwise trust to reaffirm our intentionality. Yet when those people ignore our cries, pay no heed to our evident suffering, we know that this can only be achieved by abolishing a picture of us as psychological beings. Our residual dependence on the social other to reaffirm our psychic reality causes the regression to a psychic equivalence mode of thought and the dissociative/ pretend mode of thinking which developmentally represents its counterweight. This regression widens the breach in the boundaries of the self left behind by momentary experiences of inescapable, though probably inadvertent, attacks on intentionality within all infant-caregiver relationships. Individuals with relatively minor disorganisation within their attachment system we expect to withstand trauma more effectively but it is unlikely that anyone is immune. Once opened, this gap takes perhaps many generations to heal, and through it pass images of horror, including confusions of identity between victim and torturer, guilt and shame, paranoia and helplessness. Yet once inherited, they acquire meaning in terms of the individual's current psychic reality, and need to be dealt with in the here and now, not the there and then. The third generation survivor may, however, require unusual care from the analyst to ensure that the intentionality of the patient is fostered specifically in the domains where the intactness of the patient's subjectivity has been so deeply compromised.

Notes

1. The psychoanalytic literature on the Holocaust is vast and a comprehensive review is beyond the scope of this paper and this author's competence. The interested reader is referred to reviews by Jucovy (1992) or Moses (1993).
2. The Consultant was the late Marion Burgner, whose enormous help with this case I am pleased to acknowledge.

CHAPTER TWENTY ONE

The holocaust and the power of powerlessness: survivor guilt an unhealed wound

Alfred Garwood

Reading the psychodynamic literature on Holocaust survivors, my increasing sense of dissatisfaction prompted the writing of this paper. Numerous authors present deeply moving material from survivors' lives and then offer some explanation of psychic function. The theoretical bases of these explanations were usually derived from classical psychoanalytic theory. It became increasingly clear that current theory did not satisfactorily explain Holocaust trauma and its psychic consequences which led me to the new formulations offered. There is an implicit but unstated belief that only material obtained from the clinical setting has value or reliability. This view asks us to believe that behaviour in everyday life is not motivated by the same emotions and psychic processes demonstrated in the therapeutic setting and that survivors only allow their true selves in therapy? In the standard literature material from therapy or psychoanalysis is presented: the context and interpersonal setting are often needed to give it solidity but are lacking. It is for this reason I have drawn on my experience of being a child survivor of the Holocaust, a child of survivors, as well as the many subsequent years of contact with the world of survivors to attempt to make the mental processes of the

Holocaust survivor more accessible and comprehensible. None of the material is presented as though derived from the clinical setting. This is a considered choice. If compared with clinical material in the now extensive literature it will be seen that there is no qualitative significant difference. There are strikingly few detailed case histories and reports on psychotherapeutic work available (Grubrich-Simitis, 1981). Almost all the material presented was taken from my family's direct experience in which I have been a participant as well as a witness. My survivor relatives, like the vast majority of survivors, would not seek therapy or psychoanalysis. However, much of the material was presented during my own analyses. In my attempts to understand my own psychic processes and formative experiences, both during and after the Holocaust, I have had what I believe is a rare if not an unique opportunity—to explore, as a participant, an analysand and a psychoanalytic psychotherapist, a complete nuclear survivor family's entire post-Holocaust life and their struggle with their massive psychic trauma, which would never have become available for study as clinical material. It is unlikely that in the clinical setting the precise chronology, and completeness of detail, as well as the complex interactions described, which are open to verification, would ever have come to light. These efforts have produced the ideas and conclusions presented. In traumatised families one member often takes the role of the healer. It is in this spirit that this paper was written.

When psychoanalysis and psychotherapists attempt to understand the effects of the Nazi Holocaust on its survivors they are faced with inherent difficulties. The experiences of the survivors are unimaginable. Even if the survivor's suffering is graphically described, the listener's self-protective conscious and unconscious defences prevent them subjecting themselves to that degree of suffering. Thus the Holocaust survivors' experiences and psychological processes tend to be imbued with a mysticism and fear that may inhibit full and free analysis. As the survivor is so often held in awe, what tends to be overlooked is that they entered the nightmare world of the Holocaust as ordinary human beings and were forced to endure extraordinary events. The mental mechanisms available to them were no different from those available to all human beings. Although the full intensity of the experiences and suffering of the survivor is unimaginable, it may still be examined and understood.

Survivor guilt

It should be stated clearly that not all survivors suffer guilt nor has the extent to which it is suffered been fully investigated. There appears to be little consensus as to the psychic determinants of its formation or the mental mechanisms involved. This has confused the efforts and compounded the well-recognised difficulties of those working with Holocaust survivors (Chodoff, 1980; Danieli, 1981; Kren, 1989). Survivor guilt does not fit classical theory which maintains that the creation of neurotic guilt is related to the fulfilment or feared fulfilment of instinctual impulses or infantile unconscious wishes (Rycroft, 1995). Thus survivor guilt has been widely viewed as being guilt for behaviour Holocaust survivors would not have engaged in under ordinary circumstances (Ornstein, 1989). The important early theories were Anna Freud's (1937) concept of 'identification with the aggressor'. This proposes that identification with the aggressor reinforces and increases the intensity of the guilt. Bettelheim (1943), a psychoanalyst who spent a year in Dachau and Buchenwald in 1938, was an important but misleading influence. His description of behaviour in the camp was unremittingly negative and denigratory in tone, omitting the important place of reciprocity described by Frankl (1987) and others. Most recent theorists have held the classical view that survivor guilt is a form of pathological mourning in which the individual felt guilty for aggressive feelings towards the lost object, these feelings being suppressed. These death wishes became linked with the actual destruction of the object. Niederland (1981) later suggested that survivor guilt was a reaction to simply having survived. More recent views have considered its adaptive aspect. Distinction has been made between various types of guilt. Carmelly (1975) distinguished passive carriers who felt guilty about their survival from those who felt guilty about actual immoral acts. Robert Jay Lifton (1967) studies Hiroshima survivors coining the term, 'death guilt'. Lifton (1979) later differentiated between moral and psychological guilt and considered classical writing as having described the latter. He viewed moral guilt as an adaptive experience that helps individuals see their shortcomings which, when not worked through, can lead to psychopathology. Grubrich-Simitis (1981) suggests extreme trauma can be cumulative (Khan,

1974), causing permanent changes in psychic structures through deprivation of external narcissistic supplies leading to narcissistic depletion, which causes grave and permanent changes to the ego ideal. Klein (1984) considered that guilt maintained a link to the Holocaust survivors' past and those they lost, thereby serving a healthy adaptive purpose in maintaining a sense of belonging to their lost family and to the Jewish people.

Survivor guilt development

All the above theories appear to offer some degree of understanding of survivor guilt, the more recent adaptive theories being of greatest value. However they do not adequately explain its perplexingly high incidence in survivors nor its formation, intensity and persistence. Some were forced to act in ways for which guilt was entirely appropriate. For them, all causes of guilt will be linked and add to the intensity of the guilt. The classical theories of guilt direct thinking away from the actual experience and towards the phantasies generated in the unconscious. These may intensify and reinforce the response to the experience but did not determine the psychic mechanisms and consequences. In the formation of the established views the existing theories have been inadequate and new hypotheses are required and are offered below. It may be that the manifest horror of the concentration camp experience obstructed clear analysis and distracted from the pre-camp experience which gives the clues enabling the survivor guilt puzzle to be solved. It is also essential to the understanding of the survivors' post-Holocaust functioning.

The four essential components to Holocaust survivors' trauma are: (1) *threat of annihilation*, (2) *powerlessness*, (3) *object loss* and (4) *torture*. The latter would be considered by some to be a combination of powerlessness and threat of annihilation. All four reinforce one another but powerlessness in the fact of annihilation threat is of the greatest importance.

The majority of Nazi Holocaust survivors were confirmed in the *ghettos* of Eastern Europe. Many were the fitter younger Jewish inhabitants of the thousands of adjacent smaller communities, their parents and younger siblings having been murdered. The ghettos were formed in the major towns adjacent to the railway and were walled off from the non-Jewish part of the town. They were inhumanely overcrowded and unsanitary. Anyone attempting to leave was shot on the spot. A *Judenrat*, a Jewish administration of Jewish elders, was immediately formed by order of the Nazis. They were made to maintain lists of the ghetto's population from which they were forced to make the selections for deportations to camps or for immediate murder by shooting. Some elders resisted, well aware of the fatal consequences (Freiwald & Mendelsohn, 1994). They were forced to distribute the progressively reduced starvation rations leading to death from malnutrition and disease.

> Death from 'natural causes' such as starvation and typhoid fever was the norm. Early mornings brought the sight of those that had thus died together with victims of random shootings and hangings by one or two Gestapo who had dropped in for a visit the previous evening. In the distorted faces of these adults and children strewn around, I would recognise those of kin, friends and teachers ... '*Aktions*' or raids were routine and culminated in the victims being murdered by machine-gunning, were succeeded by the more 'efficient' deportation to the death camps. Although the fate of those deported was not known for certain, though suspected by those left behind, a deep depression always hung on the emptied ghetto streets for days after. [Rosenbloom, 1988]

These carefully planned and developed programmes of systematic terrorisation, ghettoisation and concentration camp internment—intended to impoverish, humiliate, deceive and enslave—made the Jews feel they were in part responsible for their own fate. They were led to believe that if they obeyed, worked and were useful they could buy a little more time and survive. The true purpose of these systems was to ensure that virtually no Jew had enough food, luck or resourcefulness to escape death. To have survived despite all this, the survivors were made to feel they had had more than their fair share of luck, usefulness, resourcefulness or food (Leon *et al.*, 1980). Thus they were made to feel they had survived by eating the food or using the lucky chance that might have kept their loved ones from death—that the price of their survival was the death of their loved ones and fellow Jews.

In the fact of their cumulative losses and these inescapable yet impossible choices, of the mental mechanisms available to adopt or defend against their powerlessness, *self blame* and consequential guilt were almost inevitable. It is my view that *'survivor self blame'* had the initial primary and principal function of reducing the pain and anguish of intolerable powerlessness in the face of annihilation risk and overwhelming loss. Being forced to be totally passive and helpless in the face of the Holocaust was perhaps the most devastating experience for the survivor.

Resistance to healing and mourning

Survivor guilt has persisted primarily because survivors are unable to grieve and mourn their losses successfully. Whenever losses are remembered, the overwhelming feelings of powerlessness and annihilation fears that were experienced at the time of the events together with the highly effective defence of self-blame are mobilised with others described below. These effectively obstruct working through and thus the mourning process. The unconscious tension between the fundamental need to mourn and the overwhelming feelings of powerlessness and annihilation anxiety that would then have to be endured generate effective defences to alleviate the psychic pain. It can be seen that, if effective defences are not mobilised, then the unremitting intensity of feelings of self-blame and guilt would be likely to cause intense and possibly psychotic depression with suicidal feelings, culminating in suicide which, sadly, has been observed.

The effective mourning of loss has long been understood as fundamental to mental health. It is well established that the mourning of a single important loss can be difficult, often needs facilitation and frequently, when to some degree unsuccessful, leads to psychopathology. When the losses were unnatural, cruel, often unprepared for, and frequently multiple, then the difficulties of mourning are increased exponentially. Mourning at the time of the losses was virtually impossible as survivors were involved in their own life and death struggle. On liberation the understandable priority was to rebuild their lives; and they were encouraged to look forward and put the past behind them. Delay in mourning is known to increase the difficulty and reduce the likelihood of success. It may be that "the mourning cannot be finished in one lifetime. It will take generations. Over six million Jews died, the enormity staggers one" (Kestenberg, 1995, personal communication).

Powerlessness and self-blame

In order to explain survivor self-blame and traumatic stress properly a new primal developmental theory is proposed (Garwood, 1996). In the post-partum period the neonate is totally dependent on its carer for survival. Until memory is developed internalisation of the carer as a protective object cannot take place. All significant discomforts such as hunger, pain and cold will be experienced as possible abandonment which will provoke instinctual fear of annihilation with attendant instinctually driven anxiety derived from the self-preservation instinct. Hunger implies mother's failure to feed and potential starvation; cold implies the absence of mother's protective and warmth-providing care; and pain implies an attack on the body's integrity. This early experience of annihilation threat and helplessness produces what may be described as primal agony which is encapsulated (Hopper, 1991) and becomes hidden by infant amnesia. The biological instinct for self-preservation generates psychic energy which is both more powerful than, and reinforces and underpins the sexual drive as it is a prerequisite that the individual must survive to attain sexual maturity in order to preserve the species. Powerlessness in later life evokes unconscious memories of this earliest vulnerable state and primal agony, accompanied by overwhelming emotions, mobilising powerful defences, often self-blame and consequential guilt. The power and effect in later life of this neonatal experience have been underestimated. Permanent loss, bereavement, is a psychic trauma which forces us to confront our mortality and thus resurrects these earliest instinctual annihilation anxieties. This gives grief its extraordinary psychic power. Thus loss, powerlessness and annihilation anxiety are instinctually and psychically linked. Self-blame in the face of powerlessness is a commonly observed phenomenon. Those confronted with the death of a loved one frequently turn to self-blame or blame of the medical profession as a defence against their powerlessness and the finality of the loss. Young children, when faced with the break-up of their parents' marriage, are observed to promise to be good and to behave better in future if only their parents would stay together. Self-blame and consequential guilt, though still causing great psychic pain, are less emotionally painful, anxiety-provoking and overwhelming than powerlessness. They create a self-empowering omnipotent phantasy which presupposes responsibility and the power, ability and possibility to exercise it. Self-blame implies "I chose wrongly: I could have done something: I can do something and if I only try hard enough I will find what it is" (Danieli, 1988). Self-blame and survivor guilt are observed in many survivors of life-threatening traumata other than the Nazi Holocaust. A young man in his early twenties developed acute myeloid leukaemia and needed a bone-marrow transplant to survive. He was admitted to a specialist ward with nine other young men all undergoing similar transplants. Three years later he consulted his general practitioner in great distress. He was the sole survivor. Having seen them die, one by one, he was consumed by intolerable and overwhelming guilt. His feelings at times were so overwhelming and painful that he preferred to die with the others even though he had a young wife and child.

A survivor of a Polish ghetto showed great courage by regularly escaping, risking death to purchase food, and continuing even after narrowly escaping execution. Subsequently he was taken to Bergen-Belsen with his wife and two young children, all of whom survived. In his later years he expressed a willingness to go back to Belsen, the site of their terrible ordeal and triumphant survival. Asked if he would go back to Poland he said that 'he could not possibly bear the dreadful memories which this would bring'. The pain he expected was far greater than from returning to Belsen. For him, the effect of the ghetto was greater than two years in Belsen, even though he had shown defiance and resistance, his spirit unbroken.

When his wife's parents, whom he loved dearly, were 'selected' in the ghetto, his wife, five months pregnant, handed him their three-year-old daughter and attempted to go with them to her virtually certain death. She preferred to die rather than suffer this dreadful loss. She was prevented, not by her husband, but by an SS officer who ordered her back. Her husband knew he was totally powerless to stop her and, without the Nazi's intervention, he would have lost his wife and unborn child. To a man of action and fearlessness in the face of death, his powerlessness during these vents evoked unbearable psychic pain and then later the defence of self-blame and guilt. Twenty years after liberation he stated: "I still have nightmares. I dream they are coming to take my wife and children away from me". Soon after liberation he met a Belsen survivor who said of him to one of his relatives that in Belsen 'he had had it good'. He had been a *Lager Friseur*, a camp barber, a needed trade, which meant he was able to earn extra food. Thus he had some advantage. There are a number of survivors who tell of his sharing his bread and saving their lives at the risk of being shot. He also risked his life obtaining costume jewellery to make into jewellery that appears to be of great value 'to sweeten' the notorious SS guard, Irma Grese. She had a Dobermann dog which she used to set on the camp inmates for her pleasure. These 'gifts' were known to reduce her ferocious brutality. Thus he saved lives at risk of his own. Yet he took the remark that 'he had had it good' as implying he had collaborated and never forgot the insult. For over 40 years he avoided contact with this precious remnant of his family—choosing virtual isolation rather than face this accusation and his own survivor self-blame and guilt.

A unifying hypothesis

The classically based theories of survivor guilt are largely of the superego. These include oedipal murderous phantasies towards lost objects, identification with the aggressor (Anna Freud) and cumulative trauma damaging the ego ideal (Grubrich-Simitis). The separation of moral and psychological guilt (Lifton) separates conscience and superego, and is self contradictory. Guilt for simply having survived (Niederland) or death guilt (Lifton) is descriptive rather than explanatory. Most of the remaining theories are separative-adaptive theories maintaining links to the lost past (Klein). At first glance powerlessness in the face of loss has little obvious connection with the classic concepts of oedipal murderous phantasies or identification with the aggressor and the other reparative adaptive theories. However, further examination reveals links. The postulate that the central traumatising experiences were powerlessness in the face of annihilation risk, reinforced by object loss, would lead one to predict that the defences generated would be primarily omnipotent phantasies as a response to powerlessness, encapsulation as a response to annihilation threat and anxiety and attempted reparation of losses. The psychic self-empowerment necessary for self-blame is achieved through omnipotent phantasy. Both oedipal murderous phantasies and identification with the aggressor may be viewed as defensive omnipotence. Cumulative trauma and damaged ego ideal imply regression to a primitive malleable state. The traumata, undefined in the writings of Khan and Grubrich-Simitis, producing psychic changes through altered internal objects and ego ideal, are congruent with the unifying hypothesis. The intense psychic energy generated by the unconscious memories of annihilation threat will be directed into any defence or psychic process at any level which will diffuse it. Self-blame is the response to memories of primal powerlessness, which will cause guilt at the level of the superego and ego ideal, and remembered actions or humiliations will be found to become its vehicle.

The important issues of rage and shame deserve some discussion. When an annihilation threat is experienced, the instinctive reflex response of fight or flight (Cannon & De LePaz, 1911) is generated. In a neonate neither flight nor fight is possible nor can internalisation of an object occur until memory develops. This increases the intensity of the instinctual fear generated. Primal psychic agony is experienced which sensitises the individual to powerlessness, and annihilation threat in later life is postulated as a new developmental hypothesis (Garwood, 1996). In the adult Holocaust victim the rage generated by the fight response to annihilation threat could not be expressed without increasing the threat and anxiety (Danieli, 1995). This it was invariably directed towards self (Woodmansey, 1966)—by intensifying the self-blame and guilt. The super-ego is conceived as deriving its energy from the child's own aggression: as a result the sense of guilt is influenced directly by the extent to which the individual expresses his aggressive feelings by taking it out on himself in moral condemnation (Rycroft)—or by identification with the aggressor. Many survivors suffer feelings of shame. Self-blame and shame are functions of the self-observing aspect of the psyche, the super-ego and the ego ideal. Survivors, when attempting to integrate the humiliation and degradation they suffered, will find remembered experiences of denigration to act as vehicles for self-blame causing shame.

The traumata

It is a commonly held belief that the concentration camp was the most traumatising Nazi Holocaust experience due to its manifest dreadfulness and was presumed to be the major aetiological experience of the so-called survivor syndrome and survivor guilt. It is observed that the dreadful screaming nightmares together with the other florid symptoms commonly suffered by concentration camp survivors diminish in frequency and intensity with time. However, the memory of their losses usually remains unbearably painful. Eitinger (1971) studied 227 non-Jewish Norwegian concentration camp survivors and found that guilt was not a significant characteristic in his subjects. He suggested that the absence of a hero's welcome for the Jewish survivors accounted for their survivor guilt. This may have had some reinforcing effect but does not provide a convincing explanation.

Although the great majority of the European Jewish population were concentrated in the East and were forced into ghettos, many survivors came from Holland, France, Belgium and Denmark, where ghettos were the exception. The Jews of Germany and Austria never suffered ghettoisation during this period. However, many suffer survivor guilt.

I have proposed that powerlessness in the fact of annihilation risk and loss are the essential traumata required to generate the defence of self-blame and thus survivor guilt. These traumata can readily be found in the experience of the Jews of Northern and Western Europe. In Germany and Austria increasingly anti-Jewish laws and public humiliation were intended to disempower, impoverish and terrorise. Ten thousand Kindertransport children from Germany, Austria and Czechoslovakia were torn from their families and put on trains to Britain by anguished parents desperate to save their children's lives. In the other occupied countries deportation to camps took place rapidly without formation of ghettos. In the camps disempowerment infantalisation, humiliation, starvation, torture and murder wee the daily fare. Many children were hidden in these countries and were totally dependent for their survival on the protectors. Most suffered the loss of one or both parents. Thus the combination of powerlessness, annihilation and loss can be found in experiences of survivors of ghettos, the camps, hiding, Kindertransports and refugees from Germany and Austria.

Adaptive and maladaptive defensive behaviour

Survivors' post-Holocaust behaviour shows successful adaptive as well as maladaptive defensive patterns. These may be defensive, reparative and adaptive at the same time. They can be described as *searching, silence, living in the past, readiness for disaster, overprotectiveness, intrusiveness, boundarylessness, dependence phobia and control excess*. These have been described separately for the sake of clarity but may be seen to coexist and overlap.

In the survivor family previously described, the man and woman showed two well-recognised patterns of behaviour. He, characteristically, turned to action and was constantly searching for survivors. There is a well-described post-Holocaust symptom-free interval in the survivor syndrome. Williams & Kestenberg (1974) suggested this was due to survivors still hoping and waiting to find some remnant of their families in fantasy thereby delaying the full impact of the losses. This observation would support the thesis of the effectiveness of the denial and the attempted reparation in actively searching together with the other defences used to minimise the attendant anguish in this initial post-Holocaust period when the losses had to be faced.

In his constant searching, the man had discovered on one of their many trips to Israel that there might be a surviving *Landsmann*, a fellow exile from their home community, who was a pre-war friend and a ghetto policeman living in Paris. Forty-five years after their liberation they found him. On meeting, the conversation was entirely between the men, with the wife a silent onlooker. Their conversation was confined to the confirmation of who had died, how they had died. Eventually they came to the death of his wife's parents. Although the ghetto policeman had reported having seen her father's body in the square, she was unable to retain this. She became confused and, on later questioning, said that she could not remember what he had said. Her husband was most careful to protect her from this affirmation of her losses, being uncharacteristically gentle and sensitive, allowing her her defence.

The defensive behaviour of searching is common. It is not usually seen by the survivor as consciously searching for surviving family members but logically must include that possibility. It is clearly reparative bringing a reduction of the sense of loss and, if the *Landsmann* knew their family, it brings an affirmation of their pre-Holocaust family and life. This may facilitate a degree of healing nostalgia and is generally felt to be of great comfort. However, whilst searching goes on, powerlessness and loss are denied and mourning is to some degree blocked.

His wife behaved in an entirely different manner showing passive stillness, silence and avoidance of anything to do with her losses, avoiding any mention of her murdered parents, sister and brothers. This silence was so complete that their children were not told the names of their murdered grandparents, aunts and uncles until some 45 years after the war. The survivor who never talks of the Holocaust or their lost family is repeatedly described in the literature. The example given typifies this behaviour which demonstrates the defence mechanisms of repression, confusion and denial. It may also demonstrate encapsulation of annihilation anxiety (Hopper, 1991). Both survivors described were always highly protective towards one another when dealing with any loss. The serious illness or death of a friend or acquaintance would be carefully kept from one another for as long as possible, sometimes permanently, in a clear manoeuvre to protect the other's feelings and perhaps their own. The link to the avoidance of facing loss is clear.

A couple survived in hiding for 11 months in a camouflaged cellar, often starving and losing their first-born son in a fire. They live in the past, maintaining the same lifestyle since the Holocaust. The husband had learnt whilst under the Russian occupation of Poland that working in a hospital kitchen meant he and his family never went hungry. His post-war daily routine would begin at dawn when he would prepare food for the day. He made soup, a meat dish with vegetable dishes—always enough to feed his family with much to spare. His conversation was almost solely on the subjects of his exploits and experiences whilst the personal slave of the SS commander of his town, the recently convicted Joseph

Schwamberger (Freiwald & Mendelsohn, 1994), and whilst in hiding. His wife would also talk of little else other than the ghetto, her home community and her murdered family. They seemed to be living as though still in the ghetto, frozen in time. They believed the cause of any illness was due to 'bad' or inadequate food and the cure, his special cooking.

Holocaust survivors are commonly observed to hoard food, hide money, jewellery and valuables, living with a suitcase packed and ready to flee from disaster (the Nazis). This is another form of living in the past. The freezing of the Holocaust lifestyle expressed in readiness for disaster can be seen as an attempt to avoid the finality of these massive and cumulative losses as well as a defence against annihilation anxiety. If the Holocaust has not ended, then, in fantasy, there is still a chance that some relative may return. Whereas if the reality is of 50 years having passed without the return of the loved one, then their loss must be faced.

Many married survivors are inseparable from their spouses. The extent to which they are never parted, almost fused together, is underestimated or goes unrecognised. There are numerous descriptions in the literature of survivors marrying quickly after their liberation and living unhappily but inseparably. The large and growing literature on the second generation frequently describes the overprotectiveness of survivor parents. Difficulties of physical as well as psychological separation are significant and often central problems. Intrusiveness and the lack of boundaries are also frequently described. Fusion, clinging and physical proximity as protection from danger are all defences against annihilation anxiety, separation and loss.

Powerlessness being one of, if not the most traumatic experience of the Holocaust then empowerment if not omnipotence may be sought by the achievement of wealth and financial independence as well as control within the survivors' lives. Many if not most survivors are self-employed. Often their spouses and families are involved in their business. Control can be equated with power so that control over their lives, spouses, and children avoids the return of the feelings of powerlessness. However, this is usually overcontrol due to excessive unconscious anxiety and thus brings great tensions and sometimes catastrophic rebellion in their partner or children, driving them away.

Self-healing

Many survivor responses to their traumata have been adaptive, highly successful and healing. This is achieved through *safety, effective mourning* and *the creative reparative response to loss, reparation and memorialisation*. Thus the rebuilding of a family and a place in a new community with the gathering of the surviving remnants of their community was observed to be undertaken with the intense energy.

Through searching fellow survivors were found. In Israel and New York where substantial numbers were located, *Landsmannschaften*, the Yiddish name of associations of fellow countrymen and townsmen, were formed. Most survivors will recount being implored by a dying relative or fellow Jewish victims to survive and bear witness so that they had not died in vain. The recording of their testimony then became of paramount importance. Many write an account of their experiences and of their community before the Holocaust which would be amalgamated with others and published as a *Yiskor* book, giving them permanence. *Yiskor* is the Hebrew word for remembrance. The testimonies would usually include their last contact with their murdered loved ones, memorialising them. The therapeutic value of documenting these testimonies has been eloquently described (Krell, 1985).

In the year following the liberation of Bergen-Belsen 1000 babies were born to the survivors. The formed the World Association of Bergen-Belsen Survivors and still meet annually to commemorate their liberation. In 1945 the British Government, discovering many orphaned children in the concentration camps, agreed to bring 1000 of them to England. In the event only about 730 came. They were housed in ex-army camps and children's homes (Moskowitz, 1983). They formed strong bonds, acting as surrogate siblings and parents, and formed the 45 Aid Society, keeping in close touch ever since. They were unusual in being brought over as a group. Most survivors dispersed forming small clusters. Recently they have increasingly felt the effects of their isolation. As a consequence shared experience groups have formed. In England, associations of Holocaust survivors include groups of Camp Survivors, Child Survivors, Hidden Children and Kindertransport Children. After these groups formed the need for a meeting place was recognised and a centre was founded. Shared experience groups are particularly healing. The Child Survivor Association of Great Britain exemplifies these well. Most of the members had rarely met a fellow child survivor before coming to the group. It does not replace family and community in any immediately obvious way. There is a mixture of Child Survivors, Hidden Children and Kindertransport. What is shared and especially valued is the reparation of their enforced isolation as a consequence of their attempts at normal life. The almost universally expressed feeling that they are not understood by non-survivors is addressed. They are drawn together by a usually unspoken recognition of shared wounds and losses, without shame, explanation or justification of their needs, perhaps as it could be in a healing family.

Memorials are of the greatest importance. A fourteen-year-old survivor of a community of 1100 Jews in Galicia hid when the Nazis came to his village. On returning he discovered that his entire family together with the other Jewish villagers had been taken to the Jewish cemetery and murdered. Initially he was overwhelmed and immobilised with grief. When he recovered he vowed that they should never be forgotten. He was captured by the Nazis, survived a number of camps and eventually emigrated to Israel. There he formed a *Landsmannschaft* of the handful of survivors of his community scattered around the world. Being a close community, all had been to the village school and knew each other's murdered families. As the fiftieth anniversary of the murder of his family approached he became energised and worked frantically to realise his goal. Rather than meet in Israel as in previous years he arranged to meet in the village of their birth. He organised the building of a memorial on the site of the mass grave and had a road and bridge build over the stream. He arranged a solemn ceremony in which the Israeli Ambassador and a number of Polish high officials, including the Cardinal of Galicia, participated, observed by hundreds of the Polish villagers. Finally *Kaddish*, the Jewish memorial service for relatives who had died, was recited.

At the Chamber of the Holocaust on Mount Zion, Jerusalem, Israel's first Holocaust museum, there are hundreds of plaques commemorating survivors' murdered relatives. They are understandably precious as there are no graves and few have known resting places. There are hundreds of plaques commemorating the destruction of the Jewish communities, their dates, carved in Yiddish, the language of these destroyed communities. *Yiskor*, the service of remembrance, is recited annually on the anniversary. It may be no accident that the museum is part of a *Yeshiva*, a Hebrew college where Jewish law and tradition is studied and its students supported by the community, thus replacing one of the thousands of Yeshivot. memorialisation and naming of perished family give them a permanence that combats the fear that they will be forgotten and lost forever. This act of reparation is a fundamental one, its importance recognised and ritualised in most religions and societies. Recently, the famous Nazi hunter Serge Klarsfeld (1994) published a book naming the 11,104 Jewish children deported from France, most never to return. It contains 1500 photographs. He states: "We wanted to save the memory of these children from oblivion ... It is not a book of death but a book of life."

Successive Israeli governments have clearly understood this fundamental need, many ministers and members of parliament being Holocaust survivors. In Israel a day of Holocaust commemoration, Yom Hashoa, is a solemn national day of mourning. Moving ceremonies take place including a two-minute silence which is respected throughout the country. On the roads all vehicles are found at a standstill with their passengers and drivers standing in respectful silence when the announcing sirens are sounded. In addition, for the whole day the names of some of the millions that died are read out over loudspeakers throughout the country so that their names are spoken even when the last surviving relative has died. Thus they are never lost to oblivion. These are creative responses to the massive losses, which for some Holocaust survivors will be sufficient to enable adequate healing.

Yad Vashem, the Israeli Holocaust memorial and museum, has a Hall of Remembrance and a Hall of Names. The latter is where the names of those whose death had been witness is inscribed in books and treated with great reverence. Recently, a new memorial, the Valley of the Lost Communities, has been built. The deep significance of these memorials can be seen on the faces of the survivors present.

The Hassidic Jewish community, recognised by their black hats, long coats and sidelocks, frequently used to depict the archetypal Jew, continue to use Yiddish as their day-to-day language. it is believed that this community includes many Holocaust survivors. Little is known of them. However, it may be speculated that in this historically frozen, highly protective community where every aspect of their day-to-day life is laid down by Jewish law and tradition, Holocaust survivors may effectively insulate themselves from the past as well as slowly heal through the many rituals in the Jewish liturgy for mourning and loss. The history of the Jewish people includes many periods of great suffering which are commemorated in the liturgy, thereby giving numerous opportunities to mourn. It is the view of some writers that the ability to retain a strong religious belief has a powerful effect in assisting self-healing (Marcus & Rosenberg, 1989). Although this has not generally been linked with the psychic process of alignment with a deity, an omnipotent power may be seen as a defence against powerlessness and annihilation anxiety.

Therapeutic implications

Working as a psychoanalytic psychotherapist with those who have suffered severe traumatisation as well as many severely borderline psychotics has been of great benefit in considering the therapeutic implications for those working with survivors and their children. The proposed additions to psychodynamic theory offered and their therapeutic implications merit discussion. Therapists will be presented with the difficulty of containing and working with the affects associated with annihilation anxiety, powerlessness and multiple losses. These echo the neonatal dependent state and generate the most primitive and painful of emotions, and the most difficult to endure, for the patient and therapist. The countertransference may be so powerful as to be overwhelming and crippling (Danieli, 1981).

The taking of a history may be essential to establish and communicate that the Holocaust trauma and its importance in the current difficulties are recognised by the therapist. This avoids the conspiracy of silence invariably complained of by survivors who complain that their Holocaust experiences were avoided or barely touched on during their analyses. The initial task of making the therapeutic setting a safe one will inevitably be more difficult.

Consistency will be of greater than usual importance. Survivors have learnt not to trust too quickly as the price for error could be death. They are invariably extremely watchful with finely tuned antennae. This annihilation anxiety will colour the therapy from its onset. The defences developed at a time of existential annihilation threat will not readily be challenged nor relinquished. Focusing on and communicating the recognition of these feelings and the reasons for them are likely to speed the development of the therapeutic alliance.

The start, end and breaks between sessions are likely to be the centre of a struggle for control as they may be painfully experienced as a reminder of past powerlessness and thus be deeply persecuting. Trust and dependency are likely to be slow to develop and, when it does, the dependency is likely to be of great intensity. Thus breaks between sessions as well as longer breaks will be experienced with the attendant anxiety and power given them by the actual object losses experienced in the Holocaust. Defensive pre-empting and lengthening of the breaks may be more common than usual. The pain of powerlessness will need to be focused on repeatedly in its various manifestations. If feelings of loss and mourning are generated, then the attendant anguish, rage, hatred and desire for revenge will be present in the transference, of greater than usual intensity and much more difficult to bear in the countertransference.

The success of the working through of this intense grief may largely depend on the capacity of the therapist to tolerate, contain and work through the projected countertransference powerlessness, annihilation anxiety and feelings of loss. Many, if not most, attempts at therapy with survivors do not succeed.

At a conference a therapist despondently gave the example of a child survivor who asked "How can you help me if you cannot bring my mother and father back?" The psychotherapist expressed feelings of helplessness and of being deskilled. He may well have felt in his countertransference the survivor's overwhelming powerlessness and despair. Another psychotherapist, a Hidden Child Survivor, described treating a child survivor who at nine years of age had thrown herself into a ditch to avoid being shot with her family, hiding there for some days, immobilised with fear. The therapist described an attempt at psychodrama in which he offered his hand to help her out of the ditch in which she was still metaphorically hiding. He repeatedly implored her to take his hand but she was unable to do so. Her annihilation anxiety may simply have been too great. Had the countertransference powerlessness led him to need to be active? Would recognising the patient's annihilation anxiety and powerlessness, and communicating this to her and persisting with this approach, have been more effective and helped her psychically leave the ditch? Focusing on the survivor's powerlessness and annihilation anxiety in all its manifestations is probably only possible if the analyst or psychotherapist is able to recognise its place in the traumatisation, and thus in the countertransference, and thereby free themselves of its paralysing and deskilling effects.

In a large group the author held with children of survivors, the focus being on guilt, traumatic and painful material was presented of parental suffering and traumatising behaviour towards the participants. The tension in the group rose as successive participants related their experiences and expressed their feelings of guilt (and unconscious powerlessness). Nearing the end of the session when the tension had risen to a great intensity, the author offered the interpretation that their intense guilt was a response to their powerlessness in the face of the immense burden they felt in the face of their parents' loss and suffering. The tension in the group diffused almost instantaneously as though the valve of a pressure cooker had been released.

Self-styled specialists in working with Holocaust survivors are appearing. They often offer eclectic and short-term contract therapy. The idea that these psychological traumata can be treated by short-term therapy can clearly be seen to be unrealistic for the reasons given. The term 'eclectic therapy' may be a rationalisation of the therapist's 'acting in' as a consequence of their inability to tolerate the countertransference powerlessness. Without the foundation of an appropriate qualifying training, together with considerable skill and experience and probably supportive supervision, therapy is likely to fail. As survivors are likely to be easily disillusioned and then despair of help ever being available, particularly as they usually come to therapy only with great difficulty and often in crisis, never to return if let down, then referral for therapy should be restricted to those appropriately trained and experienced.

Discussion

It might well be asked why is a paper on the psychological effects of the Holocaust being written 50 years after its end? When so many survivors have died and most of those remaining will not come to therapy or are probably too old to benefit from it? What is its relevance today? Part of the answer is self-evident. The extensive specialist literature reflects how ill understood the effects of the Holocaust have been. This is particularly true of survivor guilt. There are relatively few detailed accounts of lengthy analyses or therapies of survivors. During my researches I discovered papers which stood up well to examination in the light of survivor's experience. Some added significantly to my understanding. Most presented moving experiences of survivors and then offered little or no insight or understanding. Some authors engaged in veritable intellectual contortionism attempting to use classical theory to explain survivor guilt. Most survivors complained of the conspiracy of silence during their psychotherapy which avoided their Holocaust experiences. It also seemed self evident that the only likely source of understanding of Holocaust trauma would come from psychoanalytic and psychodynamic concepts as non-psychodynamic theories seemed superficial and largely descriptive rather than explanatory. Detailed discussion of the application of psychodynamic or psychoanalytic theory or of mental mechanisms was invariably superficial, and discussion of technical implications was conspicuous by its absence. These conflicting observations led me to believe there were fundamental omissions in current psychoanalytic theory and thus prompted my attempt to identify clearly the essential traumatising experiences and the nature of the difficulties of understanding them and their psychological consequences. The question of why these traumatising experiences—annihilation threat, powerlessness, object loss and torture—were so powerfully traumatising led me to the omnipotent defence of self-blame and consequential survivor guilt, as well as the new developmental theory of the sensitising experience of neonatal powerlessness, annihilation threat, pain, cold and hunger and their link with the self-preservative instinct and primal agony.

It became increasingly apparent that these explanations could and should help explain the psychological sequelae of other traumata such as birth of a sibling, bereavement, rape (Hill & Zautra, 1989), incest, sexual abuse and other forms of post-traumatic stress. Sadly, history is repeating itself. The wars, genocides and human rights abuses of Korea, Vietnam, the former Yugoslavia, South Africa, South America and Rwanda have produced many traumatised survivors.

With the passage of 50 years the numbers of Holocaust survivors are dwindling. The child survivors will be the last witnesses of the Holocaust. Fortunately, they seem more open to psychodynamic therapies. The literature on survivors and the transgenerational effect is substantial and growing (Eitinger & Krell, 1985). The avoidance of powerlessness and loss is usually transmitted. The subject of therapy for survivors and the transgenerational effects, although discussed briefly, is one that requires lengthy and separate consideration. However, the issues of powerlessness, annihilation anxiety, loss and self-blame as a response are likely to be central. The extent of the transmission to subsequent generations is now recognised (Bergmann & Jucovy, 1982), and the massive task of mourning is passed on (Wardi, 1992). Thus, sadly, this paper may have particular relevance for many generations.

Acknowledgements

I must pay special tribute to my wife Yvonne without whose support this paper would not have been written. For their encouragement and helpful comments on earlier drafts of this article, I am indebted to Yael Danieli, Marvin Hurvich, Earl Hopper, Ann Karpf, Judith Kestenberg, Robert Krell, Sarah Maskovitz and to my colleagues, Anthony Garelick, Bron Lipkin, Kannan Navaratnem and David Vincent.

CHAPTER TWENTY TWO

Exile and bereavement

Barbara Hart

Introduction

It has been pointed out by Grubrich-Simitis (1984) in relation to the survivors of the Holocaust, that whereas in psychosis a disruption of inner reality is experienced, for the survivor the catastrophe is an actually experienced external event, though with massive effect on the internal reality. It is the collision of external and internal realities which I will examine in considering the impact of bereavement in the context of the multiple traumas of exile. While this collision is a feature of bereavement in general, there are particular factors, internal and external, which have an effect on the mourning process in exile and increase its difficulty.

Psychological implications of exile

The experience of exile itself has been characterised as one of multiple bereavement (de Wind, 1971; Munoz, 1981; Grubrich-Simitis, 1984) in terms of loss of country, status, activity, cultural reference points, social networks, and, above all, of family.

There is also the commonly experienced sense of 'lost time', i.e. hopes, ambitions, expected life-pattern disrupted, for example, by periods of imprisonment or being in hiding, or by discriminatory laws. These losses are often experienced simultaneously as a massive, pervasive trauma, or cumulatively.

The difficulty of achieving deferred hopes and expectations in exile leads to demoralisation. Freire (1980/82) describes the phenomenon of 'delayed arrival': denial of loss followed by the shock of the reality of exile.

Pre-flight periods frequently include severely traumatising experiences such as imprisonment, rape, and other forms of torture; by long periods of responding to external dangers, and of concomitant fear, anxiety, and necessarily sustained states of hyper-alertness.

These pre-flight experiences are often extended into the period of exile by the real or perceived threat of continued surveillance and pursuit, of deportation, and by the difficulty of meeting the basic needs for survival—food, housing, communication—while contending with an unfamiliar and often actively hostile environment.

The additional experience of bereavement in these circumstances is one of loss within a situation of pervasive loss, and in a context where both external and internal resources are severely depleted, so that the sense of self is already threatened, and in a state of increased vulnerability to further trauma.

In the case of pre-flight bereavement, it is common that, at the time, the event could not be adequately responded to, either in terms of traditional observance, or in terms of the individual's inner acknowledgement of the loss. Where self-preservation was the overriding imperative, to have mourned openly would have been to invite external danger (i.e. as a result of political repression). To have mourned inwardly would have exposed the self to feelings of depression and apathy, and inhibited the ability to respond to danger, so that affective response had to be denied, repressed or split off. Alternatively, response may already be numbed by reaction to pre-existing trauma. Bettelheim (1990a,b) gives an eloquent description of such circumstances in relation to orphaned child-survivors of the Holocaust.

The circumstances of a loved-one's death may in themselves have prevented both public expression of grief or its private acceptance; for example, where the death has occurred in prison, particularly after torture, the corpse is often withheld from relatives.

If any of these conditions obtain, the loss is carried, unmourned, into exile, if at all. This is well illustrated in the dream of a patient who had physically survived such an experience:

> I was cycling, with some friends, and on the back of my bicycle I was carrying a coffin: we were going to bury the person, but we came to a crossroads, and I had to go on alone, with the coffin ...

In the case of children in exile, the parents or surviving parent may exclude for them the possibility of mourning by denial of the event in an attempt to shield the child (and themselves) from the reality. Through the parents' inability to mourn, the task of mourning is displaced onto the children. This phenomenon is well documented in the literature concerning the second generation of Holocaust survivors (Pines, 1986; Winnik, 1968; Grubrich-Simitis, 1984).

In my own practice this was an important factor in the disturbance of two South East Asian adolescents I worked with, where there had been an attempt by the parents to shield the children from memory or discussion of the immediate pre-flight and flight experiences. This led to an alienating effect, in terms of cutting the children off from their past, and exacerbated intergenerational conflicts over cultural identity arising during a prolonged exile.

Once in exile, whether the bereavement occurred before or after the flight, the bereaved are unable to mourn successfully because of a number of both external and internal factors militating against this. Typically these are: (1) difficulty of reality-testing and (2) lack of containment and loss of socio-cultural structures.

Difficulties of reality testing

The impairment of reality-testing in reaction to trauma is compounded by the difficulty of how to differentiate a general and particular sense of loss, of how to verify the loss if a death is only reported to the bereaved, and the corpse or grave are unseen.

A frequent comment is: 'If only I could see for myself ... I don't feel he/she is dead.' It may be difficult to verify a death because the act of communicating with friends or relatives at home might endanger them, or it may be feared that this might be the case. Alternatively, communication may be possible, but rendered unreliable through censorship, interception, or by accepted custom in which relatives will temporise, and break bad news slowly or indirectly.

In these circumstances, there is frequently an unrealistic demand by surviving family members at home that the exiled person should return to take part in funerals or should contribute financially to the ceremonies, the maintenance of orphans; or, more painfully still, a feeling that they should have paid for medicines or otherwise prevented the death. Such demands feed into feelings of guilt and regret, and often there is no redress, no possibility of exculpation; or even explanation, because of the inherent objective difficulties of communication.

The difficulty of obtaining news of relatives left behind feeds into fantasies of their fate which are often more or less reality-based. One patient said: "My best hope is that my wife and the children are in prison but not yet dead." This person oscillates between the hope that they are alive, and despair that they are dead. He cannot be sure, and exists in a limbo in which he cannot, with any confidence, plan a future with them; but he cannot mourn them either, and is distressed by the conflict between his loyalty towards them and his own wish to live: "I do not know if I may marry again." In effect he is still in his own internal prison within himself, in his own mind—a predicament which commonly reflects subjectively the objective world experience.

Lack of a containing space

This applies in external terms as literally lack of private space in which to mourn (for example, in an overcrowded room in a bed-and-breakfast hostel), and societally.

In terms of the internal world, severely traumatised individuals experience a diminution of psychic space as a result of the experienced failure of external reality to provide adequate containment of projections, a phenomenon described by Reyes (1989).

A further aspect of lack of containment is the absence of the social structure of family and friends which would normally serve to facilitate and support mourning, and the absence of common cultural observance. This deprivation is particularly significant because mourning rituals universally contain, explicitly or implicitly, both explanatory and/or blaming components and reparative elements. That is to say, they require acknowledgement of loss and they facilitate reinstatement of the lost object. Such rituals both sanction a culturally acceptable expression of grief, and delimit it, setting the expectation of a gradual return to normal activity after the prescribed period of mourning. Frequently, they include physically holding the bereaved, restraining them from self-harm, sharing ritual mourning and offering comfort, bringing food to the house, and so on. The effect is to provide containment for grief, safety for the period of withdrawal from activity.

In the absence of either the comfort of ritual, or of family, or of friends, there may be no permission to grieve, no sense of safety in doing so, and no permission to cease grieving. Furthermore, the failure to carry out customary rites carries its own burden of guilty and in many cultures (see Harrell-Bond & Wilson, 1990, and clinical material below) incurs specific punishments such as possession by the spirit of the dead, and death curses: accurate metaphors for unaccomplished mourning.

Clinical implications

The difficulties of writing about, or clinically working with, bereavement in traumatised people reflects the dilemma with which they themselves are faced. When trauma is itself essentially an experience of profound loss, and the bereavement itself traumatic, is it possible to differentiate, to disentangle the experiences? To address the one without the other?

In the context of an already traumatised individual, the experience of bereavement serves to confirm other losses. For example the loss of mother would be seen as final confirmation of an irretrievable loss which began with loss of motherland. So that the inner resonance would be that whereas the good object had somehow been preserved up until this point (as evidenced by the very fact of survival), bereavement may be experienced as its final loss. This creates a sense of utter hopelessness, confirms the loss of home country "there is nothing there (—or anywhere?) for me now". It foreshadows the subject's own death, and suggests the probability of its occurring in exile, this embodying the feared finality and irreparability of the whole experience.

One strategy to defend against this is the 'immobilisation of the object' described by Auerhahn and Laub (1984). Some describe not so much a sense of irretrievable loss as a prolonged searching for the lost object far beyond the normal duration of this phase. An inner void may be experienced, leading to a 'provisional existence' movingly described in the testimonies of Claudine Vegh's interviewees, who had been unable to acknowledge or to mourn their parents' death in the Holocaust, secretly hoping, even thirty-five years later that they might still return. The acknowledgement was dreaded as an unthinkable betrayal; and yet the realisation of the death, as a result of the interviews, brought considerable relief.

It is possible to work through the losses, it may go some way to resolving the experience as a whole. However, the mourning process is greatly complicated by the heightened likelihood of guilt and ambivalence present in relation to survival and exile. Niederland (1968b) defines 'survivor guilt' as "a form of unresolved grief and mourning"—and this is further complicated by the very unconscious strategies which have enabled survival. These may range from denial and repression to more severely impaired functioning.

The psychoanalytic literature concerning survivors of the Holocaust and other 'man-made' disasters describes the phenomenon of regression as a response to trauma (see Lorenzer, 1968; Grubrich-Simitis, 1984; Simenauer, 1968; Jaffe, 1962). A recent study of adult refugees (Bathai, 1992) has shown a correlation between severity of reaction to trauma in adulthood and exposure to traumatic experience in childhood.

Factors such as preparedness for the event, the degree of violence involved, and the mental state and personality development of the individual at the time, play a part in determining the severity of the outcome.

The experience of severe trauma is likely to have even more profoundly disturbing effects on children and adolescents (Fink, 1968) because of the disruption of psychic development. There is the possible collision of reality and aggressive fantasy analogous to the impact of sexual or other abuse in other contexts; or in the impact of the death of the same-sex parent (Gill, 1986). Fantasies of having somehow caused the event may of course serve as an attempt, by retrospectively gaining control over the situation, to ward off trauma.

The effects are likely to be seen in an increase in sadomasochistic or narcissistic functioning, with increased use of splitting and projection, or with the use of obsessional, controlling defences as a protection against further regression. Krystal (1988) describes "patchy regression" in which some features of various levels of regression may be present, but without wholly impaired functioning.

Such defences may be seen as protecting against the state of 'psychic death': that of the 'Mussulmen' of the Nazi concentration camps, the 'dokhodyagi' of the Gulags, in which the trauma has extended beyond the surrender stage to the onset of "automatic anxiety" (Freud, 1926) and is a precursor of death.

Defences which serve the purpose of survival in intolerable circumstances are a source of difficulty once the external danger has passed (for example, in identification with the aggressor). They give rise to anxiety, depression, psychosomatic disorders, self-isolation, and by their very nature interfere with the formation of new object relationships.

Complaints of confusional states, and the experience of 'dual reality' are common. This experience is in itself distressing when perceived by the subject as an anomaly, and may give rise to fears of madness and disintegration, as do the severe anxiety states and near psychotic intensity of post-traumatic flashback experiences. Reyes (1989) describes this confusion as regression to a state of 'ambiguity' in which past and present are experienced as simultaneous, and a loss of differentiation between live and dead occurs. This allows a simultaneous acknowledgement and denial of the experience, so that working through implies consigning the event to the past. Auerhahn & Laub (1984), mention the difficulty of historicising, i.e. of disentangling pre-trauma memories when both past and present are felt to be ineradicably contaminated and depleted by the profound losses experienced in trauma.

In the state described by Reyes, an inner fragmentation has occurred, which gives rise to a substitutive use of objects to stand in for the lost object—'symbolic equation' (Segal, 1957)—and to loss of distinction between inner and outer reality, and of subject/object differentiation. Similar confusion of identity is described both in survivors and the children of survivors (Grubrich-Simitis, 1984; Jaffe, 1962; Winnik, 1968; Klein, H., 1971)—a form of projective identification. Reyes suggests that mourning is avoided as equated with the subject's death. At the same time, it is the inability to mourn which perpetuates a deathly state, whether due to guilt, fear of overwhelming affects, or denial of the death (so that to mourn would be to betray the object). Whereas the mourning process would accomplish a re-differentiation of self and object, a means to reintegration of the self.

A commonly seen reaction is that of 'psychic closure' (Reyes, 1989; McDougall, 1989; Adamo, 1988; Lifton, 1967), in which affects are not merely repressed, but excluded completely, and expressed instead through somatisation. Typical symptoms are headaches, gastric complaints, skin disorders, generalised malaise, asthma, and in two of my patients the specific complaint of 'dry eyes' (with no conscious connection on their part with the inability to weep). Somatisation is accompanied by concrete thinking and desymbolisation 'unavailability of metaphor' (Pines, 1986; Krystal, 1971) as a way of defending against overwhelming affects. Lifton sees extreme desymbolisation as a form of identification with the dead. Krystal (1988) posits a fear of all affect as signalling the imminent return or repetition of the trauma.

A closely related factor favouring pathological reactions to loss in survivors is extreme fear of and denial of aggression. To have expressed anger at their own suffering, or in protest against the death of those close to them would have invited reprisal, usually their own death, and there may be present the sense of guilt and humiliation at that perceived failure. Conversely, some extremely traumatised individuals avoid depression, but find themselves in the grip of uncontrollable rage.

De Wind calls attention to the necessity of addressing both the infantile and adult trauma and its fantasy aspect. Aggressive wishes towards the object may be felt as having caused the death; dread of the fantasised destructive abilities may lead to self-isolation, the avoidance of new relationships and to the avoidance of fantasy.

Grubrich-Simitis regards all such manifestations as an attempt to regulate aggression by turning against the self. The repression in itself may give rise to guilt if felt as a form of acquiescence. Similarly, Krystal (1988) describes the elderly survivor's difficulty with acceptance of their past as equated with collusion or acquiescence. Krystal takes the view that mourning in such circumstances can never be fully accomplished, and that, rather, a continuous re-editing of the past takes place, in an attempt to integrate the experience.

Technical implications

The difficulties in working through losses in severely traumatised states raise questions regarding appropriate intervention: in other words, about the advisability of working with the defences or of working in a more ego-supportive way. Grubrich-Simitis emphasises the importance of accepting transference phenomena however primitive. Attention is drawn (Pines, Krystal) to the danger of re-enacting and therefore re-activating a traumatising situation, and to the importance of avoiding collusion with the compulsion to repeat arising from the difficulty of working through or even representing the experience. Transference is likely to be experienced in terms of persecutor or protector (Pines, 1986); and both Pines and Grubrich-Simitis acknowledge the difficulty of the countertransference.

The therapeutic task may then be seen as a particular version of how to facilitate the patient's mourning, where affects are frozen, somatised, or felt to be overwhelmingly threatening to the ego.

Niederland, Hoppe, de Wind and Grubrich-Simitis all favour psychotherapy of a supportive nature. De Wind proposes the therapist as 'auxiliary ego', a view supported by Pines in terms of the ability to acknowledge the external reality, and of being able to verbalise, to speak the unspeakable until the patient is able to do so.

Adamo (1988), and Auerhahn & Laub (1984) in different contexts mention the main feature of the dynamic as pressure on the therapist to share the experience and at the same time of the need for the therapist to be able to keep a distance from it as a means of regaining access to the pre-trauma experience. Adequate words may be unavailable and a degree of acting-out may be the only possible means of communication, and should be understood as such.

The process as a whole may be seen as one of regaining access to symbolisation, and to fantasy, thus to the ability to distinguish between reality and fantasy—'disentangling', and to verbalisation. Therapy provides the opportunity for containment otherwise denied, and the possibility of "regaining trust in an external object" (Klein, 1940) and therefore reintrojection, and reinstatement, of the lost object.

The clinical material

> That which cannot be spoken cannot be treated; if they are not treated, these wounds will continue to ulcerate from generation to generation. [Bettelheim, 1979, my translation]

I should like to present some clinical material which illustrates some of the themes mentioned, and to discuss and contrast reactions to bereavement in two traumatised individuals. It will be noted that, as often occurs, multiple bereavements are involved in the recent past, and that the recent bereavements may repeat earlier losses through violent death.

Case 1

> Mrs A, a woman in her early forties, had been forced to flee her country in Francophone Africa clandestinely following the imprisonment, torture, and murder of her husband by the government for his political activities, and her own imprisonment during which she was tortured to reveal names, but resisted. It was only after her 'provisional' release that she learned of her husband's death: she went with her oldest child to the prison to hand in clothes and food for him, and heard the details from a prison warder. It was a particular source of grief to her that his last request, to write to her and the children, had been denied. He had been hanged, and his body thrown into the river "like a dog". She immediately went into hiding and made arrangements to leave. The only documents she was able to obtain showed children of similar ages to three of her children. The two other children had been left in the care of her brother, who was subsequently murdered in a massacre by the army. It was this last event which precipitated the referral for therapy.

Mrs A presented in a state of extreme distress, clutching the letter which, as it turned out later, had told her of her brother's death. She was dressed in mourning. For the first two sessions she was unable to give any account of what had happened, apart from a recent incident in which she had left some cornmeal cooking, which had set the kitchen alight, while she went to weep in the bathroom. This had frightened her very badly, as I think she had had a glimpse of her suicidal and destructive impulses. She frequently referred to herself as "bizarre". It was only in later sessions that she was able to verbalise her suicidal thoughts. Instead she howled her grief, which she also expressed physically in paroxysmic states: her head thrown back, arms outstretched in supplication, body rigid; or she would throw herself onto the floor and crawl weeping into a corner, where she would curl up in a foetal position. In subsequent sessions she would arrive in a state of greater self-possession, and was able to tell parts of the story, but when the pain was unbearable, and words inadequate, she would revert to enactments, which in themselves gradually became more coherent, and accompanied by commentary: crawling on the floor and pawing it, "Where is he? Where? How can I bury him? I don't even know where he is." This was a very concrete enactment of the searching phase of bereavement, and of her dilemma. Eventually she enacted a scene with gestures of wild despair, and complaint, kneeling, arms and head thrown back, lamenting her husband, which seemed unmistakably that of ritual, graveside mourning, so that I as therapist was co-opted as witness to stand in for family and friends who would have accompanied and held her, insofar as I was able to recognise and contain what was occurring.

It was only after this session that Mrs A was able to express her concerns for the children left behind, and to express some of her ambivalent feelings for her husband, who had until then been very much idealised, apart from the complaint that he had abandoned them by dying: a fate which seemed much preferable to her own. It became clear that she wore black from head to foot not only as a token of mourning, but as a quite explicit identification with her husband who was dressed in black for his execution, and she intended to wear it for ever. She frequently repeated "I'm dead, I'm dead" using the masculine form of the word.

She also became able to verbalise her anger towards the perpetrators, and at this stage oscillated between a desire to protect the children from any further danger, and a wish that they would one day fulfil her thirst for revenge: a wish she felt she had to deny in the next breath.

She reproached herself, seeing her grief as something that set her apart, made her unacceptable, and for the abandonment of her other children. It was only with the greatest difficulty that she was able to recognise the courage with which she had acted, having regarded this as her husband's prerogative; that is, she recognised as her own the qualities she had projected onto her husband. In reality she had long had the major responsibility for the family finances and the children's upbringing.

In the transference I was at times experienced as the abandoning mother. For example, after the first two-week break, she began the session by reproaching me for abandoning her, addressing me as Maman, expressing both her own feelings of abandonment, and as I thought, identifying with her own abandoned daughter. She did in fact then begin a conversation with her daughter, answering for her: "What does she think? She can't reason. Everybody has left me."

She then told me how she had begun to sleep on the floor, to leave the bed empty for her missing daughter, and would talk to her at night, and sing the daughter's songs—which she proceeded to do, in a child's voice.

This led her to recall her own feelings of abandonment when her parents had been murdered in an earlier political conflict, and she and her brother had been taken to live at a mission, at a time when she was of an age similar to her daughter's at this time. Only in the following session was she able to mention for the first time her younger sister who had died in the mission (of a snake-bite), and the grief at seeing her buried. She felt that she had failed as a mother to her sister, her brother, and her own children. However, her recall of the funeral that really had taken place seemed important, possibly because it introduced the idea of finality, limits. She later described the normal period of mourning: three days of ritual mourning, and the burial on the third day, after which the relatives would put on mourning clothes and desist from all usual activities for forty days.

Now she modified her ideas about wearing black, saying that she would end her mourning if she could get her daughter back. She was in great uncertainty and fear about whether the two children were still alive. Her identification with her daughter, the hardships she imposed on herself, seemed a form of self-substitution (for example she deprived herself of the food the children would have eaten) as a way of preserving her, and perhaps magically making restitution.

Shortly after this, her son rejoined the family. She was at first in conflict over her relief that he was safe, and simultaneous anger with him for also abandoning her daughter. However, she was able to contain these feelings and to understand his anger towards her. By displacing some of her self-reproach onto him, and eventually forgiving him, she was also able to forgive herself. His arrival seemed to restore her faith in herself as a mother; she resumed her protective role towards the children, and was able to consider their needs and functioning. She started to speak of the future, and make plans to study and to work.

Around this time, she also acceded to the children's request that she should cease mourning "although I still weep inside". Accordingly she put on her best clothes, make-up, and jewellery, went out and bought cake and wine, and provided them with the equivalent of the *'retraite de deuil'* the feast formally marking the end of mourning.

Several months later, her daughter was reunited with her, and only then was she able to say "I no longer weep when I'm cooking" with its resonance to the fire in the kitchen; that is, ostensibly because she no longer weeps for the abandoned hungry children, they are reunited; but also perhaps because the abandoned and angrily destructive parts of herself have been reintegrated, and her maternal function, both towards the children and herself, reinstated.

Case 2

Mr B was referred due to a range of psychosomatic complaints, including headaches and dry eyes, and anxiety states. She had suffered multiple bereavements in the previous three years, including both his father, then his mother two years later. The parents, his uncle and two close friends were all shot. He had been present at the death of one of the friends in an ambush. He had suffered constant harassment by the military; and after an arrest, went into hiding and was eventually forced to flee.

He presented with the conviction that he was physically sick, an explanation which he found both anxiety-provoking and at the same time strangely comforting. This reaction seemed to serve as a defence against the threat of overwhelming grief and guilt. He described a confusional state in which he lost concentration, and felt as though he were involved in two simultaneous conversations. An experience of *déja vu* shocked him and he asked friends "Can a person experience the same thing twice?"; his thought had been "Does this mean my parents are still alive and must die again?"

He later told me that he was very much afraid that other people would notice his confusion and see that he was sick, and from this infer his badness and guilt. On that occasion he was also able to tell me that he feared that that was how I saw him. It became clear that he had been unable to mourn these deaths at the time, with the possible exception of his father. In the case of the friend killed in the ambush, the friend's family considered that, as host, he was responsible for his friend's safety, and blamed him, chasing him away from the funeral with threats against his own life. He angrily denied responsibility in the matter. In the case of his mother, her death occurred at a time when the paramount concern was to find a place of safety for himself and his younger sister.

His anxiety symptoms lessened after he was able to tell me of particular feelings of guilt towards his mother: because of the circumstances, he had been unable to carry out the customary rites. Although this is a clan responsibility, failure to do so results in a death curse on the children. He thus expected, and experienced pursuit by the Furies and believed his own death to be inevitable. However, reflecting on this, he told me of a similar story, where the rites had been carried out some years after the event, yet no ill had befallen the children. This thought surprised him. Shortly after this he met an old friend of his mother's, and worked out a way of sending at least a token offering home, in partial fulfilment of the rites.

His insistence on physical expression of pain also derived both from a fear of madness (seen traditionally as a form of possession), and from a fear of being overwhelmed by emotional pain. The session above had begun with a complaint that he had been unable to sleep because of his dry eyes, and when I mentioned a link with his inability to weep he said: "Oh I would only cry about something really important."

After telling me about his mother, he also began to tell me his dreams, which he saw as prophetic. These were at first of a catastrophic nature often involving massacre, some based on actual occurrences, then a dream in which he found himself stranded in his home country where figures connected with his mother at first tried to disobey him, but then respected his authority. This seemed ambiguous in that on the one hand she was seen as acknowledging him as an adult; on the other, his command had been that she should not go to the defence of a child who was being attacked. This he interpreted as his conflict over his health. By now he had begun to regain access to metaphor. The next dream was the one quoted above, of fleeing, but having to take the coffin with him. He became able to consider his feelings as they were evoked through the series of dreams, and they also provided us with a framework for examining the transference. An example was a dream in which

> he was sitting by a roadside in his home country, and speaking to a boy and girl resting on the bank. Opposite was a clinic. Perplexed, Mr B asked 'What is the doctor doing?' 'The doctor is seeing a patient.' The patient emerges, looking disappointed and holding some tablets in his hand.

Mr B's associations to this were that in the countryside at home, as in many cultures, the only trusted treatment is an injection, and these are often given as placebos using sterile water. This was why the patient was disappointed. I pointed out the transference content and his disappointment that I was not furnishing him with a magical cure. He agreed. He went on to tell me some more of the dream, and said, remembering with surprise, "The funny thing is, the man was fit and well."

He became more aware of the affective content of the anxiety and confusional states, particularly massive rage, which caused him to avoid others for fear of harming them. We have linked this with his view of himself as dangerous and destructive to his objects: he told me with great sadness, how after his first friend was killed, another school-friend had joked that it was bad luck to be his friend. He seemed to have experienced this as a self-fulfilling prophecy. We have also linked these states to the extreme rage and anguish he experienced when he was powerless to express it, humiliated and tortured during his interrogation.

The dilemma for Mr B is the fear of being overwhelmed by intolerable affects—re-traumatised, on the one hand, while, on the other, experiencing a deeply persecutory defence system, in which aggression had been turned against himself through somatisation.

In both of these cases, although very different in presentation, crucial factors appear to have been the containing function of the therapy: the ability to make use of transference, to make some connection between the bereavement and traditional practice, and to make symbolic use of that practice.

Conclusion

In conclusion I would like to mention some factors in positive outcome. In terms of external structures and support, the existence and use of family networks or exile religious or secular organisations can be helpful. In terms of assessment, the usual criteria apply, but there is a particular need for sensitive appraisal of the cumulative trauma and sequelae. An extended assessment period may be appropriate. Regarding treatment, I feel there is a need for flexibility in technique. The witnessing and acknowledging of the trauma and losses and their impact are an important part of the process. I have found that sensitivity to traditional mourning practices and their symbolic value is very facilitative. It is important to be aware of the transitional use of substitution, of non-verbal communication and the use of the transference. The aim should be to provide adequate containment and the availability of the therapist as auxiliary ego/transference object, for a successful mourning process to be possible, with the reinstatement of the good object, and renewal of, and return to life. These are, after all, surely the aim of therapeutic intervention.

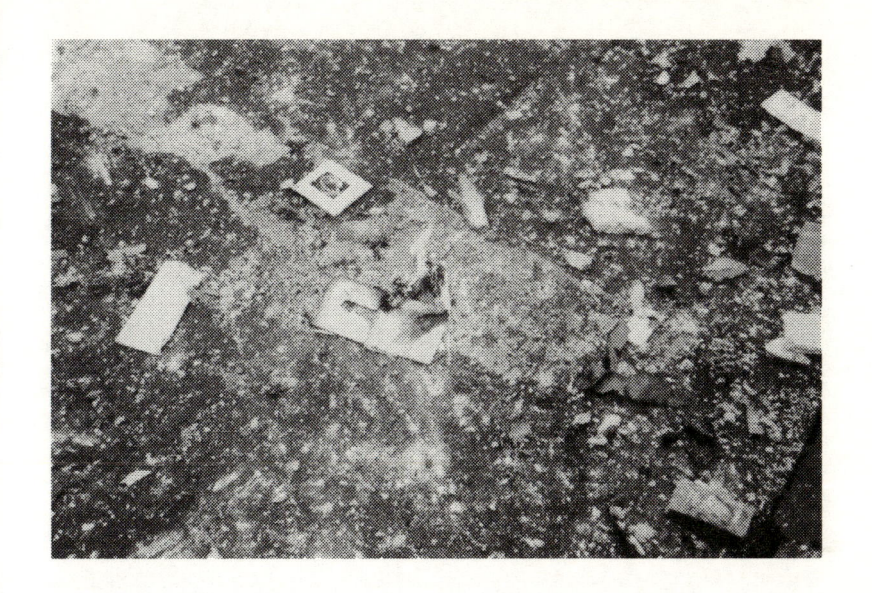

Forget

"Forget the suffering
You caused others.
Forget the suffering
Others caused you.
The waters run and run,
Springs sparkle and are done,
You walk the earth you are forgetting.

Sometimes you hear a distant refrain.
What does it mean, you ask, who is singing?
A childlike sun grows warm.
A grandson and a great-grandson are born.
You are led by the hand once again.

The names of the rivers remain with you.
How endless those rivers seem!
Your fields lie fallow,
The city towers are not as they were.
You stand at the threshold mute."

Czeslaw Milosz
(Translated from the Polish by Jessica Fisher and Bozena Gilewska)

GLOSSARY*

For those who find some of the terms we have used confusing or who do not have access to more formal psychoanalytic texts (e.g. Rycroft, 1968; Moore & Fine, 1968; Laplanche & Pontalis, 1973; Hinshelwood, 1989, from whom we have borrowed) we offer a brief glossary of terms to be encountered in this book and elsewhere, with related comments.

Claustro-agoraphobia

Pathological fears of closed or open spaces are relatively common and like many other phobias may respond to behavioural methods of treatment. However, some cases are resistant to such treatment and can prove extremely disabling. This disturbance can be explained more or less satisfactorily as the expression of a state of mind brought about by the excessive use of projective identification, which confers a particularly severe quality of anxiety. This dynamic can be described as a phantasy of *being trapped inside an object*, or

---

*With acknowledgments to Murray Jackson and Paul Williams, authors of "Unimaginable Storms: a search for meaning in psychosis" (Karnac Books).

else of being threatened by psychic disintegration when outside it, as a result of its total loss.

Containment

This term is often used loosely and it is therefore important to be clear about what is being referred to, about whom and in what context. Broadly, it signifies actions necessary to protect the acutely disturbed patient from harm to himself or others, usually involving admission to a suitable containing structure, typically a psychiatric hospital ward, where he will find people who will try to "contain" him. This means controlling dangerous or self-destructive behaviour: reassuring him as far as possible by words and behaviour: talking with him if this can be done in order to understand what he is experiencing: and if these anxiety-alleviating measures prove insufficient, administering appropriate tranquillizing medication. When the acute disturbance subsides, a further level of containment then becomes possible, facilitated by the understanding, withstanding, accepting, and enquiring attitude described. A final sense of the word is to be found in the process whereby the helper may at times detect that the patient is attempting to recruit him into acting a role in his inner drama. This definition of containment refers to being able to accept and emotionally digest the patient's projections in the service of understanding him. Elucidation of the drama being revealed in the therapeutic relationship can help him to recognize, tolerate, *work through* and ultimately find improved solutions to the (often unconscious) inner impulses and desires being lived out. Nursing staff can play an important part in this revelatory process, and it requires them to differentiate between *regressive* behaviour that is undesirable from that which represents material the patient is unwittingly bringing to the specialists to be helped. The concept of containment in this sense of a potentially growth-promoting process has been elaborated in detail by Bion in his "container–contained" theory.[1]

Delusion

In psychiatric usage, a delusion is a false but fixed belief which is impermeable to reason or logic (see Hingley, 1992; Roberts, 1992). The circumstances that give rise to it are incompletely understood.

Grandiose, persecutory, or erotic delusions are characteristic of schizophrenic, paranoid, and manic psychoses, and delusions of unworthiness of psychotic depression. Persecutory delusions, sometimes constructed around a fragment of truth, may represent the retaliatory consequences of destructive envious and acquisitive wishes (see Freeman, 1981). Delusions may appear in the psychotherapeutic transference, and depending on the circumstances and the skill of the therapist, may bring psychotherapy to a halt or, on the other hand, may be worked through to provide a unique learning experience for the patient.

Depressive position

Klein asserted that the normal infant has, by the age of three–six months, reached sufficient mental maturity to be able to integrate the previously split and opposing versions of his mother (good-providing and bad-withholding). Before this his feelings of love and hatred have been dealt with by primitive defence mechanisms, principally splitting and projective–introjective procedures. This early stage is the *paranoid–schizoid* position and the later one the *depressive* position. The latter can be regarded as a maturational achievement, the 'stage of concern' (Winnicott, 1958). The first stage is accompanied by persecutory guilt, where concern is for the survival of the self, the second by depressive guilt, where concern is for the object. Attainment of the capacity for depressive anxiety is considered a necessary quality for the forming or maintaining of mature object relationships, since it is the source of generosity, altruistic feelings, reparative wishes, and the capacity to tolerate the object's ultimateness/separateness. It is not a once and for all achievement in which the paranoid–schizoid mode is left behind, but rather a dialectic, (or diachronic) relationship between different levels of integration, continuing throughout life. Increasing maturity brings a growing capacity to function at the level of the depressive position. Such growth does not bring an idealized freedom from unhappiness, but rather brings new and different burdens, albeit of a human sort, and a potential for freedom to make responsible choices. It is not the resolution of a dilemma ... "one is stuck with it, with all its advantages and disadvantages, unless one regressively flees from it into the refuge and imprisonment of the paranoid–

schizoid position or through the use of manic defences" (Ogden, 1990).

Envy

The envious wish to possess what the object is seen or believed to have, and that the subject does not have, may generate admiration and a desire to emulate and acquire through personal effort. This constructive, life-affirming impulse represents the positive face of envy. In the case of destructive envy, sometimes referred to as primary or infantile envy, there issues a wish to deprive the object of his possession or to spoil it by devaluation or other hostile means. Klein regarded envy as an innate element in mental life, first directed at the mother's feeding breast and at the creativity this represents, and considered it to be a basic pathogenic factor in mental illness, in particular at the core of schizophrenic psychopathology. In contrast to *jealousy*, which involves three parties, envy reflects a two-party situation. The envied object is hated, not because it is bad, but because it is good, but is not in the possession of the envious subject. This carries profound implications for mental life.[2] Primary envy, according to Klein, leads in infancy to phantasies of invading and colonizing the interior of the mother's body which is felt to be the container of good things, and of destroying those contents which are felt to be bad or undesirable, such as other babies. Normal mental mechanisms, primarily splitting, projection and introjection, permit development to proceed in infancy, in the process generating feelings of love, trust and *gratitude* which overcome envious hatred.[3] An individual is rendered vulnerable to psychosis in later life by the varying degrees of failure of these normal developmental steps. This view of mental life, and of psychosis, has by no means been accepted by all psychoanalysts.[4]

Identification

Contrary to the popular sense of this term as a process of recognition, identification refers to a mental process whereby the subject comes to feel himself to be similar, the same as or identical with another person in one or more aspects. It may be a complex state and take different forms. He can achieve this by either extending his identity *into* someone else (projection), borrowing his identity *from* someone else (introjection) or by fusing or confusing his identity *with* someone else (at times believing similarity to mean equivalence). *Projective identification* refers to an unconscious belief that a part of the self or inner world, usually unwanted, can be disposed of by re-location into the mental representation of another object. This is usually regarded as a primitive form of the mental mechanism of *projection*, different in that it may involve behaviour by the subject towards the object in a way that will allow him to confirm his omnipotent suppositions. The projectively-identifying mechanism can be used for purposes of denial (of disposing of unwanted elements), or of controlling the object or of communication. In the latter case the therapist is required to attend to his own non-rational responses to the patient's communications, his *countertransference*, which will constitute an important source of information about the patient's state of mind at that moment. Many psychoanalysts hold that projective identification is a primary form of communication between mother and baby, comparable with the *attunement* described by workers in infant observation research (Stern, 1985). *Introjection* is a process of taking something into the mind (internalizing) which can sometimes felt as a bodily event (incorporating). Such elements may then be integrated, temporarily or permanently, into the ego and felt as being part of the self, thus completing the process of *introjective identification*. Since projective identification depletes the self and distorts perceptions of the object, what is introjected may also be a more or less distorted version of the actual object. Differentiation of what belongs to the subject and what to the object is held to be a fundamental process of infant mental development, and is often a major sorting-out process in psychotherapy later in life. Introjective identification is the basis of much normal learning, and normal projective identification underlies a mature capacity for *empathy* (the ability to imagine oneself in another person's place without losing awareness of one's identity). By contrast, *pathological* projective identification is conducted with omnipotence and violence (Bion, 1959) leading to a confusion of self and object and susceptibility to psychotic developments. *Splitting* is a term used to depict a normal mental activity in which the ego strives as part of its development to effect distinctions and differences. Pathological splitting is an extremely primitive defence thought to precede developmentally many others including repression.

Identity

One of the characteristics of maturity is the possession of a strong sense of identity, the stable conviction of being an individual distinguishable from all others, and an enduring sense of existing intactly in space and time. Psychoanalytic theory holds that a sense of identity has its roots in infancy on the basis of processes of identification, which gradually evolve in the course of development into a capacity for object relationships. Many psychotic symptoms develop on the basis of a fragile sense of personal identity, and certain personality disorders are characterized by a "diffusion" of identity.

Insight

This complex concept has several referents. In everyday usage it refers to self-knowledge, or self-awareness. In psychiatry it refers to the capacity to recognize that disturbing thoughts and feelings are subjective, and can be tested against reality, a capacity that is more or less absent in the psychotic. In clinical practice the assessment of insight is of central importance. Insight can be considered as a continuum, with different mechanisms responsible for impairment in individual patients.[5] In psychoanalytic usage a distinction is made between emotional and intellectual insight. The latter can be used for constructive purposes or for defence (pseudo-insight).

Interpretation

In the simplest sense this means an explanation that the therapist gives to the patient of something that he believes he has understood which would be helpful to the patient to consider at that particular time. It may concern the latent meaning of what the patient is doing or saying, and may address the mechanisms of defence, the content, the transference, or may be a direct statement about the meaning of symbols given independently of the patient's associations. As a general rule defence should be attended to before content and premature interpretation of content or symbolic expressions is usually a mistake and sometimes a serious one. In psychotherapeutic practice interpretation usually involves a long period of elucidating meanings in the material of dreams, symptoms or associations that the patient brings into the therapy. Interpretation should offer information that the patient is capable of understanding and tolerating at the particular time, in the simplest possible terms, Ill-timed, misdirected or unduly complicated interpretations may be at best ineffectual and at worst harmful.[6] Although interpretations are potentially powerful devices, open to misuse, they are not necessarily the exclusive preserve of the experienced psychotherapist. Because the term itself may suggest that the practitioner has oracular powers, the term "intervention" may often be appropriate to describe the wide variety of verbal contributions that the therapist may make.[7] In sensitive hands, not necessarily psychotherapeutic, such interventions may prove extremely helpful.

Mourning

In its normal form mourning is a response to loss of a loved object, following bereavement, accompanied by grief and pursuing a course which ultimately leads to recovery and a renewed interest in life. This healing process may be arrested or distorted in many ways, and since the time of Freud's classic work "Mourning and Melancholia" (1915c) the subject of unresolved or pathological mourning has received much attention by psychiatrists and psychoanalysts.[8] Freud was the first to consider melancholia (psychotic depression) as a pathological form of mourning, and Klein extended the term to embrace losses in the inner world of object relations, losses which may be independent of external reality. Whereas depression may be associated with grief, normal or abnormal, the "depressive position" refers to a related but dissimilar use of the term.

Object

In psychoanalytic usage an object is usually a person, part of a person or a symbol representing the whole or part person, which the subject relates to in order to achieve instinctual satisfaction. In object-relations theory priority is given to the need for persons rather than simply the wish to satisfy instinctual drives. Theoretical developments have led to the conceptualization of *internal* objects and object-relationships in the inner world of unconscious phantasy, and of *psychic,* (or *psychological*) reality. These concepts concern the interplay of mental representations, usually unconscious, with external (actual) objects in the outer world.

Precipitation

In cases of gradual onset of psychosis there may be no obvious precipitating cause, and a gradual decompensation of mental defence mechanisms may prove to be a satisfactory explanation. Where the onset is more acute the cause may be found in an inability to cope with stress, often in the external world and involving combinations of such factors as disappointment, frustration, object loss or separation. Arousal of guilt and anxiety over envious, sexual or acquisitive wishes may be involved. These anxieties sometimes take the form of threat to the sense of coherent and continuous self that they have been variously termed *traumatic anxiety, organismic panic* and *ontological anxiety* to indicate their overwhelming nature.

Predisposition

Biologically-oriented psychiatry maintains that a predisposition to schizophrenic, manic-depressive and some other psychoses exists in the form of a genetically determined biological disorder, and there is evidence for this view in a significant proportion of cases. Psychoanalytic thinking, whilst not rejecting the significance of innate biological differences, tends to view vulnerability in terms of failure of adequate formation of primitive object relations in infancy, leading to the use of mental defence mechanisms to protect the fragile core of the personality. This *defence* view contrasts with a *deficit* view held by some psychoanalytic theorists who question the Kleinian emphasis on the role of conflict in early infancy.

Prognosis

The best prognostic outlook of all is for the young person with little or no sign of previous disturbance, breaking down acutely under major stress. About one-third of acutely psychotic patients recover in a matter of weeks or months, with or without specific treatment, and experience no further attack. A similar proportion have recurrent attacks which may lead to chronicity. These first two groups are likely to be suitable subjects for psychotherapy, with or without the help of anti-psychotic medication. A further, more chronically suffering group is held to be unlikely to respond to a psychotherapeutic approach and is best helped with medication, cognitive and behavioural methods of treatment, and long-term rehabilitation and support. Even with the most refractory and chronic patients it has been shown that the long-term outcome is better than had been thought. From a psychotherapeutic point of view, it is clear that suitability for psychotherapy and early treatment are the most important prognostic factors.

Psychodynamic

Although several theoretical and clinical approaches deal with concepts of mental forces in dynamic interplay, the term *psychodynamic* is widely used to define the approach founded on basic analytical concepts of unconscious mental life, conflict and defence, internal reality, transference/countertransference, repetition-compulsion, acting-out and working through in the therapeutic process. The same considerations apply to the term *psychoanalytic psychotherapy*.

Psychoneurosis

Psychoneurosis is essentially a psychogenic condition with a range of symptoms of which anxiety, symptoms and inhibitions are prominent. It is usually differentiated from psychosis on the basis of the intactness of the sense of reality in the former. In Kleinian psychoanalytic theory, neurotic disorders may represent the belated expression of psychotic processes that have not been successfully negotiated in early life.

Psychosis, psychotic

The term psychosis refers to a broad category of mental disorders which are characterized by severe abnormalities of thought processes. These are associated with disturbance of the sense of reality and often with delusions, hallucinations, and disruption of the sense of personal identity. Psychotic elements may occur in severe neuroses, psychosomatic disorders, sexual perversions, and personality disorders. Psychoses may be *organic*, if caused by demonstrable organic disease, or *functional* if no organic pathology can be found. Functional psychoses are regarded by some as purely *psychogenic*, requiring psychological understanding and treatment. At the other extreme, some hold to the view that they are purely *biogenic*. A more integrated approach might allow for the possibility that both elements make a contribution. The concept of psychotic and non-psychotic parts of the personality in the individual, introduced by Bion, provided a new perspective to the understanding of psychosis, and an emphasis in psychotherapy on making contact with the sane part of the person, presumed to be present but often hidden in every psychotic patient.

Regression

In the face of psychological stress the individual may revert to an earlier and less mature level of functioning. This regression can be understood as a defensive retreat to infantile stages of development, stages which are never completely outgrown, and which may at times have the constructive potential of a withdrawal to a safe base where mental forces can be re-grouped. Regression occurring in the course of psychotherapy can have a beneficial effect (therapeutic regression) or a bad one (malignant regression), depending on the maturity of the patient and the skill of the therapist. Opinion is divided on the question of encouraging this process in patients with severe personality disorders.[9] In psychotic patients the use of regression as a deliberate technique is generally considered as at the very least unwise, and at the worst dangerous, with the possible exception of a few specially experienced practitioners. The psychotic patient is usually quite regressed enough, at least in the acute stage, and the problem is usually that of containing the regression within the therapy and the institution. Lehtinen (1993) believes that regression in an acute psychotic attack can be substantially alleviated by family therapy meetings on first contact.

Reparation

Melanie Klein's views on the ubiquity of aggressive phantasies and destructive desires in early life have sometimes been received with scepticism, even shock by those who have not recognized or accepted the central position accorded loving and reparative feelings in her theories of development. In her analytic work with small children she recognized the distress and guilt which accompanied destructive wishes, and observed the growth of feelings of remorse and desire to repair damage done in phantasy to ambivalently loved figures who are the target of envious and jealous hatred. Such reparative desires often take the form of obsessional activity, partly understandable as an attempt to preserve the object or to repair damage by magical means. In the course of psychotherapy with adults, failed attempts at reparation may often be discerned, and manic states may sometimes be found to contain similar strivings. Such manic reparation, like other failed attempts, does not succeed, partly because the subject is unaware of the damage he believes he has done, and perhaps is still doing, and also does not know how to go about repairing it.[10] The emergence of depressive guilt and reparative wishes marks the higher level of maturity and integration of the *depressive position*, and is regarded by Klein as the mainspring of true creative processes.[11] The application of this concept to the psychotherapy of the adult adds an optimistic note to the uncovering of such unconscious, painful, facts of mental life. Reparation can become a possibility, and it is the task of the psychotherapist to help the patient differentiate between where his personal responsibility lies, and where it does not, and to find ways of making amends. The concept of the need to repair *internal* as well as *external* objects permits the possibility of working through feelings of regret and mourning, even if the victim of the destructive wishes is long dead.

Schizophrenia

The term schizophrenia was introduced to define a group of severe psychotic disorders characterized by a dissociation or splitting of the mental functions, in contrast to an earlier view of a single specific mental disease leading to dementia (dementia praecox). It has been variously considered as an illness, a syndrome, a way of living or even as a medical fiction invented to satisfy relatives, society and psychiatrists (c.f. Szasz, 1961). It has no single agreed cause, but is best considered as a syndrome or group of disorders with a range of possible contributory or causative factors, biogenic, sociogenic, and psychogenic. The development of the detailed and complex DSM 3R classification system (the revised version of the third edition of the *Diagnostic and Statistical Manual of the American Psychiatric Association*) has gone a long way towards preventing this labelling: its "multi-axial" diagnostic procedure allows for diagnosis to be regularly revised in the light of changes in the clinical condition of the patient. Thus in a case where emotional feelings are prominent, a diagnosis of *schizo-affective psychosis* is usually deemed appropriate, and unless six months of continuous illness have passed, the diagnosis *schizophreniform* should be made. Much research work includes these two diagnoses in the category "schizophrenia". Where there is a recent precipitating stress the diagnosis *reactive psychosis* is available, and where uncertainty remains, *psychosis* (unspecified) is often used.

Self

The term self, as used in psychoanalysis, refers to the individual as a reflective *agent*, aware of his own identity. It belongs to a different frame of reference from the term *ego* with which it is sometimes confused. The latter refers to a structure in the mind, parts of which are unconscious and necessitate a degree of insight to become known to the self. The various adjectival forms commonly encountered, such as self-esteem, self-preservation, self-mutilation, self-observation, are usually regarded as referring to a *whole* self. However the concept of *part*-selves which may exist in a state of identification with other (part or whole) objects, may at times promote the question *"which* self?" or *"which* object?", particularly in the case of the psychotic person. These partial identifications may be of longstanding and have complex, condensed meanings. Rey (1994), regarding mental processes as having co-ordinates in space and time, has provided a formula to help the psychotherapist who wishes to explore the details of such a process: "What part of the subject situated where in space and time does what, with what motivation, to what part of the object situated where in space and time, with what consequences for the object and the subject?"

Symbolic and concrete thinking

Schizophrenic thinking shows a literal, "concrete" quality in which symbol and metaphor, which normally provide a mental distance from objects and processes (a *representation*), and which facilitate abstract and conceptual thinking, are not recognized as such. Symbols and metaphors are then thought about as realities. In this respect it resembles the thinking of dream-life, following the laws of *primary process*, in particular in the use of *condensation* and *displacement*. Different explanations have been advanced to account for this concreteness, which often appears to be the consequence of an impairment or diminished use of the capacity to differentiate and to classify items according to their similarities. For example, a thing that *resembles* another thing may be treated as if it were *identical* with the other. Concrete thinking can be partly understood as the regressive revival, or uncovering, of the "sensorimotor" mode of thinking held by some to be characteristic of infancy, which normally evolves into metaphorical and abstract thinking. In this view, the future psychotic has suffered a failure of this normal developmental process and remains vulnerable to its revival, with the loss of the weakly-established capacity for recognition of metaphor and symbol. Freud described this regressive process as the original "thing-presentations" replacing the higher level of organization of mental representations, the "word-presentations". Concrete thinking involves a loss of differentiation between the thing symbolized and the symbol, which is associated with a confusion between self and object, and between internal and external reality. Such confusion has been considered as the outcome of possible excessive projective identification (used as a defence against envy or separation). If the object is not sufficiently differentiated from the self, a symbol, the main functions of which is to represent the object in its absence, will remain confused with the thing symbolized.[12] This is one of the characteristics of concrete thinking.[13]

Unconscious

Mental processes are regarded as being unconscious when the subject is unaware of them. Some of these can be recalled to consciousness without great difficulty (*descriptively* unconscious, or *preconscious*), others, held in repression, cannot (*dynamically* unconscious). As a noun, the term refers to a functioning structure in the mind (the *system unconscious*), which constitutes the larger part of mental life, and follows a logic and rules of its own. Freud called these characteristics the *primary processes* of thought, in contrast to the *secondary processes* of the conscious mind, and demonstrated how they dominate the thinking of dreams and of neurotic and psychotic symptoms. The concept of the unconscious has recently been approached from the perspective of mathematical logic, as a differentiating and classifying system (Matte-Blanco, 1988). The *collective* unconscious is a term of Jung's designed to describe the realm of archetypes, universal innate ideas, or the tendency to organize experience in innately determined patterns. This usage has a conceptual connection with Klein's use of the term unconscious phantasy as the psychic expression of innate libidinal and destructive instincts which are held to underlie mental processes and to accompany all mental activity.

Notes

1. See Bion's "Container and contained transformed" in *Attention and Interpretation* (1970).
2. See "Envy in everyday life" (Joseph, 1986).
3. See "Envy and Gratitude" (Klein, 1957).
4. A detailed exposition of sources of evidence in favour of these concepts and an examination of the disagreements has been provided by Hinshelwood (1989).
5. See David (1990), Berrios & Markova (1992). The term has at times been misused to promote a "eurocentric" world view (Perkins & Moodley, 1993).
6. A psychotic patient who believes he is sane may experience such an ill-conceived intervention as an attempt by the therapist to drive him mad, or as a confession by the therapist that he is afraid of the patient.
7. See Sandler *et al.*, 1992.
8. Klein (1940), Parkes (1975), Bowlby (1980, 1988), Pedder (1982).
9. See Winnicott's concept of "false self" (1960) and Balint's "new beginning" (1952).
10. See Riviere (1936).
11. See Segal (1986).
12. See Segal on the "symbolic equation" (1981).
13. See Searles (1962), Rosenfeld (1987).

BIBLIOGRAPHY AND REFERENCES

Abraham, N., & Torok, M. (1975). The lost object—me: notes on endocryptic identification. In: *The Shell and the Kernel, Volume 1* (pp. 139–156). Chicago & London: The University of Chicago Press, 1994.

Abraham, N., & Torok, M. (1976). *The Wolf Man's Magic Word: A Cryptonymy*. Minneapolis: University of Minnesota Press, 1986.

Abrams, M. H. (1973). *Natural Supernaturalism*. New York: W. W. Norton & Co.

Adamo, S. (1988). Liquidation and working through traumatic experience: movement within a therapeutic relationship. Paper delivered at 7th Rome Conference, London, Tavistock Clinic.

Agazarian, Y. (1994). The phases of development and the systems-centred group. In: Schermer & Pines (Eds.), *Rings of Fire*. London: Routledge.

Ainsworth, M. D. S., Blehar, M. C., Waters, E., & Wall, S. (1978). *Patterns of Attachment: A Psychological Study of the Strange Situation*. Hillsdale, NJ: Erlbaum.

Akhtar, S. (1992). *Broken Structures: Severe Personality Disorders and their Treatment*. Northvale, NJ: Jason Aronson.

Akhtar, S. (1995). Some reflections on the nature of hatred and its emergence in the treatment process. In: S. Akhtar, S. Kramer & H. Parens (Eds.), *The Birth of Hatred: Developmental, Clinical, and Technical Aspects of Intense Aggression* (pp. 83–102). Northvale, NJ: Jason Aronson.

Akhtar, S. (1996). "Someday" and "if only" fantasies: pathological optimism and inordinate nostalgia as related forms of idealisation. *Journal of the American Psychoanalytic Association*, 44: 723–753.

Akhtar, S. (1999). *Inner Torment: Living Between Conflict and Fragmentation.* Northvale, NJ: Jason Aronson.

Alexander, F. (1949). *Fundamentals of Psychoanalysis*. New York: Jarold.

Alexander, F., & French, T. (1946). The principle of corrective emotional experience—the case of Jean Valjean. In: F. Alexander & T. French (Eds.), *Psychoanalytic Theory, Principles and Application* (pp. 66–70). New York: Ronald Press.

Allen, J. G. (1995). *Coping with Trauma: A Guide to Self-Understanding*. Washington, DC: American Psychiatric Press, Inc.

Amichai, Y (2000). *Open and Closed*. Chana Bloch & Chana Kronfeld (Trans.). New York: Hartcourt Inc.

Anzieu, D. (1985). *The Skin Ego: A Psychoanalytic Approach to the Self*. New Haven & London: Yale University Press, 1989.

Apfel, R. J., & Simon, B. (2000). Mitigating discontents with children in war: an ongoing psychoanalytic inquiry. In: M. Robben & M. Suarez-Orozco (Eds.), *Cultures Under Siege*. Cambridge University Press.

Askenasy, H. (1978). *Are We All Nazis?* Secaucus, NY: Lyle Stuart Inc.

Auden, W. H. (1939). *Collected Poems*. New York: Random House, 1976.

Auerhahn, N. C., & Laub, D. (1984). Annihilation and restoration: post-traumatic memory as pathway and obstacle to recovery. *International Review of Psycho-Analysis*, 11: 327–344.

Bak, R. C. (1954). The schizophrenic defence against aggression. *International Journal of Psychoanalysis*, 35: 129–134.

Baker, R. (1992). Unpublished paper.

Balint, M. (1937). Early developmental states of the ego. Primary object-love. In: *Primary Love and Psycho-Analytic Technique*. London: The Hogarth Press, 1952.

Balint, M. (1952). Early developmental stages of the ego. Primary object-love. In: *Primary Love and Psycho-Analytic Technique*. London: The Hogarth Press, 1937.

Balint, M. (1969). Trauma and object relationship. *International Journal of Psycho-Analysis*, 50: 429–435.

Barag, G. (1947). The question of Jewish monotheism. *American Imago*, 4: 8.

Baranger, M., Baranger, W., & Mom, J. M. (1988). The infantile psychic trauma from us to Freud: pure trauma, retroactivity and reconciliation. *International Journal of Psycho-Analysis*, 69: 113–128.

Barber, B. R. (1995). *Jihad vs McWorld*. New York: Ballantine Books.
Barnaby, F. (1983). *Peace Studies Paper No. 4*. Bradford: University of Bradford.
Barthes, R. (1981). *Camera Lucida*. R. Howard (Trans.). New York: Noonday Press.
Bathal, P. (1992). Refugees and trauma. Unpublished paper.
Belsky, J., Rosenberger, K., & Crnic, C. (1995). The origins of attachment security: "Classical" and contextual determinants. In: S. Goldberg, R. Muir & J. Kerr (Eds.), *John Bowlby's Attachment Theory: Historical, Clinical and Social Significance* (pp. 153–184). Hillsdale, NJ: Analytic Press.
Ben-David, Y. (1962). Confronting and deviant images of youth in a new society. In Transactions of the Fifth World Congress of Sociology. International Sociological Association. Louvain, France.
Benjamin, J. (1998). *Shadow of the Other: Intersubjectivity in Psychoanalysis*. New Haven: The Yale University Press.
Benoit, D., & Parker, K. (1994). Stability and transmission of attachment across three generations. *Child Development*, 65: 1444–1457.
Bergmann, M. S., & Jucovy, M. E. (1982). *Generations of the Holocaust*. New York: Columbia University Press.
Berman, E. (1991). From war to war: cumulative trauma. Sihot-Dialoge. *Israel Journal of Psychotherapy*, 2(1): 37–41.
Bettelheim, B. (1943). Individual and mass behaviour in extreme situations. *Journal of Abnormal Social Psychology*, 38: 417–452.
Bettelheim, B. (1960). *The Informed Heart*. New York: The Free Press [reprinted London: Peregrine Books, 1986].
Bettelheim, B. (1990a). *Je ne lui ai pas Dit au Revoir* (Postface) Vegh, 1979. Paris: Gallimard.
Bettelheim, B. (1990b). *Recollections and Reflections*. London: Thames & Hudson [reprinted New York: A. Knopf].
Bick, E. (1968). The experience of the skin in early object-relations. *International Journal of Psycho-Analysis*, 49: 484–486.
Biesel, D. (1994). Looking for enemies. *The Journal of Psychohistory*, 22(1): 1–38.
Bion, W. R. (1952). Group dynamics: a re-view. *International Journal of Psycho-Analysis*, 33: 235–247; also in *New Directions in Psychoanalysis*. Tavistock: London, 1955.
Bion, W. R. (1957). Differentiation of the psychotic from the non-psychotic personalities. In: *Second Thoughts* (pp. 43–64). New York: Jason Aronson, 1967.

Bion, W. R. (1959). Attacks on linking. *International Journal of Psycho-analysis, 40*: 308–315.
Bion, W. R. (1961). *Experiences in Groups and Other Papers*. London: Routledge.
Bion, W. R. (1962a). A theory of thinking. In: *Second Thoughts* (p. 110). New York: Jason Aronson, 1967.
Bion, W. R. (1962b). *Learning from Experience*. London: Heinemann.
Bion, W. R. (1963). *Elements of Psycho-Analysis*. London: Maresfield Reprints.
Bion, W. R. (1970). *Attention and Interpretation*. London: Tavistock Publications [reprinted London: Karnac Books, 1984].
Blake, W. (1825). *The Marriage of Heaven and Hell*. Facsimile (1927) (p. 4). London and Toronto: J. M. Dent.
Bloomfield Report. (1998). *We Will Remember Them*—a report on the victims of the troubles. Northern Ireland Office.
Bluhm, H. O. (1954). How did they survive: mechanisms of defence in Nazi concentration camps. *American Journal of Psychotherapy, 2*: 2–32.
Blum, H. P. (1995). Sanctified aggression, hate, and the alteration of standards and values. In: S. Akhtar, S. Kramer & H. Parens (Eds.), *The Birth of Hatred: Developmental, Clinical, and Technical Aspects of Intense Aggression* (pp. 15–38). Northvale, NJ.
Bodansky, Y. (1999). *Bin Laden: The Man Who Declared War on America*. California: Prima Publishing.
Bollas, C. (1992). *Being a Character: Psychoanalysis and Self Experience*. New York: Hill and Wang.
Bollas, C. (1995). The structure of evil. In: *Cracking Up*. London: Routledge.
Bouthoul, G. (1951). *Les Guerres: Elements de Polenologie*. Paris: Payot.
Bowlby, J. (1960). Grief and mourning in infancy and early childhood. *Psychoanalytic Study of the Child, 15*: 3–39.
Bowlby, J. (1969). *Attachment and Loss, Volume 1: Attachment*. London: Hogarth Press and the Institute of Psycho-Analysis.
Bowlby, J. (1973). *Attachment and Loss, Volume 2: Separation: Anxiety and Anger*. London: Hogarth Press and Institute of Psycho-Analysis.
Bowlby, J. (1988). *A Secure Base: Clinical Applications of Attachment Theory*. London: Routledge.
Bowlby, J., & Durbin, E. (1939). *Personal Aggressiveness and War*. London: Kegan.
Bracken, P. (1984). *The Command and Control of Nuclear Force*. New Haven, CT: Yale University Press.
Britton, R. (1989). The missing link: parental sexuality in the Oedipus complex. In: J. Steiner (Ed.), *The Oedipus Complex Today*. London: Karnac.

Britton, R. (1992). Fundamentalism and idolatry as transference phenomena. *Bulletin*, 28(1): 2–11.

Bromberg, P. (1998). *Standing in Places: Essays on Clinical Process, Trauma and Dissociation*. Hillsdale, NJ: The Analytic Press.

Brown, J. A. C. (1963). *Techniques of Persuasion*. London: Penguin Books.

Buber, M. (Ed.) (1965). *The Knowledge of Man* (pp. 164–184). With an introductory essay by M. Friedman. New York: Harper & Row.

Cairns, E. (1996). *Children and Political Violence*. Oxford: Blackwell.

Campbell, J., & Kapur, R. (1997). The troubles mind of Northern Ireland: the application of object relations theory to the conflict. *Changes, An International Journal of Psychology & Psychotherapy*, 15: 19–22.

Cannon, W. B., & De LaPaz, D. (1911). Emotional stimulation of adrenal secretion. *American Journal of Physiology*, 28: 64.

Caper, R. (1995). On the difficulty of making a mutative interpretation. *International Journal of Psycho-Analysis*, 76: 91–101.

Carmelly, F. (1975). Guilt feelings in concentration camp survivors? Comments of a survivor. *American Journal of Jewish Communal Services*, 52(2): 139–144.

Cassidy, J., & Marvin, R. S. (1992). Attachment organization in preschool children: Coding guidelines. Seattle: MacArthur Working Group on Attachment—Unpublished Coding Manual.

Cavell, M. (1998). Triangulation, one's own mind and objectivity. *International Journal of Psycho-Analysis*, 79, 449–467.

Chasseguet-Smirguel, J. (1990). Reflections of a psycho-analyst upon the Nazi biocracy and genocide. *International Review of Psycho-Analysis*, 17, 167–176.

Chodoff, P. (1980). Psychotherapy of the survivor. In: J. E. Dimsdale (Ed.), *Survivors, Victims, Perpetrators* (pp. 205–218). Washington: Hemisphere Publishing.

Colvard, K. (2002). Commentary: the psychology of terrorists. *British Medical Journal*, 324: 359.

Corrado, R. R. (1982). A critique of the mental disorder perspective of political terrorism. *Journal of Law & Psychiatry*, 4: 293–309.

Curran, P. S., Bell, P., Murray, A., Loughrey, G., Reddy, R., & Rocke, L. E. (1990). Psychological consequences of the Enniskillen bombing. *British Journal of Psychiatry*, 156: 479–482.

Danieli, Y. (1981). Countertransference in the treatment and study of Nazi Holocaust survivors and their children. *Victimology: An International Journal*, 5(2–4): 355–367.

Danieli, Y. (1982). Therapists' difficulties in treating survivors of the Nazi Holocaust and their children. Doctoral dissertation, New York University, 1981. University Microfilms International #949–904.

Dasberg, H. (1987). Society facing trauma (or: Psychotherapists facing survivors) Sihot-Dialoge. *Journal of Israel Psychotherapy*, *I*(2): 98–104.

Davidson, S. (1980). On relating to traumatized/persecuted people. In Israel–Netherland Symposium on the impact of persecution, No. 2, Dalfsen, Amsterdam. Ministry of Social Welfare, Rijswijk, Holland, 55–62.

Davidson, S. (1985). Forty years later. Paper presented at the First International Conference on Grief and Bereavement in Contemporary Society, Jerusalem, Israel.

de Bernières, L. (1995). *Captain Corelli's Mandolin*. London: Random House, Minerva.

de Wind, E. (1968). The confrontation with death. *International Journal of Psycho-Analysis*, *49*: 302–305.

de Wind, E. (1971). Psychotherapy after traumatization caused by persecution. In: H. Krystal & W. G. Niederland (Eds.), *Psychic Traumatisation*. Boston: Little, Brown.

Dennett, D. (1987). *The Intentional Stance*. Cambridge, Mass: MIT Press.

Dixon, N. (1976). *On the Psychology of Military Incompetence* (p. 274). London: Futura.

Eilon, A. (1981). *The Israelis*. Tel-Aviv: Adam (in Hebrew).

Einstein, A., & Freud, S. (1932). Correspondence on "Why War?". In: J. Strachey (Ed.), *Complete Psychological Works of Freud*. S.E., 12: 197–215.

Eissler, K. R. (2000). On hatred with comments on the revolutionary, the saint, and the terrorist. *The Psychoanalytic Study of the Child*, *55*: 27–44.

Eitinger, L. (1971). Acute and chronic psychiatric and psychosomatic reactions in concentration camp survivors. In: Frank M. Ochberg (Ed.), *Society, Stress and Disease*. New York: University Press.

Eitinger, L., & Krell, R. (1985). *The Psychological and Medical Effects of Concentration Camps and Related Persecutions on Survivors of the Holocaust: A Research Bibliography*. Vancouver: University of British Columbia Press.

Ellis Davidson, H. R. (1964). *Gods and Myths of Northern Europe*. London: Penguin Books.

Erikson, E. (1950). *Childhood and Society*. London: Penguin Books.

Erikson, E. (1968). *Identity—Youth and Crisis*. New York: Norton.

Erikson, E. H. (1985). Pseudospeciation in the Nuclear Age. *Political Psychology*, *6*(2): 213–217.

Erikson, K. (1996). On pseudospeciation and social speciation. In: C. B. Strozier & M. Flynn (Ed.), *War and Human Survival* (pp. 51–57). London: Rowman & Littlefield.

Ezell, D. (1995). Satan. *The 1995 Grolier Multimedia Encyclopedia*, CD Version 7.0. Grolier Inc.

Faimberg, H. (1987). Die ineinanderruckung (telescoping) der generationen. Zur genealogie gewisser identifizierungen ("Telescoping" of generations: On the genealogy of some identifications). *Jahrbuch der Psychoanalyse, 20*: 114–142.

Fairbairn, W. (1943). The war neuroses. In: *Psychoanalytic Studies of the Personality*. London: Routledge and Kegan Paul.

Fairbairn, W. (1950). *Psychoanalytic Studies of the Personality* (pp. 76–81, 256–288). London: Tavistock Publications.

Fairbairn, W. R. D. (1954). *Object Relations Theory of Personality*. New York: Basic Books.

Fairbairn, W. R. D. (1994). *From Instinct to Self. Volume 1 Clinical and Theoretical Papers*. London: Jason Aronson Inc.

Felman, S., & Laub, D. (1992). *Testimony. Crises of Witnessing in Literature, Psycho-analysis and History*. London: Routledge.

Fenichel, O. (1954). The ego and the affects. In: *The Collected Papers Second Series*. New York: W. W. Norton & Co., Inc.

Ferenczi, S. (1933). Confusion of tongues between adults and the child. In: S. Ferenczi (1955) *Final Contributions to the Problems and Methods of Psychoanalysis* (pp. 156–167) M. Balint (Ed.). New York: Basic Books.

Fink, H. F. (1968). Development arrest as a result of Nazi persecution during adolescence. *International Journal of Psycho-analysis, 49*: 327–329.

Folsom, F., & Fledderjohann, C. (1988). *The Great Peace March, Santa Fe, New Mexico*. Santa Fe, New Mexico: Ocean Tree Books.

Fonagy, P. (1997). Attachment and theory of mind: Overlapping constructs? *Association for Child Psychology and Psychiatry Occasional Papers, 14*: 31–40.

Fonagy, P., & Morgan, G. S. (1991). Two forms of psychic change in psychoanalysis. Paper read at Institute of Psychiatry, London, March 1991.

Fonagy, P., & Target, M. (1995). Towards understanding violence: The use of the body and the role of the father. *International Journal of Psychoanalysis, 76*: 487–502.

Fonagy, P., & Target, M. (1996). Playing with reality: I. Theory of mind and the normal development of psychic reality. *International Journal of Psychoanalysis, 77*: 217–233.

Fonagy, P., Redfern, S., & Charman, T. (1997). The relationship between belief-desire reasoning and a projective measure of attachment security (SAT). *British Journal of Developmental Psychology*, 15: 51–61.

Fonagy, P., Steele, H., & Steele, M. (1991b). Maternal representations of attachment during pregnancy predict the organization of infant-mother attachment at one year of age. *Child Development*, 62: 891–905.

Fonagy, P., Steele, H., Moran, G., Steele, M., & Higgitt, A. (1991a). The capacity for understanding mental states: the reflective self in parent and child and its significance for security of attachment. *Infant Mental Health Journal*, 13: 200–217.

Fonagy, P., Steele, M., Steele, H., Higgitt, A., & Target, M. (1994). The Emmanuel Miller Memorial Lecture 1992. The theory and practice of resilience. *Journal of Child Psychology and Psychiatry and Allied Disciplines*, 35: 231–257.

Fonagy, P., Steele, M., Steele, H., Leigh, T., Kennedy, R., Mattoon, G., & Target, M. (1995). The predictive validity of Mary Main's Adult Attachment Interview: A psychoanalytic and developmental perspective on the transgenerational transmission of attachment and borderline states. In: S. Goldberg, R. Muir & J. Kerr (Eds.), *Attachment Theory: Social, Developmental and Clinical Perspectives* (pp. 233–278). Hillsdale, NJ: The Analytic Press.

Fordham, M. (1974). Defences of the self. *Journal of Analytical Psychology*, 19: 192–196.

Fornari, F. (1975). *The Psychoanalysis of War*. Bloomington: University of Indiana Press.

Foulkes, S. H. (1964). *Therapeutic Group Analysis*. New York: International University Press.

Foulkes, S. H. (Ed.) (1968). *Psychiatry in a Changing Society*. London: Tavistock.

Fraiberg, S. (1982). Pathological defenses in infancy. *Psychoanalytic Quarterly*, 51: 612–635.

Frankl, V. E. (1987). *Man's Search for Meaning*. London: Hodder & Stoughton.

Franklin, J. L. (1982). The religious right and the new Apocalypse. *Boston Globe*, 2 May.

Freidman, P. (1949). Some aspects of concentration camp psychology. *American Journal of Psychiatry*, 105(8): 604.

Freire, M., & Berdishevsky, B. (1980/82). Profile of Latin American political refugees, a longitudinal study. Toronto Board of Education. Based on paper delivered at Oxford Symposium, 1989.

Freiwald, A., & Mendelsohn, M. (1994). *The Last Nazi: Joseph Schwamberger and the Nazi Past*. New York: W. W. Norton.
Freud, A. (1936). The ego and the mechanisms of defence. *Works*, 2.
Freud, A. (1937). *The Ego and the Mechanisms of Defence*. London: Hogarth Press.
Freud, A. (1960). Discussion of Dr Bowlby's paper (Grief and mourning in infancy and early childhood), *The Writings of Anna Freud* (pp. 167–186). New York: International University Press, 1969.
Freud, A., & Burlingham, D. (1945). *Infants without Families*. London: Allen & Unwin.
Freud, A., & Dann, S. (1951). An experiment in group upbringing. *Psychoanalytic Study of the Child*, 6: 127–168.
Freud, S. (1893). On the psychical mechanism of hysterical phenomena: a lecture. *S.E.*, 3.
Freud, S. (1895a). Draft G. Melancholia. *S.E.*, 1: 200–206 [reprinted London: Hogarth Press, 1966].
Freud, S. (1895b). Project for a scientific psychology. *S.E.*, 1: 281–397
Freud, S. (1904). The psychopathology of everyday life. *S.E.*, 6: 258–259.
Freud, S. (1910). Leonardo da Vinci and a memory of his childhood. *S.E.*, 11: 123.
Freud, S. (1911a). Psycho-analytic notes on an autobiographical account of a case of paranoia (dementia paranoides). *S.E.*, 12: 9–82.
Freud, S. (1911b). Formulations on the two principles of mental functioning. *S.E.*, 12.
Freud, S. (1912). *S.E.*, 11: 115–117.
Freud, S. (1913a). Totem and taboo. *S.E.*, 13.
Freud, S. (1913b). The claims of psycho-analysis to scientific interest. *S.E.*, 13.
Freud, S. (1915a). The unconscious. *S.E.*, 14: 202–204.
Freud, S. (1915b). A meta-psychological supplement to the theory of dreams. *S.E.*, 14: 230.
Freud, S. (1915c). Mourning and melancholia. *S.E.*, 14: 237–243.
Freud, S. (1915d) Thoughts for the times on war and death. *S.E.*, 14.
Freud, S. (1915e). Letter to James J. Putnam (8 July 1915). In: E. L. Freud (Ed.), T. & J. Stern (Trans.), *The Letters of Sigmund Freud* (pp. 307–309). New York: Basic Books, 1960.
Freud, S. (1917). The taboo of virginity. *S.E.*, 17.
Freud, S. (1919). A child is being beaten. *S.E.*, 17.
Freud, S. (1920). Beyond the pleasure principle. *S.E.*, 18.
Freud, S. (1921). Group psychology and the analysis of the ego. *S.E.*, 18.
Freud, S. (1923a). The ego and the id. *S.E.*, 19: 3–66.

Freud, S. (1923b). A seventeenth-century demonological neurosis. *S.E.*, 19: 69–105.
Freud, S. (1924). The economic problem of masochism. *S.E.*, 19.
Freud, S. (1926). Inhibitions, symptoms and anxiety. *S.E.*, 20.
Freud, S. (1927a). Letter to Werner Achelis (30 January 1927). In: E. L. Freud (Ed.), T. & J. Stern (Trans.), *The Letters of Sigmund Freud* (pp. 374–375). New York: Basic Books, 1960.
Freud, S. (1927b). The future of an illusion. *S.E.*, 21.
Freud, S. (1928). Dostoevsky and parricide. *S.E.*, 21.
Freud, S. (1930a). Civilisation and its discontents. *S.E.*, 21: 113.
Freud, S. (1930b). In a letter to Arnold Zweig, dated Nov 26 1930, published in E. L. Freud (Ed.), *The Letters of Sigmund Freud and Arnold Zweig*. London: Hogarth Press, 1970.
Freud, S. (1933a). New introductory lectures on psycho-analysis. *S.E.*, 22: 5–182.
Freud, S. (1933b). Why war? *S.E.*, 22.
Freud, S. (1938a). An outline of psychoanalysis. *S.E.*, 21: 152–157.
Freud, S. (1938b). Splitting of the ego in the process of defence. *S.E.*, 23: 273–278.
Freud, S. (1939). Moses and monotheism: three essays. *S.E.*, 23: 1–137.
Freud, S. (1940). An outline of psycho-analysis. *S.E.*, 23.
Freud, S. (1952). Some theoretical conclusions regarding the emotional life of the infant. In: *The Writings of Melanie Klein, Volume 3*. London: Hogarth, 1975.
Friedman, M., & Jaranson, J. (1992). The applicability of the PTSD concept to refugees. In: A. J. Marsella *et al.* (Eds.), *Amidst Peril and Pain. The Mental Health and Social Well-Being of the World's Refugees*. Washington, DC: American Psychological Association.
Fromm, E. (1984). Malignant aggression: Adolf Hitler. In: *The Anatomy of Human Destructiveness*. Harmondsworth: Penguin Books.
Frosch, J. (1983). *The Psychotic Process*. New York: International Universities Press.
Furst, S. (Ed.) (1967) *Massive Psychic Trauma*. New York: Basic Books.
Gabbard, G. (1997). A reconsideration of objectivity in the analyst. *International Journal of Psycho-Analysis*, 78: 15–26.
Galbraith, J. K., & Salinger, N. (1981). *Almost Everyone's Guide to Economics*. London: Pelican Books.
Gambini, R. (1997). The soul of underdevelopment. In: M. A. Matton (Ed.), *Open Questions in Analytical Psychology: Zurich 1995*. Einsiedeln: Daimon Verlag.

Gampel, Y. (2000). Reflections on the prevalence of the uncanny in social violence. In: M. Robbens & M. Suarez-Orozo (Eds.), *Cultures Under Siege*. Cambridge University Press.

Garwood, A. (1996). Life, death and the power of powerlessness (manuscript).

George, C., & Solomon, J. (1996). Representational models of relationships: Links between caregiving and attachment. In: C. George & J. Solomon (Eds.), *Defining the Caregiving System (Infant Mental Health Journal, 17)*. New York: John Wiley.

Gill, H. S. (1986). Oedipal determinants in differential outcomes of bereavement. *British Journal of Medical Psychology, 59*: 21–25.

Gilligan, J. (1996). *Violence, Our Deadly Epidemic and Its Causes*. New York: G P Putnams's Sons.

Gilligan, J. (2001). *Preventing Violence*. New York: Thames & Hudson.

Glover, E. (1933). *War, Sadism and Pacifism: Further Essays on Group Psychology and War*. Edinburgh: Hugh Paton & Sons.

Glover, E. (1946). *War, Sadism and Pacifism* (p. 174). London: George Allen and Unwin.

Glover, E. (1955). *The Technique of Psycho-Analysis*. New York: International Universities Press.

Goldberg, C. (1996). *Speaking with the Devil. A Dialogue with Evil*. New York: Viking/Penguin.

Green, A. (1983). *Narcissisme de vie—Narcissisme de mort*. Paris: Editions de Minuit.

Green, A. (1988). Pourquoi le mal? *La folie privée. Psychanalyse des cas-limites*. Paris: Gallimard.

Grinberg, L. et al. (1985). *Introduction to the Work of Bion*. London: Maresfield.

Grosskruth, P. (1986). *Melanie Klein: Her World and Her Work*. New York: Knopf.

Grotstein, J. S. (1990). Nothingness, meaninglessness, chaos, and the "black hole", I & II. *Contemporary Psychoanalysis, 26*: 257–290; 377–407.

Grotstein, J. S. (1991). Nothingness, meaninglessness, chaos, and the 'black hole', III. *Contemporary Psychoanalysis, 27*: 1–33.

Grotstein, J. (1997). Integrating one-person and two-person psychologies: autochthony and alterity in counterpoint. *Psychoanalytic Quarterly, LXVI*.

Grubrich-Simitis, I. (1981). Extreme traumatization as cumulative trauma: Psychoanalytic investigations of the effects of concentration camp experiences on survivors and their children. *Psychoanalytic Study of the Child, 36*: 415–450.

Grubrich-Simitis, I. (1984). From concretism to metaphor: thoughts on some theoretical and technical aspects of the psychoanalytic work with children of holocaust survivors. *Psychoanalytic Study of the Child*, 39: 301–319.

Haldane, J. B. S. (1995). Is history a fraud? In: *The Inequality of Man and Other Essays* (pp. 49–51). Philadelphia: R. West [original work published in 1932].

Harrell-Bond, B., & Wilson, K. (1990). Dealing with dying: some anthropological reflections on the need for assistance by refugee relief programmes for bereavement. *Journal of Refugee Studies*, 3: 228–243.

Haynal, A. (2001). Groups and fanaticism. In: Ethel Specter Person (Ed.), *Freud's Group Psychology and the Analysis of the Ego*. Hillsdale, NJ: Analytic Press.

Haynal, A., Molnar, M., & DePumège, G. (1983). *Fanaticism: A Historical & Psychoanalytic Study*. New York: Schocker Books.

Hazlitt, W. (1826). On the pleasure of hating. In: *The Plain Speaker. Opinions on Books, Men and Things*. London: Colburg.

Heatherton, T. F., Kleck, R. E., Hebl, M. F., & Hull, J. R. (2000). *The Social Psychology of Stigma*. New York: The Guilford Press.

Heimann, P. (1975). In: *Sacrificial Parapraxis Annual of Psycho-analysis, Volume 111*. New York: International University Press.

Hering, C. (1994). The problem of the Alien: emotional mastery or emotional fascism in contemporary film production. *Free Associations*, 4: 391–407.

Herzog, J. (1982). World beyond metaphor: Thoughts on the transmission of trauma. In: M. S. Bergmann & M. E. Jucovy (Eds.), *Generations of the Holocaust* (pp. 103–119). New York: Columbia University Press.

Hill, J. L., & Zautra, A. J. (1989). Self blame attribution and unique vulnerability as predictors of post rape demoralization. *Journal of Social and Clinical Psychology*, 8(4): 368–375.

Hill, L. B. (1938). The use of hostility as defense. *Psychoanalytic Quarterly*, VII: 254–264

Hinshelwood, R. D. (1986). Psychological defence and nuclear war. *Medicine and War*, 2(1): 29–38.

Hinshelwood, R. D. (1987a). Large group dynamics and nuclear war. *Group Analysis*, 20: 137–146.

Hinshelwood, R. D. (1987b). What happens in groups. In: *Psychoanalysis, the Individual and the Community*. London: Free Association Books.

Hinshelwood, R. D. (1989). *A Dictionary of Kleinian Thought*. London: Free Association Books.

Hinshelwood, R. D., & Manning, H. (1979). *Therapeutic Communities*. London: Routledge & Kegan Paul.

Hinze, E. (1986). The influence of historical events on psychoanalysis. *International Journal of Psycho-Analysis*, 67: 459–466.

Honig, A. M. (1988). Cumulative traumata as contributors to chronicity in schizophrenia. *Bulletin of the Menninger Clinic*, 52: 423–434.

Hopkins, J. (1984). The probable role of trauma in a case of foot and shoe fetishism: Aspects of the psychotherapy of a 6-year-old girl. *International Review of Psycho-Analysis*, 11: 79–90.

Hoppe, K. D. (1968a). Psychotherapy with concentration camp survivors. In: H. Krystal (Ed.), *Massive Psychic Trauma*. New York: International University Press.

Hoppe, K. D. (1968b). Re-somatisation of affects in survivors of persecution. *International Journal of Psycho-analysis*, 49: 324–326.

Hoppe, K. D. (1971). Aftermath of Nazi persecution reflected in recent psychoanalytic literature. In: H. Krystal & W. G. Niederland (Eds.), *Psychic Traumatisation*. Boston: Little, Brown.

Hopper, E. (1991). Encapsulation as a defence against the fear of annihilation. *International Journal of Psycho-Analysis*, 72: 607–623.

Horowitz, M. J. (1970). Psychological response to serious life events. In: V. Hamilton & D. Warburton (Eds.), *Human stress and Cognition: An Information Processing Approach*. New York: Wiley.

Humphrey, N. (1982). *Four Minutes to Midnight*. London: Menard Press.

Hunter-Brown, I. H. (1984). Some psychological factors underlying the making of War. *Journal of Medical Association for Prevention of War*, 3(12): 273–280.

Hunter-Brown, I. H. (1989). Doctors' attitudes on civil defence and nuclear issues. *Medicine and War*, 5(4): 175–180.

Ichimura, A., Nakajima, I., & Juzoji, H. (2001). Investigation and analysis of a reported incident resulting in an actual airline hijacking due to a fanatical and engrossed VR state. *Cyber Psychology and Behaviour*, 4(3): 355–363.

Ignatieff, M. (1998). *The Warrior's Honour*. New York: Viking.

Ikonen, P., & Rechardt, E. (1993). The origin of shame and its vicissitudes. *Scandinavian Psychoanalytic Review*, 16: 100–124.

Izhar, S. (1949). *Four Stories*. Tel-Aviv: Am-Oved (in Hebrew).

Jackson, M., & Williams, P. (1994) *Unimaginable Storms: A Search for Meaning in Psychosis*. London: Karnac Books.

Jacobson, E. (1953). The affects and their pleasure-unpleasure qualities in relation to the psychic discharge processes. In: R. M. Loewenstein

(Ed.), *Drives, Affects, Behavior*. New York: International Universities Press.

Jaffe, R. (1962). Dissociative phenomena in former concentration camp inmates. *International Journal of Psycho-Analysis*, 49: 310–312.

Jaques, E. (1951). *The Changing Culture of a Factory*. London: Routledge and Kegan Paul.

Jaques, E. (1955). Social systems as defence against persecutory and depressive anxiety. Klein *et al.* (Eds.), *New Directions in Psychoanalysis* (pp. 482–486). London: Tavistock Publications.

Jaques, E. (1965). Death and the mid-life crisis. *International Journal of Psycho-Analysis*, 46: 502–514.

Jones, E. (1929). Fear, guilt and hate. In: *Papers on Psychoanalysis*. Baltimore: Williams and Wilkins Co., 1950.

Jones, E. (1938). How can civilization be saved? *Essays in Applied Psychoanalysis, Volume 1*. Hogarth, 1951.

Jones, E. (1953–1957). *The Life and Work of Sigmund Freud, Volume 3*. New York: Basic Books.

Jones, H. (1953). *The Therapeutic Community*. New York: Basic Books.

Jucovy, M. (1992). Psycho-analytic contributions to holocaust studies. *International Journal of Psycho-Analysis*, 72(2): 267–282.

Jung, C. G. (1928). The Swiss line in the European spectrum. *Collected Works*, 10.

Jung, C. G. (1934/1950). Conscious, Unconscious and Individuation. *C.W.*, 9i.

Jung, C. G. (1943). Psychotherapy and a philosophy of life. *C.W.*, 16.

Jung, C. G. (1956) The battle for deliverance from the mother. *C.W.*, 5.

Jung, C. G. (1959). The Shadow. *C.W.*, 9ii.

Jung, C. G. (1963). The Conjunction. *C.W.*, 14.

Kafka, J. (1992). *Multiple Realities*. New York: International University Press.

Kahneman, D., Slovic, P., & Tversky, A. (Eds.) (1982). *Judgement Under Uncertainty: Heuristics and Biases*. Cambridge: Cambridge University Press.

Kalsched, D. (1996). *The Inner World of Trauma. Archetypal Defenses of the Personal Spirit*. London: Routledge.

Kapur, R., & Campbell, J. (2001). The troubled mind of Northern Ireland: social care, object relations theory and political conflict. *Journal of Social Work Practice* (submitted).

Keinan-Kon, N. (1998). Internal Reality, External Reality, and Denial in the Gulf War. *Journal of the American Academy of Psychoanalysis*, 26(3) Fall.

Kennedy, C. (Ed.) (2002). From *Profiles in Courage for Our Time* (p. 344). New York: Hyperion Books.

Kernberg, O. F. (1984). *Severe Personality Disorders: Psychotherapeutic Strategies.* New Haven, CT: Yale.

Kestenberg, J. S. (1982). A metapsychological assessment based on an analysis of a survivor's child. In: M. S. Bergmann & M. E. Jucovy (Eds.), *Generations of the Holocaust* (pp. 137–158). New York: Columbia University Press.

Khan, M. M. R. (1963). The concept of cumulative trauma. *Psychoanalytical Study of the Child,* 18: 283–306.

Khan, M. M. R. (1974). *The Privacy of Self* (pp. 42–68). London: Hogarth Press.

Khan, M. M. R. (1981). *The Privacy of the Self* (pp. 42–59). London: The Hogarth Press and the Institute of Psycho-analysis.

Khan, M. M. R. (1986). Introduction. In: D. W. Winnicott (1986) *Holding and Interpretation: Fragment of an Analysis.* New York: Grove Press.

Kirpal, B. N. (2002). Courts and Terrorism—the Indian Experience (unpublished).

Klarsfeld, S. (1994). *Le Mémorial des Enfants Juifs Déportés de France.* Edited and published by Les Fils et Filles des Déportés de France.

Klauber, J. et al. (1987). *Illusion and Spontaneity in Psycho-Analysis.* London: Association Books.

Klein, H. (1971). Families of Holocaust survivors in the kibbutz. In: H. Krystal & W. G. Niederland (Eds.), *Psychic Traumatisation.* Boston: Little, Brown.

Klein, H. (1973). Children of the Holocaust: Mourning and Bereavement. In: Antony and Koupernik, *The Child and His Family.*

Klein, H. (1984). The survivor's search for meaning and identity. *The Nazi Concentration Camps.* Proceedings of the Fourth Yad Vashem International Historical Conference (pp. 543–552). Jerusalem: Yad Vashem.

Klein, M. (1929). Personification in the play of children. *The Writings of Melanie Klein, Volume 1* (pp. 203–205). London: Hogarth, 1975.

Klein, M. (1940). Mourning and its relation to manic-depressive states. *International Journal of Psycho-Analysis,* 21, and in *Writings of Melanie Klein, Volume 2.* London: Hogarth 1975.

Klein, M. (1946). Notes on some schizoid mechanisms. *International Journal of Psycho-Analysis,* 27: 99–110 [reprinted in (1975) *The Writings of Melanie Klein, Volume 3* (pp. 1–24). London: The Hogarth Press].

Klein, M. (1948a). *Contributions to Psychoanalysis (1921–1945).* London: Hogarth.

Klein, M. (1948b). On the theory of anxiety and guilt. *International Journal of Psycho-Analysis, 28* [reprinted in (1975) *The Writings of Melanie Klein, Volume 3* (pp. 25–42). London: The Hogarth Press].

Klein, M. (1952). Some theoretical conclusions regarding the emotional life of the infant. *The Writings of Melanie Klein, Volume 3.* Hogarth, 1975.

Klein, S. (1980). Autistic phenomena in neurotic patients. *International Journal of Psychoanalysis, 61:* 395–402.

Kohut, H. (1971). *The Analysis of the Self.* New York: International Universities Press.

Kohut, H. (1972). Thoughts on narcissism and narcissistic rage. *Psychoanalytic Study of the Child, 27:* 360–400.

Kolev, N. (1991). *An Unknown Dimension of Paranoia: The Significance of Archaic Space.* Paper presented at the Xth International Symposium for the Psychotherapy of Schizophrenia, Stockholm, August.

Kolev, N. (1997). Introduction à l'étude de l'espace archaïque. *L'Évolution Psychiatrique, 62:* 721–742.

Kovel, J. (1983). *Against the State of Nuclear War* (p. 109). London: Pan.

Kovel, J. (1988). *The Radical Spirit—Essays on Psychoanalysis and Society.* London: Free Association Books.

Krell, R. (1985). Therapeutic value of documenting child survivors. *Journal of the American Academy of Child Psychiatry, 24*(4): 397–400.

Kren, G. M. (1989). In: P. Marcus & A. Rosenberg (Eds.), *Healing Their Wounds: Psychotherapy with Holocaust Survivors and Their Families.* New York: Springer.

Kris, E. (1956). Recovery of childhood memories in psycho-analysis. *Psychoanalytic Study of the Child, 11:* 54–89.

Krystal, H. (Ed.) (1968). *Massive Psychic Trauma.* New York: International University Press.

Krystal, H. (1971). Trauma: considerations of its intensity and chronicity. In: H. Krystal & W. G. Niederland (Eds.), *Psychic Traumatisation.* Boston: Little, Brown.

Krystal, H. *Integration and Self-healing: Affect, Trauma, Alexthemia.* New York: NJ Analytic Press.

Krystal, H., & Niederland, W. G. (1971). *Psychic Traumatisation, Aftereffects in Individuals and Communities.* Boston: Little, Brown.

Kubler-Ross, E. (1969). *On Death and Dying.* New York: Macmillan.

Lasch, C. (1978). *The Culture of Narcissism.* New York: Norton Books.

Lemlij, M. (1992). Being a psychoanalyst in violent country. *International Psychoanalytical Journal.*

Leon, G. R., Butcher, J. N., Kleinman, M., Goldberg, A., & Almagor, M. (1981). Survivors of the Holocaust and their children: current statement and adjustment. *Journal of Personality and Social Psychology,* 41: 503–516.

Levine, H. B. (1982). Toward a psychoanalytic understanding of children of survivors of the Holocaust. *The Psychoanalytic Quarterly,* 51: 70–92.

Lichtenberg, J. D. (1995). Can empirical studies of development impact on psychoanalytic theory and technique? In: T. Shapiro & R. N. Emde (Eds.), *Research in Psychoanalysis: Process, Development, Outcome* (pp. 261–276). New York: International Universities Press.

Lifton, K. J. (1967). Observations on Hiroshima survivors. In: S. Furst (Ed.), *Massive Psychic Trauma.* New York: Basic Books.

Lifton, R. J. (1967). *Death in Life? Survivors of Hiroshima.* New York: Simon and Schuster.

Lifton, R. J. (1979). Victimization and mass violence. In: *The Broken Connection.* New York: Simon and Schuster.

Lifton, R. J. (1982). *Nuclear War's Effect on the Mind.* London: Faber & Faber.

Lifton, R. J. (1985). *Nuclear Threat and the Problem of Imagination.* Paper given to the 42nd Annual Conference of the American Group Psychotherapy Association, New York.

Lifton, R. R. (1978). Advocacy and corruption in the healing profession. In: Ch. R. Figley (Ed.), *Stress Disorders Among Vietnam Veterans* (Chapter 10). New York: Brunner Mazel.

Limentani, A. (1989). The psychoanalytic movement during the years of the war (1939–1945), according to the archives of the I.P.A. *International Review of Psychoanalysis,* 16: 3–12.

Lindy, J. D. (1989). Countertransference and post-traumatic stress disorder. Sihot-Dialogue. *Israel Journal of Psychotherapy,* III(2) March: 94–101.

Liotti, G. (1992). Disorganized/disoriented attachment in the etiology of the dissociative disorders. *Dissociation,* 5: 196–204.

Liotti, G. (1995). Disorganized/disorientated attachment in the psychotherapy of the dissociative disorders. In: S. Goldberg, R. Muir & J. Kerr (Eds.), *Attachment Theory: Social, Developmental and Clinical Perspectives* (pp. 343–363). Hillsdale, NJ: Analytic Press, Inc.

Little, M. (1960). On basic unity. In: *Transference Neurosis and Transference Psychosis: Toward Basic Unity* (pp. 109–125). London: Free Association Books & Maresfield Library, 1981.

Locke, J. (1693). *Some Thoughts Concerning Education.* Cambridge: Cambridge University Press, 1902.

Loewenberg, P. (1995). *Fantasy and Reality in History*. New York: Oxford University Press.
Lorca, F. G. (1960). *Lorca: Penguin Poets*. Introduced, edited and translated by J. L. Gili. Harmondsworth: Penguin Books.
Lorenzer. (1968). Some observations on the latency of symptoms in patients suffering from persecution sequelae. *International Journal of Psycho-Analysis, 49*: 316–318.
Lyons-Ruth, K. (1996). Attachment relationships among children with aggressive behavior problems: The role of disorganized early attachment patterns. *Journal of Consulting and Clinical Psychology, 64*: 64–73.
Main, M., & Goldwyn, R. (in preparation). Adult attachment rating and classification systems. In: M. Main (Ed.), *A Typology of Human Attachment Organization Assessed in Discourse, Drawings and Interviews* (Working Title). New York: Cambridge University Press.
Main, M., & Hesse, E. (1990). Parents' unresolved traumatic experiences are related to infant disorganized attachment status: Is frightened and/or frightening parental behavior the linking mechanism? In: M. Greenberg, D. Cicchetti & E. M. Cummings (Eds.), *Attachment in the Preschool Years: Theory, Research and Intervention* (pp. 161–182). Chicago: University of Chicago Press.
Main, M., Kaplan, N., & Cassidy, J. (1985). Security in infancy, childhood, and adulthood: A move to the level of representation. *Monographs of the Society for Research in Child Development, 50*(1–2): 66–104.
Main, T. (1957). The ailment. *British Journal of Medical Psychology, 30*: 129–145.
Malcolm, N. (1994). *Bosnia. A Short History*. London: Macmillan.
Mandelstam, N. (1971). *Hope Against Hope*. London: Collins.
Marcus, P., & Rosenberg, A. (Eds.) (1989). *Healing Their Wounds: Psychotherapy with Holocaust Survivors and Their Families*. New York: Praeger.
Marsella, A. J. et al. (Eds.) (1996). *Ethnocultural Aspects of Post traumatic Stress Disorder. Issues, Research, and Clinical Applications*. Washington, DC: American Psychological Association.
Matte-Blanco, I. (1988). *Thinking, Feeling and Being*. London: Routledge.
Mayes, L., & Cohen, D. (1993). Playing and therapeutic action in child analysis. *International Journal of Psycho-Analysis, 74*: 1235–1244.
McDougall, J. (1982). *Theatres of the Mind*. Paris: Gallimard.
McDougall, J. (1989). *Theatres of the Body*. London: Free Association Books.
Meltzer, D. (1975). *Explorations in Autism*. Perth: The Clunie Press.

Menzies Lyth, I. (1988). *Containing Anxiety in Institutions*. London: Free Association Books.
Menzies, I. E. P. (1960). The functioning of social systems as a defence against anxiety. *Human Relations, 13*: 95 [republished 1970 as Tavistock Pamphlet No. 3].
Menzies, I. (1970). *The Functioning of Social Systems as a Defence against Anxiety*. London: Tavistock Institute of Human Relations.
Milgram, S. (1974). *Obedience to Authority*. New York: Harper & Row.
Mill, J. S. (1950). *Mill on Bentham and Coleridge*. (Introduction by F. R. Leavis, p. 111). London: Chatto and Windus.
Miller, A. (1980). Adolf Hitler's childhood: from hidden to manifest horror. In: *For Your Own Good. Hidden Cruelty in Child-Rearing and the Roots of Violence*. London, Boston: Faber and Faber.
Milosz, C. (1983). Ruins and Poetry. The New York Review of Books, 17 March 1983, pp. 20–23.
Molad, G. (1991). Unsealed Room: Reflections on treatment in situation of total threat. Sihot-Dialogue. *Israel*, 5 Feb.
Money-Kyrle, R. E. (1934). Descriptive notice of Edward Glover (sadism and pacifism). *British Journal of Medical Psychology, 14*: 349–353.
Money-Kyrle, R. E. (1937). The development of war. *British Journal of Psychiatry, 16*.
Money-Kyrle, R. (1978). In: D. Meltzer & E. O'Shaugnessy (Eds.), *Collected Papers* (pp. 131–160; 366–376). Strathtay, Perthshire: Clunie Press.
Moses, R. (1987). Adult psychic trauma: the question of early predisposition and some detailed mechanisms. *International Journal of Psychoanalysis, 59*: 353–364.
Moses, R. (Ed.) (1993). *The Persistent Shadows of the Holocaust: The Meaning to Those Not Directly Effected*. Madison, CT: International Universities Press.
Moskowitz, S. (1983). *Love Despite Hate: Child Survivors of the Holocaust and Their Adult Lives*. New York: Schocken Books.
Munoz, L. (1980). Exile as bereavement: socio-psychological manifestations of Chilean exiles in Great Britain. *British Journal of Medical Psychology, 53*: 227–232.
Neubauer, P. (1995). Hate and developmental sequences and group dynamics. In: S. Akhtar, S. Kramer & H. Parens (Eds.), *The Birth of Hatred: Developmental, Clinical, and Technical Aspects of Intense Aggression* (pp. 149–164). Northvale, NJ: Jason Aronson.
Niederland, W. G. (1968a). An interpretation of the psychological stresses and defences in the concentration camp life and the late

after-effects. In: H. Krystal (Ed.), *Massive Psychic Trauma* (pp. 60–70). New York: International University Press.
Niederland, W. G. (1968b). Clinical observations on the survivor syndrome. *International Journal of Psycho-Analysis, 49*: 313–315.
Niederland, W. G. (1971). Introductory notes on the concept, definition and range of psychic trauma. In: H. Krystal & W. G. Niederland (Eds.), *Psychic Traumatisation*. Boston: Little, Brown.
Niederland, W. G. (1981). The survivor syndrome: further observations and dimensions. *Journal of the American Psychoanalytic Association, 29*: 413–425.
Novey, S. A. (1959). Clinical view of affect theory. *International Journal of Psychoanalysis, XL*.
Noy, S. (2000). *Traumatic Stress Situations*. Tel-Aviv: Schocken Publishing House.
Ogden, T. (1982). *Projective Identification and Psychotherapeutic Technique*. New York: Jason Aronson.
Ogden, T. (1985). On potential space. *International Journal of Psychoanalysis, 66*: 129–141.
Ogden, T. (1986). *The Matrix of the Mind: Object Relations and the Psychoanalytic Dialogue*. New York: Aronson.
Ogden, T. (1989). Playing, dreaming, and interpreting experience: Comments on potential space. In: M. G. Fromm & B. L. Smith (Eds.), *The Facilitating Environment: Clinical Applications of Winnicott's Theory* (pp. 255–278). Madison, CT: International Universities Press.
Olden, C. (1941). About the fascinating effect of the narcissistic personality. *American Imago, 2*: 347–355.
Olds, D. (2000). A semiotic model of the mind. *Journal of the American Psychoanalytic Association, 48*(2): 497–529.
Orange, D., Atwood, G., & Stolorow, R. (1997). *Working Intersubjectively: Contextualism in Psychoanalytic Practice*. Hillsdale, NJ: The Analytic Press.
Ornstein, A. (1989). An interview. In: P. Marcus & A. Rosenberg (Eds.), *Healing Their Wounds: Psychotherapy with Holocaust Survivors and Their Families*. Sage.
Orwell, G. (1949). *Nineteen Eighty Four*. London: Secker & Warburg.
Osama bin Laden. (2001). *Financial Times*, 10th October.
Ostell, A. (1992). Absolutist thinking and emotional problems. *Counselling Psychol. Quarterly, 5*: 161–176.
Ostell, A., & Oakland, S. (1999). Absolutist thinking and health. *British Journal of Medical Psychology, 72*: 239–250.

O'Toole, M. E. (2000). *The School Shooter: A Threat Assessment Perspective.* National Centre for the Analysis of Violent Crimes FBI Academy, Quantico, VA 22135. Available at www.fbi.gov/library/school/school2.pdf.

Oxford Research Group. (1986). *How Nuclear Weapons Decisions are Made.* S. McLean (Ed.). London: Macmillan.

Papadopoulos, R. K. (1996). Therapeutic presence and witnessing. *The Tavistock Gazette Autumn*: 61–65.

Papadopoulos, R. K. (1997). Individual identity and collective narratives of conflict. *Harvest: Journal for Jungian Studies*, 43(2): 7–26.

Papadopoulos, R. K. (1998a). Jungian perspectives in new contexts. In: A. Casement (Ed.), *The Post-Jungians Today*. London: Routledge.

Papadopoulos, R. K. (1998b). The tyranny of change. *Proceedings of the Cumberland Lodge Conference, 1996.* London: The Champernowne Trust.

Papadopoulos, R. K. (in press a). Working with families of Bosnian medical evacuees: therapeutic dilemmas. *The Journal of Child Psychology and Psychiatry*.

Papadopoulos, R. K. (in press b). Individual identity in the context of collective strife. In: J. G. Donat & J. Livernois (Eds.), *Eranos Yearbook, Volume 66.* Woodstock, Connecticut: Spring Journal Books.

Papadopoulos, R., & Hildebrand, J. (1997). Is home where the heart is? Narratives of oppositional discourses in refugee families. In: R. K. Papadopoulos & J. Byng-Hall (Eds.), *Multiple Voices; Narrative in Systemic Family Psychotherapy.* London: Duckworth.

Pennebaker, T., & Harber, K. D. (1993). A social stage model of collective coping: the Lima Prieta earthquake and the Persian Gulf war. *Journal of Social Issues*, 49: 125–145.

Pentz, M. (1984). After the day after, earth's nuclear winter. *Sanity, Jan*: 9–11.

Pine, F. (1990). *Drive, Ego, Object and Self: A Synthesis for Clinical Work.* New York, NY: Basic Books.

Pines, D. (1986). Working with women survivors of the Holocaust: affective experiences in transference and countertransference. *International Journal of Psycho-Analysis*, 67: 295–307.

Plato. (1979). Battle of Gods and Giants. In: A. Flew (Ed.), *A Dictionary of Philosophy.* Plato's Sophists (p. 36). London and Birmingham: Macmillan.

Post, J. M. (1990). Terrorist psycho-logic: terrorist behaviour as a product of psychological forces. In: W. Reich (Ed.), *Origins of Terrorism: Psychologies, Ideologies, Theologies, States of Mind.* Cambridge: Cambridge University Press, 1990.

Potamianou, A. (1992). *Un Bouclier dans l'Economie des Etats Limites L'Espoir*. Paris: Presses Universitaires de France.

Proner, B. (1986). Defences of the self and envy of oneself. *The Journal of Analytical Psychology*, 31: 275–279.

Puget, J. (1980). Social violence and psychoanalysis in Argentina. *Free Associations*, 13.

Raveau, F. (1960). Neuro-psychiatric data on the state of former deportees 15 years after their liberation. Congress, Oslo, quoted in K. D. Hoppe (1968). A. Reyes (1989), The destruction of the soul, a treatable disease. *British Journal of Psychotherapy*, 6: 191–202.

Reck-Malleczewen, F. P. (1966). *Tagebuch eines Verzweifelten [von] Freidrich Percyval Reck-Malleczewen*. Mit einem Vortwort von Klaus Harpprecht. (Neuausg.) Stuttgart: Goverts.

Redfearn, J. (1992). *The Exploding Self: the Creative and Destructive Nucleus of the Personality*. Wilmette, Il: Chiron.

Renik, O. (1998). Triangulation, one's own mind and objectivity. *International Journal of Psycho-Analysis*, 79: 487–497.

Rey, H. (1994). *Universals of Psychoanalysis*. London: Free Association Books.

Richards, B. (1984). Civil defence and psychic defence. *Radical Science Journal*, 15/Free Associations: 85–97.

Ricoeur, P. (1970). *Freud and Philosophy*. New Haven: Yale Univ. Press.

Ringstrom, P. (1999) Discussion of Stolorow's The Phenomenology of Trauma and the Absolutisms of Everyday Life. 22nd Conference on the Psychology of the Self October, 1999, Toronto, Ontario.

Robben, M. (2000). The assault on basic trust: disappearance, protest, and reburial in Argentina. In: M. Robben & M. Suarez-Orozo (Eds.), *Culture under Siege*. Cambridge University Press.

Robertson, S. (1984). Nuclear states of terror. *Radical Science Journal*, 14/ No Clear Reason: 117–126.

Rosenberg, E. (1949). Anxiety and the capacity to bear it. *International Journal of Psycho-analysis*, 30: 1–12.

Rosenbloom, M. (1988). Lessons of the Holocaust for mental health practice. In: R. L. Braham (Ed.), *The Psychological Perspectives of the Holocaust and of its Aftermath*. New York: Columbia University Press.

Rosenfeld, D. (1990). Countertransference. Paper given at the Swedish Psychoanalytic Society.

Rosenfeld, D. (1992). *The Psychotic: Aspects of the Personality*. London: Karnac Books.

Rosenfeld, H. (1950). Note on the psychopathology of confusional states

in chronic schizophrenics. In: *Psychotic States: A Psychoanalytic Approach* (pp. 52–62). New York: International University Press.
Rosenfeld, H. (1987a). Destructive narcissism and the death instinct. *Impasse and Interpretation*. London and New York: Tavistock.
Rosenfeld, H. (1987b). *Impasse and Interpretation: Therapeutic and Anti-Therapeutic Factors in the Psychoanalytic Treatment of Psychotic, Borderline and Neurotic Patients*. London: Routledge.
Rosenfeld, H. (1988). Impasse and interpretation. *New Library of Psychoanalysis*. London: Routledge.
Rosenman, S. (1984). The psychoanalytic writer on the Holocaust and Bettelheim. *American Journal of Social Psychiatry*, 4(2): 65.
Ross, C., Norton, G., & Fraser, G. (1989). Evidence against the iatrogenesis of multiple personality disorder. *Dissociation Progress in the Dissociative Disorders*, 2: 61–65.
Roy, A. (1997). *The God of Small Things*. Tel-Aviv: Zmora-Bitan.
Russell, B. (1940). *Power*. New York: Basic Books.
Russell, C., & Miller, B. (1983). Profile of a terrorist. In: L. Friedman & Y. Alexander (Eds.), *Perspectives on Terrorism* (pp. 45–60). Wilmington DE: Scholarly resources.
Rustin, M. (1991). *The Good Society and the Inner World*. Verso: London.
Rycroft, C. (1995). *A Critical Dictionary of Psychoanalysis*. London: Penguin.
Salonen, S. (1989). The restitution of primary identification in psychoanalysis. *Scandinavian Psychoanalytic Review*, 12: 102–115.
Samuels, A. (1993). *The Political Psyche*. London: Routledge.
Sandler, J. (1960). The background of safety. *From Safety to Superego: Selected Papers of Joseph Sandler* (pp. 1–8). London: Karnac, 1987.
Sandler, J. (1987). *From Safety to Superego*. New York: Guilford.
Sandler, J., & Sandler, A.-M. (1998). *Object Relations Theory and Role Responsiveness*. London: Karnac Books.
Sandler, J., Dare, C., & Holder, A. (1992). *The Patient and the Analyst* (2nd edn). New York: International University Press.
Sarraj, E. (2002). *Time Magazine*, April 8th, p. 39.
Schedlinger, S. (1982). On interpretation in groups: the need for refinement. *International Journal of Group Psychotherapy*, 37: 339–353.
Schnale, A. H. (1971). Psychic trauma during bereavement. In: H. Krystal & W. G. Niederland (Eds.), *Psychic Traumatisation*. Boston: Little, Brown.
Schoenberner, G. (1969). *The Yellow Star. The Persecution of the Jews in Europe 1933–1945*. London: Corgi Books.
Schuengel, C. (1997). *Attachment, Loss, and Maternal Behavior: A Study on*

Intergenerational Transmission. Leiden, The Netherlands: University of Leiden Press.

Schur, M. (1960). Discussion of Dr John Bowlby's paper. *The Psychoanalytic Study of the Child, 15*: 63–84.

Schwartz-Salant, N. (1989). *The Borderline Personality: Vision and Healing*. Wilmette, Il: Chiron.

Schwimmer, W. (2002). Opening Speech to International Judicial Conference on "The Courts and Terrorism", Strasbourg.

Searles, H. F. (1956). The psychodynamics of vengefulness. *Psychiatry, XIX*: 31–39.

Searles, H. F. (1962). Scorn, disillusionment and adoration in the psychotherapy of schizophrenia. *Psychoanalysis and Psychoanalytic Review, XLIX*: 39–60.

Searles, H. F. (1967). The schizophrenic individual's experience of his world. In: *Countertransference and Related Subjects* (pp. 5–27). New York: International Universities Press, 1979.

Segal, H. (1957). Notes on symbol formation. In: E. B. Spillius (Ed.), *Melanie Klein Today*. London: Routledge, 1990.

Segal, H. (1958). Fear of death: notes on the analysis of an old man. *International Journal of Psycho-Analysis, 39*: 187–191 [reprinted in *The Work of Hanna Segal* (pp. 173–182). Jason Aronson, 1981].

Segal, H. (1964). *Introduction to the Work of Melanie Klein*. London: Heinemann [revised edition London: Karnac, 1988].

Segal, H. (1981). *The Work of Hanna Segal*. New York: Jason Aronson.

Segal, H. (1986). Notes on symbol formation. *The Works of Hanna Segal. A Kleinian Approach to Clinical Practice*. London: Free Association Books/Maresfield Library.

Segal, H. (1987). Silence is the real crime. *International Review of Psycho-Analysis, 14*(3): 3–11.

Segal, H. (1989). Political thinking and psycho-analysis, perspectives. In: L. Barnett & I. Lee (Eds.), *Perspectives in the Nuclear Mentality* (pp. 41–48). London: Karnac Books.

Segal, H. (1995). From Hiroshima to the Gulf War and after: a psychoanalytic perspective. In: A. Elliott & S. Frosh (Eds.), *Psychoanalysis in Contexts*. London: Routledge.

Semprun, J. (1963). *Le Grand Voyage*. Paris: Editions Gallimard

Semprun, J. (1980). *What a Beautiful Sunday!* London: Abacus, 1984.

Shapiro, D. (1965). *Neurotic Styles*. New York: Basic Books.

Shavit, A. (2001). *Ha'Aretz Newspaper*, Israel (in Hebrew), 12th October.

Shaw, E. D. (1986). Political terrorists: dangers of diagnosis and an alternative to the psychopathology model. *International Journal of Law and Psychiatry*, 8: 359–368.

Shelley, P. B. (1817). Preface. The Revolt of Islam. In: *Complete Poems of Keats and Shelley* (p. 35). New York: Modern Library, 1941.

Shengold, L. (1989). *Soul Murder: The Effects of Childhood Abuse and Deprivation*. New Haven, CT: Yale University Press.

Sidoli, M. (1993). When the meaning gets lost in the body. *Journal of Analytical Psychology*, 38: 175–190.

Sigal, J. J. (1971). Second generation effects of massive psychic trauma. In: H. Krystal & W. G. Niederland, *Psychic Traumatisation*. Boston: Little, Brown.

Simenauer, E. (1968). Late sequelae of man-made disasters. *International Journal of Psycho-Analysis*, 49: 306–309.

Spielrein, S. (1994). Destruction as the cause of coming into being. *Journal of Analytical Psychology*, 39: 155–186.

Spiro, E. (1987). *Culture and Human Nature: Theoretical Papers of Melford E. Spiro*. B. Kilbourne & L. L. Langness (Eds.). Chicago: Univ. Chicago Press.

Spitz, R. A. (1953). Aggression: its role in the establishment of object relations. In: R. M. Loewenstein (Ed.), *Drives, Affects, Behavior*. New York: International Universities Press.

Spitz, R. A. (1960). Discussion of Dr John Bowlby's paper. *The Psychoanalytic Study of the Child*, 15: 85–94.

Spitz, R. A. (1963). Ontogenesis: the proleptic function of emotion. In: P. H. Knapp (Ed.), *Expression of the Emotions in Man*. New York: International Universities Press.

Spitzer, R., & Williams, J. (Eds.) (1994). *Diagnostic and Statistical Manual of Mental Health Disorders; DSM-IV*. Washington, DC: American Psychiatric Association.

Stanton, A., & Swartz, M. (1954). *The Mental Hospital*. New York: Basic Books.

Steele, H., Steele, M., & Fonagy, P. (1996). Associations among attachment classifications of mothers, fathers, and their infants. *Child Development*, 67: 541–555.

Steiner, J. (1979). The border between the paranoid–schizoid and the depressive positions in the borderline patient. *British Journal of Medical Psychology*, 52: 385–391.

Steiner, J. (1985). Turning a blind eye: the cover-up for Oedipus. *International Review of Psychoanalysis*, 12: 161–172.

Steiner, J. (1993). *Psychic Retreats*. London and New York: Routledge.

Stern, D. (1985). *The Interpersonal World of the Infant: A View from Psychoanalysis and Developmental Psychology*. New York: Basic Books.
Stern, M. (1992). Reflections on the Gulf War. Sihot-Dialoge. *Israel Journal of Psychotherapy*, *VII*(1) December: 53–57.
Stevens, A. (1982). *Archetype. A Natural History of the Self*. London: Routledge & Kegan Paul.
Stolorow, R. (1999). The phenomenology of trauma and the absolutisms of everyday life. *Psychoanalytic Psychology*, *16*(3): 464–468.
Strachey, A. (1957). *The Unconscious Motives of War*. London: Allen and Unwin.
Strauss, R. (1962). The archetype of separation. *Proceedings from the Second International Congress of Analytical Psychology*, Zurich.
Sullivan, A. (2001). This is a religious war. *New York Times*.
Sullivan, H. S. (1956). *Clinical Studies in Psychiatry* (p. 299) H. S. Perry *et al*. (Eds.). New York: W. W. Norton.
Target, M., & Fonagy, P. (1996). Playing with reality II: The development of psychic reality from a theoretical perspective. *International Journal of Psycho-Analysis*, *77*: 459–479.
Taylor, A. J. P. (1963). *The First World War*. London: Hamilton.
Taylor, M., & Ryan, H. (1988). Fanaticism, political suicide, and terrorism. *Terrorism*, *11*: 91–111.
Terr, L. (1994). *Unchained Memories: True Stories of Traumatic Memories, Lost and Found*. New York: Basic Books.
The Barnhardt Dictionary of Etymology. (1988). New York: H. W. Wilson Co.
Torok, M. (1968). The illness of mourning and the fantasy of the exquisite corpse. In: N. Abraham & M. Torok (Eds.), *The Shell and the Kernel, Volume 1* (pp. 107–124). Chicago & London: The University of Chicago Press, 1994.
Trautman, E. C. (1971). Violence and victims in Nazi concentration camps: the psychopathology of the survivor. In: H. Krystal & W. G. Niederland (Eds.), *Psychic Traumatisation*. Boston: Little, Brown.
Tronick, E. (1989). Emotions and emotional communication in infants. *American Psychologist*, *44*: 112–119.
Turquet, P. (1975). Threats to identity on the large group. In: Kreeger (Ed.), *The Large Group*. London: Constable.
Tustin, F. (1986). *Autistic Barriers in Neurotic Patients*. London: Karnac Books.
Tustin, F. (1990). *The Protective Shell in Children and Adults*. London & New York: Karnac Books.
Twain, M. (1995). *The Mysterious Stranger*. UK: Prometheus Books.

Twemlow, S. W. (1999). A psychoanalytic dialectical model for sexual and other forms of workplace harassment. *Journal of Applied Psychoanalytic Studies*, 1(3): 249–270.

Twemlow, S. W. (2001). Modifying violent communities by enhancing altruism: a vision of possibilities. *Journal of Applied Psychoanalytic Studies*, 3(4): 431–462.

Twemlow, S. W., & Sacco, F. C. (1996). Peacekeeping and peacemaking: the conceptual foundations of a plan to reduce violence and improve the quality of life in a mid-sized community in Jamaica. *Psychiatry*, 59: 156–174.

Twemlow, S. W., & Sacco, F. C. (1999). A multilevel conceptual framework for understanding the violent community. In: H. V. Hall & L. C. Whitaker (Eds.), *Collective Violence: Effective Strategies for Assessing & Interviewing in Fatal Group and Institutional Aggression* (pp. 566–599). New York: CRC Press.

Twemlow, S. W., Fonagy P., & Sacco, F. C. (in press,a). Feeling safe in school. *Smith College Studies in Social Work*.

Twemlow, S. W., Fonagy P., Sacco, F. C., & Vernberg, E. (in press,b). Assessing adolescents who threaten homicide in schools. *American Journal of Psychoanalysis*.

Twemlow, S. W., Fonagy P., Sacco, F. C., O'Toole, M., & Vernberg, E. (2002). Premeditated mass shootings in schools: threat assessment. *Journal of American Academy of Child and Adolescent Psychiatry*, 41(4): 475–477.

USA Today. (2001). 7th July.

Van de Kolk, B. S., & Van de Hart, O. (1989). Pierre Janet and the breakdown of adaptation in psychological trauma. *American Journal of Psychiatry*, 146: 1530–1540.

van der Kolk, B. (1994). The body keeps the score: memory and the evolving psychobiology of post-traumatic stress. *Harvard Review of Psychiatry*, 1: 253–265.

van IJzendoorn, M. H. (1995). Adult attachment representations, parental responsiveness, and infant attachment: A meta-analysis on the predictive validity of the Adult Attachment Interview. *Psychological Bulletin*, 117: 387–403.

Vegh, C. (1972). *Je ne lui ai pas Dit au Revoir*. Paris: Gallimard, 1972.

Volkan, V. (1988). *The Need to have Enemies and Allies*. Northvale, NJ: Jason Aronson.

Volkan, V. (1997). *Blood Ties: From Ethnic Pride to Ethnic Terrorism*. West View Press; New York: Farrar, Straus, and Giroux.

Volkan, V. (1999). Psychoanalysis and diplomacy: Part I: Individual and large group identity. *Journal of Applied Psychoanalytic Studies*, 1(1): 29–55.

Volkan, V., & Itzkowitz, N. (2000). Modern Greek and Turkish identities and the psychodynamics of Greek–Turkish relations. In: M. Robbens & M. Suarez-Orozco (Eds.), *Culture under Siege*. Chicago: University of Chicago Press.

Vossekuil, B., Reddy, M., & Fein, R. (2000). *USSS Safe School Initiative: An Interim Report on the Prevention of Targeted Violence in Schools*. National threat Assessment Centre, US Secret Service, 950 H. Street, N.S., Suite 9100, Washington, D.C. Available at www.treas.gov/usss/ntac.

Vygotsky, L. S. (1967). Play and its role in the mental development of the child. *Soviet Psychology*, 5: 6–18.

Wardi, D. (1992). *Memorial Candles: Children of The Holocaust*. London, New York: Tavistock/Routledge.

Websters 3rd New International Dictionary. (1993). Springfield, MA: Merriam-Webster Inc.

West, M., & George, C. (in press). Abuse and violence in intimate adult relationships: New perspectives from attachment theory. In: D. G. Dutton (Ed.), *Treatment of Assaultiveness*. New York: Guilford.

Wiesel, E. (1961). *Le Jour*. Paris: Editions du Seuil.

Williams, M., & Kestenberg, J. (1974). Introduction and discussion in workshop on children of survivors. *Journal of American Psychoanalytic Association*, 22: 200–204.

Wilson, J. P. (1989). *Trauma, Transformation and Healing*. New York: Brunner-Mazel.

Winnicott, D. W. (1949). Mind and its relation to psyche-soma. In: *Collected Papers: Through Paediatrics to Psycho-Analysis*. London: Tavistock.

Winnicott, D. W. (1953). Transitional objects and transitional phenomena. *International Journal of Psycho-Analysis*, 34(2).

Winnicott, D. W. (1960). The theory of the parent–infant relationship. In: *The Maturational Processes and the Facilitating Environment* (p. 46). London: Hogarth, 1965.

Winnicott, D. W. (1965). *The Maturational Process and the Facilitating Environment*. London: Hogarth Press.

Winnicott, D. W. (1967). Mirror-role of the mother and family in child development. In: P. Lomas (Ed.), *The Predicament of the Family: A Psycho-Analytical Symposium* (pp. 26–33). London: Hogarth.

Winnik, H. Z. (1968). Contribution to a symposium on psychic traumatization through social catastrophe. *International Journal of Psycho-Analysis*, 49: 298–301.

Wittels, F. (1929). Grosse Hasser. *Psychoanalytische Bewegung*, 1: 320–343.

Woodmansey, A. C. (1966). The internalisation of external conflict. *International Journal of Psycho-Analysis*, 47: 349–355.

Yalom, I. F. (1985). *The Theory and Practice of Group Psychotherapy* (2nd edition). New York: Basic Books.

Young, R. (2001). Fundamentalism. In: I. Pitchford & R. Young (Eds.), *The Human Nature Review*.